Long-Term Health Effects of the 9/11 Disaster

Long-Term Health Effects of the 9/11 Disaster

Special Issue Editors

Robert M. Brackbill
Judith M. Graber
W. Allen Robison

MDPI • Basel • Beijing • Wuhan • Barcelona • Belgrade

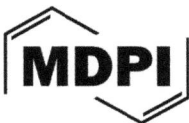

MDPI

Special Issue Editors
Robert M. Brackbill
World Trade Center Health Registry
USA

Judith M. Graber
Environmental and Occupational Health Sciences Institute, Pisca
USA

W. Allen Robison
The National Institute for Occupational Safety and Health, (NIOSH)
USA

Editorial Office
MDPI
St. Alban-Anlage 66
4052 Basel, Switzerland

This is a reprint of articles from the Special Issue published online in the open access journal *International Journal of Environmental Research and Public Health* (ISSN 1660-4601) in 2019 (available at: https://www.mdpi.com/journal/ijerph/special_issues/9-11_Disaster).

For citation purposes, cite each article independently as indicated on the article page online and as indicated below:

LastName, A.A.; LastName, B.B.; LastName, C.C. Article Title. *Journal Name* **Year**, *Article Number*, Page Range.

ISBN 978-3-03921-812-7 (Pbk)
ISBN 978-3-03921-813-4 (PDF)

Contents

About the Special Issue Editors

Robert M. Brackbill, Ph.D., MPH trained at University of Minnesota where he received a Ph.D. in experimental psychology and University of California at Berkeley, where he received an MPH in Epidemiology. Dr. Brackbill was scientist with the Centers for Disease Control and Prevention up until 2011. He was the founding Principle Investigator for World Trade Center Health Registry and currently serves as Director of Research for Registry located in the Division of Epidemiology in the New York City Department of Health and Mental Hygiene. He has over 100 publications in a wide range of areas of public health with a focus on behavioral aspects of physical and mental health.

Judith M. Graber is an occupational and environmental epidemiologist in the Rutgers School of Public Health where she is an Associate Professor and the Director of the Epidemiology Concentration. She trained at the University of Illinois, School of Public Health where she received her Ph.D. in Epidemiology (2012). Prior to her doctoral work, she worked at the Centers for Disease Control and Prevention (CDC) and the Maine Bureau of Health (now Maine CDC) for 15 years. Dr. Graber's current research examines the interconnected contributions of occupational and behaviors risk factors to cancer incidence. Her research with World Trade Center (WTC) first responders investigates risk factors and mechanisms for head and neck cancer. This work specifically explores causal pathways wherein exposure to the WTC pollutants may moderate or mediate associations between well-established risk factors for head and neck cancer incidence. These risk factors include smoking tobacco, excess alcohol use, and oral infection with the human papilloma virus (HPV). She is also currently spearheading the New Jersey Firefighters Cancer Prevention Project, looking at cancer risk among New Jersey volunteer and career firefighters. The long-term goal of this work is to reduce cancer incidence and mortality among firefighters. Dr. Graber serves on CDC grant review panels and New Jersey Department of Health advisory boards including the Biomonitoring Commission. She has over 40 peer-reviewed publications.

W. Allen Robison received his Ph.D. in Toxicology from the University of Kentucky in 1998, an MS in Biology from Western Kentucky University in 1980, and a BS in Natural Resources Management from the University of Tennessee Martin in 1977. Prior to arriving at NIOSH in 2006, Dr. Robison worked for ATSDR doing health assessments for Superfund sites, the US Fish and Wildlife Service assessing environmental contaminants, and the Commonwealth of Kentucky (air quality, laboratory QA/QA, and water quality). He has a broad science background. Dr. Robison managed a variety of extramural portfolios prior to becoming the Director of the office.

International Journal of
*Environmental Research
and Public Health*

MDPI

Editorial

Editorial for "Long-Term Health Effects of the 9/11 Disaster" in *International Journal of Environmental Research and Public Health*, 2019

Robert M. Brackbill [1,*], Judith M. Graber [2] and William A. (Allen) Robison [3]

[1]   World Trade Center Health Registry, New York City Department of Health and Mental Hygiene,
    New York, NY 10013, USA
[2]   Epidemiology Concentration Director, Department of Biostatistics and Epidemiology,
    Rutgers School of Public Health, Piscataway, NJ 08854, USA
[3]   Office of Extramural Research, National Institute for Occupational Safety and Health, Atlanta,
    GA 30329-4027, USA
*   Correspondence: rbrackbi@health.nyc.gov

Received: 2 September 2019; Accepted: 4 September 2019; Published: 7 September 2019

The call for articles on the long term health effects of the 11 September 2001 terrorist attacks (9/11) has resulted in twenty-three papers that add a significant amount of information to the growing body of research on the effects of the World Trade Center (WTC) disaster almost two decades later. The attacks on 9/11 were a paradigm altering event in US history and have had major repercussions in the political landscape and response to terrorism. The toll of 9/11 includes the continued impact of accumulated health effects among those who were directly exposed to either the air pollution or re-suspended material that resulted from the collapse of the two WTC towers, and physical injuries or psychological trauma. This includes a wide range of physical and mental health disorders that continue to plague thousands of people 18 years later as well as newly identified conditions emerging as a result of prolonged disease latency. This was recently highlighted by the addition of "The Memorial Glade" at the WTC site that acknowledges illnesses and deaths years after the towers collapsed [1].

The articles in this special issue also demonstrate the importance of the medical monitoring of the wide range of populations exposed to unprecedented levels of physical and psychological insult from the 9/11 attacks. As such, the reports in this issue represent research findings from the clinics supported by World Trade Center Health Programs and the epidemiological follow-up by the World Trade Center Health Registry. Although the majority of the articles represent rescue, recovery, and clean-up workers (12), some other non-rescue recovery groups included in the special issue are residents of Chinatown, just 10 blocks from ground zero (Kung et al. 2019 [2]), and other residents of lower Manhattan (Antao et al. 2019 [3]).

Respiratory and lung problems are among the most prevalent and highly persistent physical health problems arising from 9/11 exposure to dust clouds from the collapsing building and the subsequent re-suspension of dust (Aldrich, 2010 [4]). In this issue, there are nine respiratory-related papers that provide new insights into the long term consequences of lung damage from 9/11 exposure not reported in previous research. These papers highlight the chronic and still emerging health sequela of 9/11 exposure. An analysis of cleaning practices by residents in lower Manhattan showed that cleaning with dry methods was associated with more types of respiratory symptoms than other cleaning methods (Antao, 2019 [3]). Other papers delved into the underlying physical and biological aspects of pulmonary illness among persons exposed to 9/11 (Liu, 2019 [5]; Kwon, 2019 [6]; Pradhan, 2019 [7]). Liu et al. (2019) used chest tomography (CT) and reported that firefighters with high intensity exposure on 9/11 had increased risk of bronchial wall thickening, emphysema, and air trapping. They correlated the CT-identified abnormalities with respiratory symptoms. A second paper also evaluated the role of metabolic syndrome biomarkers (MSBs) among firefighters (e.g., elevated systolic blood pressure and insulin resistance) in airway hyperactivity (Kwon, 2019 [6]). They reported that given 9/11 exposure, having three or more MSBs increased airway hyperactivity beyond that associated with 9/11 exposure. Another paper that evaluated the bronchodilator response among community members exposed to 9/11 found that a proportion of small airway problems were irreversible, which was predicted by the bronchodilator response at initial visits (Pradhan, 2019 [7]). Two other papers evaluated the increased risk of asthma control issues and quality of life as a function of indoor allergens (Rojano, 2019 [8]) and air pollution/irritants (Yung, 2019 [9]). In addition, an emerging respiratory condition, pulmonary fibrosis (PF)—a common long term sequelae of occupational dust exposure—was documented in a paper based on data from the World Trade Center Health Registry for which there was evidence of a dose-response relationship with the level of exposure among rescue/recovery and other 9/11 workers and the likelihood of PF (Li, 2019 [10]).

Three other papers reported additional findings on a condition known as sarcoidosis (Cleven, 2019 [11]; Hena, 2019 [12]) and sarcoid-like granulomatous (Sunil, 2019). Sarcoidosis is a rare autoimmune disease that can affect any organ, but among rescue, recovery, clean-up workers, it has been previously reported as granulomatous disease involving the thoracic organs (Izbicki, 2007 [13]; Jordan, 2011 [14]), primarily among firefighters or other rescue, recovery, or clean-up workers arriving early at the WTC site. One paper in this issue describes sarcoidosis among community members who were patients at the WTC Environmental Health Center (Hena, 2019 [12]). Another paper focused on the genetic predisposition for sarcoidosis in a case control study (Cleven, 2019 [11]). Sunil (Sunil, 2019 [15]) reported a detailed pathology review of sarcoid like granulomatous disease (SGD). Out of seven cases, five were definite SGD and had high exposure to 9/11 WTC dust.

In addition to respiratory disease, other long term adverse health outcomes of WTC-related exposure include neurologic conditions and cancer. Papers in this issue focused on these emerging conditions including peripheral neuropathy (Colbeth, 2019 [16]), paresthesia (Thawani, 2019 [17]), and thyroid cancer (van Gerwen, 2019 [18]; Tuminello, 2019 [19], see Gargano, 2018 [20] for a review of non-respiratory physical health conditions). Two studies focused on neuropathic conditions that included peripheral neuropathy among New York City firefighters and emergency medical workers (Colbeth, 2019 [16]) and parenthesia among community survivors who received treatment at one of the WTC Health programs (Thawani, 2019 [17]). Potential exposures for neuropathic conditions on 9/11/2001 and afterward included heavy metals and complex hydrocarbons. Both studies used the self-reporting of unusual and painful sensations such prickling, burning, or aching pain in the limbs. Colbeth et al. reported a 35% increase in the likelihood of peripheral neuropathy symptoms among those with the highest 9/11 exposure versus low/no exposure. Similarly, Thawani et al. reported a significant hazard ratio of 1.4 for parenthesia among persons who had a job that required cleaning-up materials resulting from building fires and buildings collapsing. The physical health outcome of cancer was represented by two papers on thyroid cancer (Tuminello, 2019 [19]; van Gerwen, 2019 [18]). Thyroid cancer has been identified as a cancer with a higher expected incidence among potential WTC-exposed persons (Zeig-Owens, 2011 [21]; Li, 2016 [22]; Solan et al., 2013 [23]). Tuminello (2019) evaluated the possibility that increased surveillance for thyroid cancer among WTC survivors could account for the elevated thyroid cancer incidence. In another study (van Gerwin, 2019 [18]) that evaluated thyroid cancers derived from the same population, the authors compared the pathological characteristics of cancer tumors of WTC exposed to non-WTC cases in order to assess whether there were more false positives among the WTC exposed that would suggest a surveillance bias.

The high prevalence of adverse mental health, especially post-traumatic stress disorder (PTSD), has been documented among survivors of 9/11 (Brackbill, 2009 [24]; Stellman, 2008 [25]), in addition to the persistence of PTSD (Pietrzak, 2014 [26]; Maslow, 2015 [27]; Welch, 2016 [28]). A number of papers in this issue addressed the characteristics of those receiving or not adequately receiving mental health treatment and some measurement of the effectiveness of treatment (Jacobson, 2019 [29]; Kung, 2019 [2]; Rosen, 2019 [30]; Bellehsen, 2019 [31]). Based on data from the World Trade Center Health Registry (WTCHR), 38% of enrollees reported they had utilized mental health counseling or therapy sometime in the 15 years after 9/11, with younger persons more likely to seek counseling, but older persons perceiving treatment to be helpful (Jacobson, 2019). Those with persistent PTSD perceived treatment to be less helpful. Another paper also used WTCHR information to characterize unmet mental health care needs for a specific sub-group of Asian WTCHR enrollees, who typically underutilize mental health services (Kung, 2019 [2]). Among the 2300 Asian WTCHR enrollees included in the study, 12% said that they had an unmet mental health care need, for whom 69% reported attitudinal barriers (e.g., I do not need to see a doctor) to utilizing mental health care, 36% said there were cost barriers (e.g., lack of health insurance), and 28% had access barriers (e.g., where to go for doctor, childcare, transportation issues). Two other 9/11 mental health papers used information on patients enrolled in a community WTC Health Program (Rosen, 2019 [30]) and rescue/recovery worker health program (Bellehsen, 2019 [31]). Among patients who reached the criteria for PTSD at the first visit, 77% continued to meet the criteria for PTSD 3 to 4 years later (Rosen, 2019 [30]). Further analysis indicated that some reduction in PTSD symptoms was associated with treatment. The second paper evaluated the extent to which patients were receiving evidence-based treatment (EBT) by community health providers. Like the Rosen et al. paper, they employed baseline and follow-up information in addition to providers reporting their use of EBT. However, after an independent review, 12% of the patients were likely to have received full EBT, and another 40% received some elements of EBT.

Some papers in this issue fittingly addressed the long-term effects of 9/11 exposure on both physical and mental functioning. For instance, Brackbill et al. (2019) [32] assessed the self-reported physical and mental health functioning of persons who were injured on 9/11 15 years after the attack. The severity of injury was associated with physical functioning, but not with mental health functioning; PTSD history also had a significant additive influence on the effect of injury on physical functioning. Using a more objective measure of functionality referred to as handgrip strength, which is a measure of general health status and biomarker of aging, Mukherjee (2019 [33]) reported that rescue/recovery workers with probable PTSD had significantly lower HGS than those without PTSD or depression. Apart from functionality and physical loss, there is concern that persons exposed to 9/11 could be at greater risk of cognitive impairment, memory loss, or confusion at a faster rate than would be expected normally with age. Seil (2019) [34], using the WTC Health Registry data, derived levels of protective factor or cognitive reserve (based on educational level, employed or not, social support, and level of physical activity) for cognitive impairment and found that higher levels of cognitive reserve were associated with less self-reported memory loss for both persons with and without a history of PTSD. Two other aspects of quality of life are represented by papers on early retirement and post-2019 (Yu, 2019 [35]). Among the Lower Manhattan residents and area workers, a history of PTSD and the number of 9/11 related chronic conditions were associated with early retirement (retired before 60). In addition, income loss among those who retired was more likely among those with the highest level of exposure. In the quality of sleep study, it was reported that 9/11 related co-morbidities including gastroesophageal reflux disease, chronic rhinosinusitis, PTSD, anxiety, and depression were associated with a great proportion of sleep related complaints (Ayappa, 2019 [36]). With the presence of these co-morbidities, apnea had no significant impact on sleep quality.

The papers in this special issue clearly document the continued long term effects of the September 11, 2001 WTC disaster on a wide range of health and quality of life issues. They underscore the need for ongoing health monitoring of these highly exposed populations while also representing the cutting edge research on subject areas from the biological underpinnings of 9/11 related respiratory disease to the effectiveness of treatment for mental health problems related to 9/11. This work continues to inform the World Trade Center Health Program for those most affected by the disaster. While this is a uniquely exposed population, this large body research will inform responses to, and the monitoring of, populations exposed to future human caused and natural disasters.

Funding: This research received no external funding.

Conflicts of Interest: The views in this editorial are those of the authors and do not necessarily represent the official position of the World Trade Center Health Program, the National Institute for Occupational Safety and Health, and the Centers for Disease Control and Prevention.

References

1. Rojas, R. Unsung 9/11 Heroes Finally Get their Own Memorial. *New York Times*, 31 May 2019; A1.
2. Kung, W.W.; Wang, X.; Liu, X.; Goldmann, E.; Huang, D. Unmet Mental Health Care Needs among Asian Americans 10–11 Years After Exposure to the World Trade Center Attack. *Int. J. Environ. Res. Public Health* **2019**, *16*, 1302. [CrossRef] [PubMed]
3. Antao, V.C.; Pallos, L.L.; Graham, S.L.; Shim, Y.K.; Sapp, J.H.; Lewis, B.; Bullard, S.; Alper, H.E.; Cone, J.E.; Farfel, M.R.; et al. 9/11 Residential Exposures: The Impact of World Trade Center Dust on Respiratory Outcomes of Lower Manhattan Residents. *Int. J. Environ. Res. Public Health* **2019**, *16*, 798. [CrossRef] [PubMed]
4. Aldrich, T.K.; Gustave, J.; Hall, C.B.; Cohen, H.W.; Webber, M.P.; Zeig-Owens, R.; Cosenza, K.; Christodoulou, V.; Glass, L.; Al-Othman, F.; et al. Lung function in rescue workers at the World Trade Center after 7 years. *N. Engl. J. Med.* **2010**, *362*, 1263–1272. [CrossRef] [PubMed]
5. Liu, C.; Putman, B.; Singh, A.; Zeig-Owens, R.; Hall, C.B.; Schwartz, T.; Webber, M.P.; Cohen, H.W.; Fazzari, M.J.; Prezant, D.J.; et al. Abnormalities on Chest Computed Tomography and Lung Function Following an Intense Dust Exposure: A 17-Year Longitudinal Study. *Int. J. Environ. Res. Public Health* **2019**, *16*, 1655. [CrossRef] [PubMed]
6. Kwon, S.; Crowley, G.; Mikhail, M.; Lam, R.; Clementi, E.; Zeig-Owens, R.; Schwartz, T.M.; Liu, M.; Prezant, D.J.; Nolan, A. Metabolic Syndrome Biomarkers of World Trade Center Airway Hyperreactivity: A 16-Year Prospective Cohort Study. *Int. J. Environ. Res. Public Health* **2019**, *16*, 1486. [CrossRef]
7. Pradhan, D.; Xu, N.; Reibman, J.; Goldring, R.M.; Shao, Y.; Liu, M.; Berger, K.I. Bronchodilator Response Predicts Longitudinal Improvement in Small Airway Function in World Trade Center Dust Exposed Community Members. *Int. J. Environ. Res. Public Health* **2019**, *16*, 1421. [CrossRef]
8. Rojano, B.; West, E.; Ferdermann, E.; Markowitz, S.; Harrison, D.; Crowley, L.; Busse, P.; Federman, A.D.; Wisnivesky, J.P. Allergen Sensitization and Asthma Outcomes among World Trade Center Rescue and Recovery Workers. *Int. J. Environ. Res. Public Health* **2019**, *16*, 737. [CrossRef]
9. Yung, J.; Osahan, S.; Friedman, S.M.; Li, J.; Cone, J.E. Air Pollution/Irritants, Asthma Control, and Health-Related Quality of Life among 9/11-Exposed Individuals with Asthma. *Int. J. Environ. Res. Public Health* **2019**, *16*, 1924. [CrossRef]
10. Li, J.; Cone, J.E.; Brackbill, R.M.; Giesinger, I.; Yung, J.; Farfel, M.R. Pulmonary Fibrosis among World Trade Center Responders: Results from the WTC Health Registry Cohort. *Int. J. Environ. Res. Public Health* **2019**, *16*, 825. [CrossRef]
11. Cleven, K.L.; Ye, K.; Zeig-Owens, R.; Hena, K.M.; Montagna, C.; Shan, J.; Hosgood, H.D.; Jaber, N.; Weiden, M.D.; Colbeth, H.L.; et al. Genetic Variants Associated with FDNY WTC-Related Sarcoidosis. *Int. J. Environ. Res. Public Health* **2019**, *16*, 1830. [CrossRef]
12. Hena, K.M.; Murphy, S.; Zhang, Y.; Shao, Y.; Kazeros, A.; Reibman, J. Clinical Evaluation of Sarcoidosis in Community Members with World Trade Center Dust Exposure. *Int. J. Environ. Res. Public Health* **2019**, *16*, 1291. [CrossRef] [PubMed]
13. Izbicki, G.; Chavko, R.; Banauch, G.I.; Weiden, M.D.; Berger, K.I.; Aldrich, T.K.; Hall, C.; Kelly, K.J.; Prezant, D.J. World Trade Center "Sarcoid-Like" Granulomatous Pulmonary Disease in New York City Fire Department Rescue Workers. *Chest* **2007**, *131*, 1414–1423. [CrossRef] [PubMed]
14. Jordan, H.T.; Stellman, S.D.; Prezant, D.; Teirstein, A.; Osahan, S.S.; Cone, J.E. Sarcoidosis Diagnosed After September 11, 2001, Among Adults Exposed to the World Trade Center Disaster. *J. Occup. Environ. Med.* **2011**, *53*, 966–974. [CrossRef] [PubMed]
15. Sunil, V.R.; Radbel, J.; Hussain, S.; Vayas, K.N.; Cervelli, J.; Deen, M.; Kipen, H.; Udasin, I.; Laumbach, R.; Sunderram, J.; et al. Sarcoid-Like Granulomatous Disease: Pathologic Case Series in World Trade Center Dust Exposed Rescue and Recovery Workers. *Int. J. Environ. Res. Public Health* **2019**, *16*, 815. [CrossRef] [PubMed]

16. Colbeth, H.L.; Zeig-Owens, R.; Webber, M.P.; Goldfarb, D.G.; Schwartz, T.M.; Hall, C.B.; Prezant, D.J. Post-9/11 Peripheral Neuropathy Symptoms among World Trade Center-Exposed Firefighters and Emergency Medical Service Workers. *Int. J. Environ. Res. Public Health* **2019**, *16*, 1727. [CrossRef] [PubMed]

17. Thawani, S.; Wang, B.; Shao, Y.; Reibman, J.; Marmor, M. Time to Onset of Paresthesia Among Community Members Exposed to the World Trade Center Disaster. *Int. J. Environ. Res. Public Health* **2019**, *16*, 1429. [CrossRef] [PubMed]

18. van Gerwen, M.A.; Tuminello, S.; Riggins, G.J.; Mendes, T.B.; Donovan, M.; Benn, E.K.; Genden, E.; Cerutti, J.M.; Taioli, E. Molecular Study of Thyroid Cancer in World Trade Center Responders. *Int. J. Environ. Res. Public Health* **2019**, *16*, 1600. [CrossRef] [PubMed]

19. Tuminello, S.; van Gerwen, M.A.; Genden, E.; Crane, M.; Lieberman-Cribbin, W.; Taioli, E. Increased Incidence of Thyroid Cancer among World Trade Center First Responders: A Descriptive Epidemiological Assessment. *Int. J. Environ. Res. Public Health* **2019**, *16*, 1258. [CrossRef] [PubMed]

20. Gargano, L.; Mantilla, K.; Fairclough, M.; Yu, S.; Brackbill, R. Review of Non-Respiratory, Non-Cancer Physical Health Conditions from Exposure to the World Trade Center Disaster. *Int. J. Environ. Res. Public Health* **2018**, *15*, 253. [CrossRef]

21. Zeig-Owens, R.; Webber, M.P.; Hall, C.B.; Schwartz, T.; Jaber, N.; Weakley, J.; Rohan, T.E.; Cohen, H.W.; Derman, O.; Aldrich, T.K.; et al. Early assessment of cancer outcomes in New York City firefighters after the 9/11 attacks: An observational cohort study. *Lancet (Lond. Engl.)* **2011**, *378*, 898–905. [CrossRef]

22. Li, J.; Brackbill, R.M.; Liao, T.S.; Qiao, B.; Cone, J.E.; Farfel, M.R.; Hadler, J.L.; Kahn, A.R.; Konty, K.J.; Stayner, L.T.; et al. Ten-year cancer incidence in rescue/recovery workers and civilians exposed to the September 11, 2001 terrorist attacks on the World Trade Center. *Am. J. Ind. Med.* **2016**, *59*, 709–721. [CrossRef] [PubMed]

23. Solan, S.; Wallenstein, S.; Shapiro, M.; Teitelbaum, S.L.; Stevenson, L.; Kochman, A.; Kaplan, J.; Dellenbaugh, C.; Kahn, A.; Biro, F.N.; et al. Cancer incidence in world trade center rescue and recovery workers, 2001–2008. *Environ. Health Perspect.* **2013**, *121*, 699–704. [CrossRef] [PubMed]

24. Brackbill, R.M.; Hadler, J.L.; DiGrande, L.; Ekenga, C.C.; Farfel, M.R.; Friedman, S.; Perlman, S.E.; Stellman, S.D.; Walker, D.J.; Wu, D.; et al. Asthma and Posttraumatic Stress Symptoms 5 to 6 Years Following Exposure to the World Trade Center Terrorist Attack. *JAMA* **2009**, *302*, 502–516. [CrossRef] [PubMed]

25. Stellman, J.M.; Smith, R.P.; Katz, C.L.; Sharma, V.; Charney, D.S.; Herbert, R.; Moline, J.; Luft, B.J.; Markowitz, S.; Udasin, I.; et al. Enduring Mental Health Morbidity and Social Function Impairment in World Trade Center Rescue, Recovery, and Cleanup Workers: The Psychological Dimension of an Environmental Health Disaster. *Environ. Health Perspect.* **2008**, *116*, 1248–1253. [CrossRef] [PubMed]

26. Pietrzak, R.H.; Feder, A.; Singh, R.; Schechter, C.B.; Bromet, E.J.; Katz, C.L.; Reissman, D.B.; Ozbay, F.; Sharma, V.; Crane, M.; et al. Trajectories of PTSD risk and resilience in World Trade Center responders: An 8-year prospective cohort study. *Psychol. Med.* **2014**, *44*, 205–219. [CrossRef] [PubMed]

27. Maslow, C.B.; Caramanica, K.; Welch, A.E.; Stellman, S.D.; Brackbill, R.M.; Farfel, M.R. Trajectories of Scores on a Screening Instrument for PTSD Among World Trade Center Rescue, Recovery, and Clean-Up Workers. *J. Trauma. Stress* **2015**, *28*, 198–205. [CrossRef]

28. Welch, A.E.; Caramanica, K.; Maslow, C.B.; Brackbill, R.M.; Stellman, S.D.; Farfel, M.R. Trajectories of PTSD Among Lower Manhattan Residents and Area Workers Following the 2001 World Trade Center Disaster, 2003–2012. *J. Trauma. Stress* **2016**, *29*, 158–166. [CrossRef]

29. Jacobson, M.H.; Norman, C.; Sadler, P.; Petrsoric, L.J.; Brackbill, R.M. Characterizing Mental Health Treatment Utilization among Individuals Exposed to the 2001 World Trade Center Terrorist Attacks 14–15 Years Post-Disaster. *Int. J. Environ. Res. Public Health* **2019**, *16*, 626. [CrossRef]

30. Rosen, R.; Zhu, Z.; Shao, Y.; Liu, M.; Bao, J.; Levy-Carrick, N.; Reibman, J. Longitudinal Change of PTSD Symptoms in Community Members after the World Trade Center Destruction. *Int. J. Environ. Res. Public Health* **2019**, *16*, 1215. [CrossRef]

31. Bellehsen, M.; Moline, J.; Rasul, R.; Bevilacqua, K.; Schneider, S.; Kornrich, J.; Schwartz, R.M. A Quality Improvement Assessment of the Delivery of Mental Health Services among WTC Responders Treated in the Community. *Int. J. Environ. Res. Public Health* **2019**, *16*, 1536. [CrossRef]

32. Brackbill, R.M.; Alper, H.E.; Frazier, P.; Gargano, L.M.; Jacobson, M.H.; Solomon, A. An Assessment of Long-Term Physical and Emotional Quality of Life of Persons Injured on 9/11/2001. *Int. J. Environ. Res. Public Health* **2019**, *16*, 1054. [CrossRef] [PubMed]

33. Mukherjee, S.; Clouston, S.; Kotov, R.; Bromet, E.; Luft, B. Handgrip Strength of World Trade Center (WTC) Responders: The Role of Re-Experiencing Posttraumatic Stress Disorder (PTSD) Symptoms. *Int. J. Environ. Res. Public Health* **2019**, *16*, 1128. [CrossRef] [PubMed]

34. Seil, K.; Yu, S.; Alper, H. A Cognitive Reserve and Social Support-Focused Latent Class Analysis to Predict Self-Reported Confusion or Memory Loss among Middle-Aged World Trade Center Health Registry Enrollees. *Int. J. Environ. Res. Public Health* **2019**, *16*, 1401. [CrossRef] [PubMed]

35. Yu, S.; Seil, K.; Maqsood, J. Impact of Health on Early Retirement and Post-Retirement Income Loss among Survivors of the 11 September 2001 World Trade Center Disaster. *Int. J. Environ. Res. Public Health* **2019**, *16*, 1177. [CrossRef] [PubMed]

36. Ayappa, I.; Chen, Y.; Bagchi, N.; Sanders, H.; Black, K.; Twumasi, A.; Rapoport, D.M.; Lu, S.E.; Sunderram, J. The Association between Health Conditions in World Trade Center Responders and Sleep-Related Quality of Life and Sleep Complaints. *Int. J. Environ. Res. Public Health* **2019**, *16*, 1229. [CrossRef]

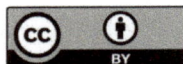

International Journal of
Environmental Research and Public Health

MDPI

Article

Characterizing Mental Health Treatment Utilization among Individuals Exposed to the 2001 World Trade Center Terrorist Attacks 14–15 Years Post-Disaster

Melanie H. Jacobson [1], Christina Norman [2], Pablo Sadler [2], Lysa J. Petrsoric [1] and Robert M. Brackbill [1,*]

[1] World Trade Center Health Registry, Division of Epidemiology, New York City Department of Health and Mental Hygiene, New York, NY 10013, USA; Melanie.E.Jacobson@gmail.com (M.H.J.); lsilverstein@health.nyc.gov (L.J.P.)

[2] Division of Mental Hygiene, New York City Department of Health and Mental Hygiene, Queens, NY 11101, USA; cnorman@health.nyc.gov (C.N.); psadler@health.nyc.gov (P.S.)

* Correspondence: rbrackbi@health.nyc.gov; Tel.: +1-646-639-6609

Received: 10 January 2019; Accepted: 15 February 2019; Published: 20 February 2019

Abstract: Following the World Trade Center (WTC) attacks in New York City (NYC) on 11 September 2001 (9/11), thousands in NYC experienced significant stress reactions and disorders, presenting an immediate need for counseling and treatment. While other studies documented post-9/11 mental health treatment utilization, none have data more than two years post-disaster. We used data from 35,629 enrollees of the WTC Health Registry, a longitudinal cohort study of those exposed to the WTC attacks, to examine predictors of counseling after 9/11, the types of practitioners seen, and the perceived helpfulness of therapy up to 15 years post-disaster. Among enrollees, 37.7% reported receiving counseling at some time after 9/11. Predictors of seeking counseling included race/ethnicity, age at 9/11, education level, exposure to the WTC attacks, other traumatic experiences, mental health symptomology, and pre-9/11 counseling. Whites and Hispanics, those who were children on 9/11, and those with high levels of exposure to the WTC attacks sought counseling soonest after 9/11. Among those who sought counseling, Blacks, Asians, and those with lower education and income were less likely to see mental health specialists and more likely to see general practitioners or religious advisors. Finally, among those who sought recent counseling, women, Blacks, those aged ≥65 years, and those with very high WTC exposures were more likely to rate their recent counseling as very helpful. This study used data up to 15 years post-disaster to document mental health treatment utilization patterns, trends, and disparities that have implications for future preparedness plans and needs assessments.

Keywords: counseling; post-disaster; psychotherapy; mental health treatment; treatment utilization

1. Introduction

The World Trade Center (WTC) terrorist attacks in New York City (NYC) on 11 September 2001 (9/11) resulted in thousands of casualties and, among the survivor population in NYC, a substantial mental health burden [1], primarily consisting of stress disorders [2,3]. Specifically, similar to the aftermath of other natural or human-made disasters, posttraumatic stress disorder (PTSD) was the most common mental health condition that resulted from the attacks [4]. This mental health burden translated into a need for crisis counseling and treatment [1]. In response, several mental health programs in New York City were established after 9/11, such as Project Liberty [5]. Project Liberty was a mental health screening and treatment program with a bilateral approach. The first tier was a general outreach program to communities affected by the attacks, providing free short-term counseling and education on coping methods for typical stress reactions. In addition, it included delivery of counseling to children in schools [6]. Secondly, individuals were screened for more severe and/or prolonged symptoms and then referred to specialized mental health treatment. Separately, mental health treatment was also offered through a program initially designed to monitor and treat those who participated in the rescue and recovery efforts [7]. Subsequently, treatment for mental health conditions was also made available to community members (i.e., those who were not involved in the rescue and recovery work) [8]. Together, these programs are collectively referred to as the WTC Health Program. Despite these established programs, it was consistently documented that receipt of these mental healthcare services was less than expected given the number of affected individuals and magnitude of the situation [9,10], which is common among populations who experience different types of mass trauma, such as natural disasters [11,12].

Several studies examined mental health treatment use after 9/11 and documented predictors of treatment receipt [9,13–17]. These studies reported that those with the greatest levels of exposure to the WTC attacks and those who had experienced peri-event panic attacks were the most likely to use mental health services after 9/11. Individuals who were Black and those without a regular doctor were less likely to use mental health services, including therapy and medication. However, these studies were conducted between six months and up to two years after the attacks, and data on longer-term or delayed utilization are sparse. Furthermore, studies generally lack specific details on the type of practitioner sought and the perceived degree of benefit of counseling.

The main objective of this study was to describe post-9/11 mental health treatment utilization, specifically counseling and therapy among individuals exposed to the WTC attacks up to 15 years post-disaster. Firstly, we examined predictors (e.g., demographics and exposure to the WTC attacks) of seeking counseling after 9/11, and then compared the characteristics of individuals who sought different types of practitioners for such counseling. Secondly, we assessed determinants of perceived benefit of recent counseling. Lastly, we evaluated the distributions of time to first counseling after 9/11 by several factors.

2. Materials and Methods

Study Population. The World Trade Center Health Registry (Registry) is a longitudinal cohort study of persons exposed to the WTC terrorist attacks on 9/11 [18]. Those who lived, worked, went to school, or were otherwise present in lower Manhattan on 9/11 and/or those who participated in the rescue and recovery efforts were eligible to enroll. The Registry was established in order to track the short and long-term potential health effects of 9/11.

The study design, eligibility, and enrollment methods of the Registry were previously described [18]. Briefly, in 2003–2004, 71,426 individuals who were exposed to the WTC attacks on 9/11 either as rescue and recovery workers or community members, were enrolled into the Registry and completed a baseline questionnaire (Wave 1). This was followed in subsequent years by Wave 2 (2006–2007), Wave 3 (2011–2012), and Wave 4 (2015–2016). The Institutional Review Boards of the Centers for Disease Control Prevention and the New York City Department of Health and Mental Hygiene approved the Registry protocol.

For this study, enrollees had to complete the Wave 4 questionnaire (N = 36,862), which included questions on their mental health treatment history, and were required to not be missing data on date of birth (N = 18) or missing a response to the question about whether the enrollee had at least one session of counseling or therapy after 9/11 (N = 1215). This yielded a final sample of 35,629.

Mental health treatment. On the Wave 4 survey, enrollees were asked about their mental healthcare-seeking behavior ever, after 9/11, and in the last 12 months. Firstly, enrollees were asked whether they had ever had a session of counseling or therapy lasting 30 minutes or longer and, if so, at what age the first session of counseling occurred, and whether any counseling was sought after 9/11. Among those who reported seeking care after 9/11, questions were asked about the conditions for which counseling was sought (e.g., depression, PTSD, anxiety, among others) and what types of practitioners were sought (e.g., psychologist, psychiatrist, social worker, clergy member, among others). Lastly, among those who reported seeking counseling in the last 12 months, questions were asked about medical indications for counseling, frequency of counseling, and perceived benefit. Whether any counseling was sought in relation to the events of 9/11 was not explicitly asked in the questionnaire.

Explanatory variables. Questionnaire data consisted of details on demographics and social factors, WTC-related exposures and experiences, health-related and care-seeking behaviors, and mental and physical health symptoms and conditions over time. Demographic information included sex, age, race and ethnicity, household income, and education. For this study focusing on mental health, exposure to the WTC attacks was operationalized using data on several traumatic experiences on and directly after 9/11 that were asked about on Waves 1 and 2. Based on work by Adams and Boscarino [19], Brackbill et al. derived a composite score consisting of 11 questions about traumatic experiences such as being in the North or South World Trade Center (WTC) towers at the time of the attack, witnessing three or more events (seeing planes hit the buildings, people fall or jump from buildings, people injured, or people running), being injured on 9/11; having a relative killed on 9/11, and being displaced from home due to 9/11 [20]. These items were summed (range = 0–11) and the score was then categorized as none/low (0–1 exposures), medium (2–3), high (4–5), and very high ($\geq$6). In addition, another measure of "exposure" to the WTC attacks was the Registry eligibility group. Enrollees were categorized with regard to how they originally became eligible for the Registry: rescue and recovery workers, lower Manhattan residents or lower Manhattan area workers, passersby, or students. Because these groups were not mutually exclusive, those who met the criteria for more than one category were placed in the category considered to be more highly exposed to 9/11, such that rescue and recovery workers had greater levels of WTC exposure than residents, who had greater exposures than area workers, passersby, and students.

Mental health measures. PTSD symptoms were assessed at each wave (Waves 1–4) using the 9/11-specific PTSD Checklist (PCL)-17 [21–23]. The PCL is a self-administered questionnaire based on *Diagnostic and Statistical Manual of Mental Disorders* (DSM)-IV criteria [24] and its validity was established [25]. Total scores $\geq$44 were considered to be indicative of probable PTSD [21]. PTSD status was summarized across time as ever (scores $\geq$44 on at least one wave) or never (scores <44 on all waves). Persistent PTSD was defined as those who had scores $\geq$44 at all four waves.

Depressive symptoms were assessed using the Patient Health Questionnaire (PHQ)-8 [26] at Waves 3 and 4 only. This self-administered and validated instrument contains eight of the nine criteria that constitute the DSM-IV diagnosis of depressive disorders [24,27]. Scores $\geq$10 were considered to be indicative of moderate to severe depression [28].

Enrollees were also asked whether they had ever been diagnosed by a doctor or other medical professional with various mental health conditions, such as depression, PTSD, or anxiety.

Statistical Analysis. Firstly, we evaluated the distribution of personal characteristics, WTC exposures, and mental health symptomology by whether enrollees sought counseling at some time after 9/11. In order to identify predictors of seeking counseling, we then fit multivariable log binomial models to estimate associations between these factors and seeking counseling after 9/11. In these models, we did not include factors that required a doctor diagnosis (e.g., doctor-diagnosed depression), since these diagnoses could have been received through such counseling visits. Instead, we included PTSD and depression symptoms as measured by the PCL-17 and PHQ-8, respectively. We fit these models among everyone in the sample, and then conducted a sensitivity analysis restricting the sample to those who had a history of PTSD (Waves 1–4) or depression (Waves 3–4) via threshold PCL-17 and PHQ-8 scores, respectively, in order to examine those with the most theoretical clinical need for counseling. Next, among those who sought counseling, we then examined the types of practitioners sought, and the distributions of personal characteristics, WTC exposures, and mental health symptomology across practitioner type. Again, we did this in the total sample, and subsequently just among those with a history of PTSD or depression. Next, among those who had sought counseling in the last 12 months prior to completing the Wave 4 questionnaire, we explored the determinants of perceived helpfulness of therapy. We fit log binomial models estimating adjusted risk ratios (aRR) and 95% confidence intervals (CI) to identify predictors of perceiving recent counseling as "very helpful" compared with all other ratings (i.e., collapsing all other categories: somewhat, slightly, and not at all). Demographic characteristics, WTC-related exposures, mental health symptomology, and variables related to care-seeking were examined simultaneously in models. Finally, among those who did not seek counseling before 9/11, we assessed the distributions of time elapsed between 9/11 and first seeking counseling (i.e., time to first counseling after 9/11) by several covariates, such as demographics and WTC exposures using unadjusted Kaplan–Meier curves.

3. Results

The study population was majority male (60.6%), White (70.0%), and had at least a college education (53.2%) (Table 1). There was approximately equal representation of rescue and recovery workers (46.3%) and community members (residents, area workers, passersby, and students; 53.7%) in the sample. Mental health conditions were common: 27.1% screened positive for PTSD on at least one Wave according to PCL-17 scores over time and 16.3% reported ever being diagnosed with PTSD by a medical professional. Likewise, although only 18.5% of individuals reported seeking counseling before 9/11, 37.7% reported counseling at some time after 9/11. Among those who sought treatment for the first time after 9/11, counseling was sought consistently throughout the 15 years after 9/11, with the largest increase observed in the first year after 9/11 (Figure 1).

Table 1. Distributions of personal characteristics, World Trade Center (WTC) exposures, and mental health symptomology by seeking counseling post 11 September 2001 (9/11) and adjusted risk ratios (aRR) and 95% Confidence Intervals (CI). GED—General Education Development; PTSD—posttraumatic stress disorder.

	Total (N = 35,629)		Sought Counseling (N = 13,435, 37.7%)		No Counseling (N = 22,194, 62.3%)		aRR [a]	95% CI	
	N	%	N	%	N	%			
Sex									
Men	21586	60.6	7240	33.5	14346	66.5	1.00	Reference	
Women	14043	39.4	6195	44.1	7848	55.9	1.01	0.99	1.03
Race/Ethnicity									
White	24939	70.0	9857	39.5	15082	60.5	1.00	Reference	
Black	3416	9.6	1045	30.6	2371	69.4	0.83	0.76	0.90
Hispanic	4046	11.4	1550	38.3	2496	61.7	0.98	0.94	1.02
Asian	2002	5.6	470	23.5	1532	76.5	0.72	0.63	0.82
Other race	1226	3.4	513	41.8	713	58.2	1.00	0.99	1.02
Education at Wave 1									
≤High school/GED	7857	22.2	2619	33.3	5238	66.7	0.94	0.90	0.99
Some college	8704	24.6	3138	36.1	5566	63.9	0.99	0.96	1.02
College	11423	32.3	4470	39.1	6953	60.9	0.99	0.98	1.00
Graduate degree	7376	20.9	3115	42.2	4261	57.8	1.00	Reference	
Income at Wave 1									
<$50,000	8876	27.6	3632	40.9	5244	59.1	1.00	0.98	1.01
≥$50,000 to <$150,000	19249	59.8	6974	36.2	12275	63.8	0.99	0.98	1.00
≥$150,000	4050	12.6	1623	40.1	2427	59.9	1.00	Reference	
Age at 9/11 (years)									
0–17	852	2.4	438	51.4	414	48.6	2.44	1.86	3.20
18–24	1720	4.8	845	49.1	875	50.9	2.42	1.84	3.17
25–44	18212	51.1	7442	40.9	10770	59.1	2.37	1.81	3.11
45–64	14010	39.3	4551	32.5	9459	67.5	2.08	1.58	2.73
≥65	835	2.3	159	19.0	676	81.0	1.00	Reference	

Table 1. *Cont.*

	Total (N = 35,629)		Sought Counseling (N = 13,435, 37.7%)		No Counseling (N = 22,194, 62.3%)		aRR [a]	95% CI	
	N	%	N	%	N	%			
Eligibility group									
Rescue/recovery worker	16480	46.3	5732	34.8	10748	65.2	1.00	0.98	1.01
Lower Manhattan resident	5103	14.3	2266	44.4	2837	55.6	0.99	0.95	1.02
Lower Manhattan area worker/passerby	14046	39.4	5437	38.7	8609	61.3	1.00	Reference	
WTC exposure score									
None/low	15620	43.8	5083	32.5	10537	67.5	1.00	Reference	
Medium	11923	33.5	4518	37.9	7405	62.1	1.08	1.04	1.12
High	6203	17.4	2743	44.2	3460	55.8	1.09	1.04	1.13
Very high	1883	5.3	1091	57.9	792	42.1	1.10	1.06	1.14
Traumatic experiences after 9/11 [b]									
No	21859	61.4	6700	30.7	15159	69.3	1.00	Reference	
Yes	13770	38.6	6735	48.9	7035	51.1	1.08	1.05	1.12
Ever-PTSD [c]									
No	17572	72.9	5156	29.3	12416	70.7	1.00	Reference	
Yes	6543	27.1	3726	56.9	2817	43.1	1.27	1.20	1.33
Ever-Depression [d]									
No	22209	77.5	6691	30.1	15518	69.9	1.00	Reference	
Yes	6451	22.5	3973	61.6	2478	38.4	1.17	1.11	1.23
Counseling before 9/11									
No	27971	81.5	7460	26.7	20511	73.3	1.00	Reference	
Yes	6340	18.5	4810	75.9	1530	24.1	2.25	2.16	2.34
Doctor-diagnosed depression (ever)									
No	28099	78.9	7366	26.2	20733	73.8	-	-	
Yes	7530	21.1	6069	80.6	1461	19.4	-	-	
Doctor-diagnosed PTSD (ever)									
No	29816	83.7	8490	28.5	21326	71.5	-	-	
Yes	5813	16.3	4945	85.1	868	14.9	-	-	
Doctor-diagnosed anxiety (ever)									
No	30950	86.9	9695	31.3	21255	68.7	-	-	
Yes	4679	13.1	3740	79.9	939	20.1	-	-	

[a] Risk ratio represents the comparison of seeking counseling vs. not seeking counseling (reference). [b] Traumatic experiences were defined as one or more of the following: experiencing a serious accident (e.g., in a car or a fall), an intentional attack with or without a weapon, forceful unwanted sexual contact, and serious family or work problems. [c] As measured by a score of ≥ 44 on the 9/11-specific PTSD Checklist (PCL)-17 on at least one wave (Waves 1–4). [d] As measured by a score of ≥ 10 on Patient Health Questionnaire (PHQ)-8 on at least one wave (Waves 3–4).

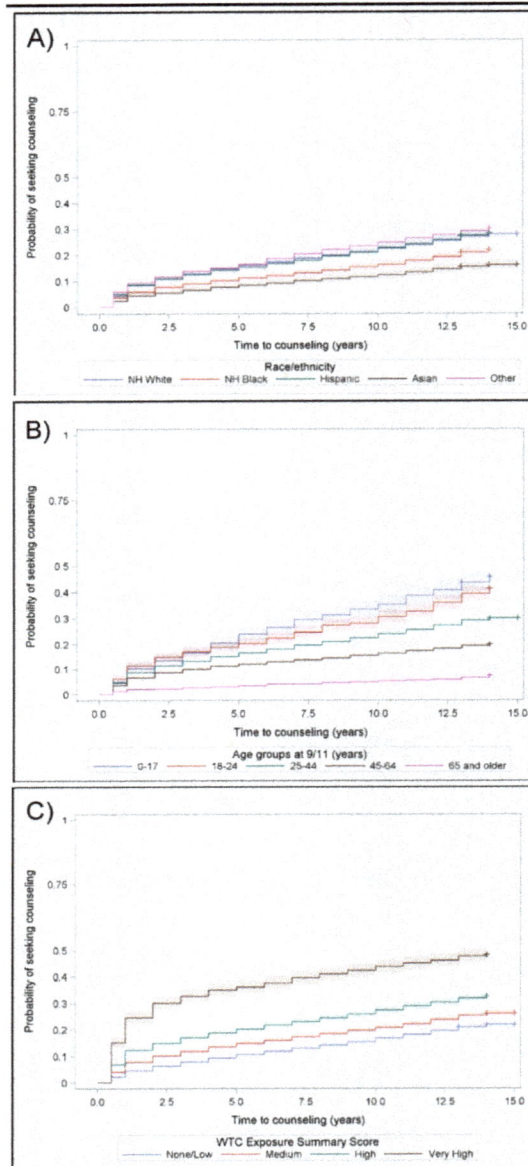

Figure 1. Unadjusted Kaplan–Meier curves and 95% confidence intervals of time to first counseling after 11 September 2001 (9/11) among those who had not sought counseling before 9/11 (N = 27,971), World Trade Center (WTC) Health Registry, 2003–2016: (**A**) by race/ethnicity; (**B**) by age at 9/11; (**C**) by WTC exposure summary score.

Females were more likely to seek counseling compared with males (44.1% vs. 33.5%, although in adjusted models, sex was not a predictor of counseling (aRR = 1.01, 95% CI: 0.99, 1.03). While Blacks (aRR = 0.83, 95% CI: 0.76, 0.90) and Asians (aRR = 0.72, 95% CI: 0.63, 0.82) were less likely to seek counseling compared with Whites, Hispanics and those of other races were equally likely to seek counseling compared with Whites. This was also apparent in the examination of time to counseling (Figure 1A). Asians were the most likely to delay counseling after 9/11 (i.e., had the longest times to counseling) compared with those of other races (i.e., who had the shortest times). Age at 9/11 was a strong predictor of counseling. Those who were younger at 9/11, especially those aged 0–17 years, were the most likely to seek counseling compared with those aged 65 years and older (Table 1). This observation was consistent in the distributions of times to counseling (Figure 1B). Those who were children (0–17 years) at the time of 9/11 sought counseling sooner than those who were older. This relationship between age at 9/11 and time to counseling was monotonically positive such that, as age increased, the delay in seeking counseling also increased (i.e., longer times). Other demographic characteristics showed mixed associations with seeking counseling; while those with less than a high school education were slightly less likely to seek counseling compared with those with a graduate degree, income was not associated with seeking counseling (Table 1).

Measures of exposure to the WTC attacks, other post-9/11 traumatic experiences, and mental health symptomology were positively associated with seeking counseling. For example, those with very high scores of WTC exposure were more likely to seek counseling compared with those with none or low exposure (aRR = 1.10, 95% CI: 1.06, 1.14), and again this pattern was visible when times to counseling were considered (Figure 1C). Those who experienced the greatest number of traumatic exposures on 9/11 sought counseling soonest, such that there was a negative dose–response relationship between the WTC exposure summary score and time to counseling; the greater the number of exposures, the sooner counseling was sought (i.e., shorter times). Other traumatic experiences after 9/11 were similarly associated with an increased likelihood of seeking counseling (aRR = 1.08, 95% CI: 1.05, 1.12)

Although residents were the most likely to seek counseling (44.4%) compared with rescue and recovery workers (34.8%) or area workers and passersby (38.7%) in bivariate analyses, all were equally likely to seek counseling in adjusted models (Table 1). Those who had threshold PTSD symptoms at any wave (ever-PTSD), as well as those who had threshold depressive symptoms at Waves 3 and/or 4 (ever-depression), were more likely to seek counseling after 9/11 compared with those who did not meet symptom thresholds for each condition. Although not included in models, those who received diagnoses of depression, PTSD, and anxiety were more much more likely to have sought counseling compared with those without diagnoses. Finally, having sought counseling before 9/11 was a strong predictor of seeking counseling after 9/11 (aRR = 2.25, 95% CI: 2.16, 2.34).

When this analysis was conducted among those with PTSD or depression symptoms (N = 9391), results did not change (data not shown). Although the prevalence of having sought counseling after 9/11 was greater among those with PTSD or depression symptoms over time (57.1%) compared to the total (37.7%), the associations between enrollee characteristics and seeking counseling did not materially vary.

Among those who sought counseling after 9/11, psychiatrists (40.2%), psychologists (50.0%), and/or other mental health professionals (i.e., social worker, therapist, or counselor) (47.3%) were the most common types of practitioners sought (Table 2). Type of practitioners sought varied across most demographic characteristics, but did not vary by sex. Whites, Hispanics, and those of other races were more likely to see psychiatrists or psychologists compared with Blacks or Asians. However, Blacks and those of other races were more likely to seek counseling from nurses/occupational therapists or religious or spiritual advisors than Whites or Asians. Finally, Asians were the most likely to report seeking general practitioners for counseling compared with other race/ethnicity groups. In addition, although seeing a psychiatrist did not vary by education or income, these demographic characteristics were positively associated with seeing a psychologist such that those with the highest level of education or income were more likely to see a psychologist compared with those with lower levels. In contrast, those with lower education or income were more likely to see a general practitioner, nurse/occupational therapist, or religious advisor compared with those more educated and/or who earned more income.

Table 2. Distributions of personal characteristics, WTC exposures, and mental health symptomology among those that sought counseling post-9/11 by type of practitioner.

	Total (N = 13,435)		Psychiatrist (N = 5399, 40.2%)[a]		Psychologist (N = 6720, 50.0%)[a]		Other Mental Health Professional (N = 6360, 47.3%)[a,b]		General Practitioner/Doctor (N = 3082, 22.9%)[a]		Nurse/Occupational Therapist (N = 726, 5.4%)[a]		Religious or Spiritual Advisor (N = 2092, 15.6%)[a]	
	N	%	N	%	N	%	N	%	N	%	N	%	N	%
Sex														
Men	7240	53.9	3009	41.6	3591	49.6	3376	46.6	1650	22.8	404	5.6	1155	16.0
Women	6195	46.1	2390	38.6	3129	50.5	2984	48.2	1432	23.1	322	5.2	937	15.1
Race/Ethnicity														
White	9857	73.4	3998	40.6	5140	52.1	4759	48.3	2118	21.5	432	4.4	1362	13.8
Black	1045	7.8	369	35.3	419	40.1	458	43.8	272	26.0	95	9.1	240	23.0
Hispanic	1550	11.5	649	41.9	703	45.4	713	46.0	408	26.3	123	7.9	308	19.9
Asian	470	3.5	142	30.2	178	37.9	186	39.6	143	30.4	32	6.8	48	10.2
Other race	513	3.8	241	47.0	280	54.6	244	47.6	141	27.5	44	8.6	134	26.1
Education at Wave 1														
≤High school/GED	2619	19.6	1126	43.0	1156	44.1	1115	42.6	726	27.7	209	8.0	419	16.0
Some college	3138	23.5	1293	41.2	1513	48.2	1578	50.3	805	25.7	197	6.3	575	18.3
College	4470	33.5	1729	38.7	2328	52.1	2142	47.9	936	20.9	203	4.5	650	14.5
Graduate degree	3115	23.4	1215	39.0	1686	54.1	1481	47.5	585	18.8	109	3.5	420	13.5
Income at Wave 1														
<$50,000	3632	29.7	1521	41.9	1718	47.3	1778	49.0	1007	27.7	300	8.3	676	18.6
≥$50,000 to <$150,000	6974	57.0	2729	39.1	3523	50.5	3399	48.7	1548	22.2	327	4.7	1064	15.3
≥$150,000	1623	13.3	659	40.6	881	54.3	651	40.1	282	17.4	38	2.3	185	11.4
Age at 9/11 (years)														
0–17	438	3.3	203	46.3	258	58.9	232	53.1	50	11.4	22	5.0	40	9.2
18–24	845	6.3	331	39.2	468	55.4	442	52.3	157	18.6	32	3.8	114	13.5
25–44	7442	55.4	3033	40.8	3787	50.9	3726	50.1	1686	22.7	384	5.2	1270	17.1
45–64	4551	33.9	1791	39.4	2168	47.6	1922	42.2	1141	25.1	268	5.9	656	14.4
≥65	159	1.2	41	25.8	39	24.5	38	23.9	48	30.2	20	12.6	12	7.5
Eligibility group														
Rescue/recovery worker	5732	42.7	2287	39.9	2811	49.0	2910	50.8	1361	23.7	354	6.2	1059	18.5
Lower Manhattan resident	2266	16.9	956	42.2	1217	53.7	978	43.2	457	20.2	120	5.3	205	9.0
Lower Manhattan area worker/passerby	5437	40.5	2156	39.7	2692	49.5	2472	45.5	1264	23.2	252	4.6	828	15.2
WTC exposure score														
None/low	5083	37.8	1901	37.4	2416	47.5	2364	46.5	1092	21.5	238	4.7	769	15.1
Medium	4518	33.6	1797	39.8	2227	49.3	2098	46.4	918	20.3	213	4.7	585	12.9
High	2743	20.4	1141	41.6	1464	53.4	1320	48.1	705	25.7	161	5.9	487	17.8
Very high	1091	8.1	560	51.3	613	56.2	578	53.0	367	33.6	114	10.4	251	23.0

Table 2. *Cont.*

	Total (N = 13,435)		Psychiatrist (N = 5399, 40.2%)[a]		Psychologist (N = 6720, 50.0%)[a]		Other Mental Health Professional (N = 6360, 47.3%)[a,b]		General Practitioner/ Doctor (N = 3082, 22.9%)[a]		Nurse/ Occupational Therapist (N = 726, 5.4%)[a]		Religious or Spiritual Advisor (N = 2092, 15.6%)[a]	
	N	%	N	%	N	%	N	%	N	%	N	%	N	%
Ever-PTSD [c]														
No	5156	58.1	1544	29.9	2361	45.8	2445	47.4	709	13.8	132	2.6	561	10.9
Yes	3726	42.0	1962	52.7	2122	57.0	1872	50.2	1201	32.2	288	7.7	744	20.0
Ever-Depression [d]														
No	6691	62.7	2018	30.2	3105	46.4	3103	46.4	1011	15.1	195	2.9	821	12.3
Yes	3973	37.3	2241	56.4	2290	57.6	2033	51.2	1359	34.2	342	8.6	803	20.2
Counseling before 9/11														
No	7460	60.8	3014	40.4	3811	51.1	3576	47.9	1624	21.8	414	5.5	1137	15.2
Yes	4810	39.2	2105	43.8	2612	54.3	2476	51.5	1086	22.6	233	4.8	760	15.8
Doctor-diagnosed depression (ever)														
No	7366	54.8	1642	22.3	3098	42.1	3245	44.1	1088	14.8	240	3.3	973	13.2
Yes	6069	45.2	3757	61.9	3622	59.7	3115	51.3	1994	32.9	486	8.0	1119	18.4
Doctor-diagnosed PTSD (ever)														
No	8490	63.2	2568	30.2	3690	43.5	3645	42.9	1511	17.8	304	3.6	1065	12.5
Yes	4945	36.8	2831	57.2	3030	61.3	2715	54.9	1571	31.8	422	8.5	1027	20.8
Doctor-diagnosed anxiety (ever)														
No	9695	72.2	3030	31.3	4463	46.0	4414	45.5	1706	17.6	363	3.7	1400	14.4
Yes	3740	27.8	2369	63.3	2257	60.3	1946	52.0	1376	36.8	363	9.7	692	18.5
Conditions for which received counseling [a]														
Depression	6421	47.8	3944	61.4	3892	60.6	3383	52.7	2037	31.7	497	7.7	1199	18.7
PTSD	4768	35.5	2751	57.7	3020	63.3	2704	56.7	1490	31.3	409	8.6	1005	21.1
Anxiety disorder	3990	29.7	2506	62.8	2447	61.3	2139	53.6	1463	36.7	392	9.8	755	18.9
Other mental health problem	3773	28.1	1848	49.0	2215	58.7	2136	56.6	1153	30.6	390	10.3	771	20.4
Alcohol/drug problems	833	6.2	509	61.1	485	58.2	559	67.1	345	41.4	116	13.9	225	27.0
Any ≥2 conditions	5734	42.7	3619	63.1	3607	62.9	3222	56.2	1962	34.2	518	9.0	1170	20.4
None of the above	3095	23.0	329	10.6	899	29.0	1067	34.5	360	11.6	73	2.4	348	11.2

[a] Respondents could select all that apply; thus, counts sum to greater than the total and percentages sum to greater than 100%. [b] Other mental health professional, such as a social worker, counselor, or therapist. [c] As measured by a score of ≥44 on PCL-17 on at least one wave (Waves 1–4). [d] As measured by a score of ≥10 on PHQ-8 on at least one wave (Waves 3–4).

Those who were children (aged 0–17 years) at 9/11 were more likely to seek counseling from mental health specialists (e.g., psychologists, psychiatrists, or other mental health professionals) compared with those who were older. However, older individuals, especially those 65 years and older, were more likely to seek general practitioners and nurses for counseling compared with those of younger age groups, whereas middle aged individuals were the most likely to see religious advisors. Rescue and recovery workers, residents, and area workers/passersby generally saw different practitioners with similar frequencies, although residents were the least likely to seek counseling from religious or spiritual advisors (9.0%) compared with rescue and recovery workers (18.5%) or area workers/passersby (15.2%).

Those with high WTC exposures were more likely to see all types of practitioners compared with those with lower exposures. The most common practitioners sought overall were psychologists; 56.2% of those with high WTC exposures reported seeing a psychologist for counseling. Similarly, those with threshold PTSD or depression symptoms were more likely to seek counseling from all types of practitioners compared with those without symptoms, although these differences were smallest for seeking counseling from other mental health professionals. Specifically, 47.4% of those who never had threshold PTSD symptoms reported seeking counseling from other mental health professionals compared with 50.2% of those who did have threshold PTSD symptoms. This pattern was similar across those who reported receiving a formal diagnosis of depression, PTSD, or anxiety compared with those who did not. There was also little difference between the types of practitioners sought comparing those who had sought counseling before 9/11 and those who had not. Finally, the conditions for which individuals sought counseling affected the type of practitioner they sought. Specifically, more of those who sought counseling for alcohol or drug problems saw all types of practitioners other than psychiatrists or psychologists, such as general practitioners, nurses/occupational therapists, and religious advisors, compared to those who sought counseling for other conditions. Overall, these trends did not change when the sample was restricted to those who experienced PTSD or depression symptoms over time (data not shown).

Lastly, among those who reported receipt of counseling within the last 12 months ($N = 5429$), the vast majority (79.3%) reported that the counseling was at least somewhat helpful (Table 3). Women (vs. men), Blacks (vs. all other race/ethnicities), and those aged ≥ 65 years at 9/11 (vs. all younger age groups) were more likely to report that therapy was very helpful. In bivariate analysis, similar distributions of perceived helpfulness were observed across eligibility groups and WTC exposure levels; however, in adjusted models, those with very high WTC exposure scores (aRR = 1.21, 95% CI: 1.07, 1.36) were more likely to rate their recent counseling as very helpful compared with those with none or low levels of WTC exposures.

Table 3. Distributions of personal characteristics, WTC exposures, mental health symptomology, and care-seeking determinants among those that sought counseling in the last 12 months by perceived helpfulness of therapy and adjusted risk ratios (aRR) and 95% confidence intervals (CI).

	Total (N = 5429)		Very (N = 2192)		aRR [a]	95% CI		Somewhat (N = 2029)		Slightly (N = 883)		Not at all (N = 217)	
	N	%	N	% [b]				N	% [b]	N	% [b]	N	% [b]
Sex													
Men	2934	54.0	1045	36.3	1.00	Reference		1165	40.5	535	18.6	132	4.6
Women	2495	46.0	1147	46.9	1.29	1.18	1.40	864	35.4	348	14.2	85	3.5
Race													
White	4073	75.0	1657	41.3	1.00	Reference		1549	38.6	650	16.2	157	3.9
Black	379	7.0	172	47.1	1.25	1.09	1.43	124	34.0	50	13.7	19	5.2
Hispanic	586	10.8	241	42.6	1.05	0.91	1.20	199	35.2	101	17.8	25	4.4
Asian	170	3.1	51	31.5	0.88	0.64	1.19	67	41.4	35	21.6	9	5.6
Other race	221	4.1	71	33.0	0.72	0.53	0.98	90	41.9	47	21.9	7	3.3
Education at Wave 4													
≤High school/GED	690	12.8	231	34.7	0.91	0.77	1.09	249	37.4	130	19.5	55	8.3
Some college	1428	26.6	513	36.9	0.95	0.85	1.05	538	38.6	271	19.5	70	5.0
College	1594	29.6	671	42.6	0.96	0.88	1.04	598	38.0	254	16.1	51	3.2
Graduate degree	1667	31.0	757	46.1	1.00	Reference		623	38.0	224	13.7	37	2.3
Income at Wave 4													
<$50,000	1360	26.2	517	39.2	1.11	0.98	1.25	481	36.5	241	18.3	80	6.1
≥$50,000 to <$150,000	2499	48.1	1016	41.3	1.04	0.95	1.14	914	37.2	430	17.5	98	4.0
≥$150,000	1340	25.8	569	43.1	1.00	Reference		547	41.4	172	13.0	32	2.4
Age at Wave 4 (years)													
18–44	1175	21.6	484	41.7	0.82	0.73	0.93	435	37.4	199	17.1	44	3.8
45–64	3366	62.0	1325	40.1	0.86	0.79	0.94	1281	38.8	563	17.0	136	4.1
≥65	888	16.4	383	44.8	1.00	Reference		313	36.7	121	14.2	37	4.3
Eligibility group													
Rescue/recovery worker	2429	44.7	944	39.8	1.08	0.98	1.18	904	38.1	413	17.4	112	4.7
Lower Manhattan resident	948	17.5	411	44.1	1.03	0.93	1.14	343	36.8	143	15.4	34	3.7
Lower Manhattan area worker/passerby	2052	37.8	837	41.5	1.00	Reference		782	38.8	327	16.2	71	3.5
WTC exposure score													
None/low	2096	38.6	861	42.2	1.00	Reference		770	37.7	322	15.8	89	4.4
Medium	1867	34.4	765	41.7	1.05	0.96	1.14	687	37.5	320	17.5	61	3.3
High	1013	18.7	365	36.6	0.96	0.86	1.08	407	40.8	179	17.9	47	4.7
Very high	453	8.3	201	44.9	1.21	1.07	1.36	165	36.8	62	13.8	20	4.5
Persistent PTSD [c]													
Never PTSD	1824	51.1	882	49.0	1.00	Reference		658	36.5	222	12.3	39	2.2
Non-persistent [d]	1295	36.3	454	35.7	0.76	0.68	0.83	518	40.7	245	19.2	56	4.4
Yes	450	12.6	159	35.7	0.68	0.58	0.81	165	37.1	97	21.8	24	5.4

Table 3. Cont.

	Total (N = 5429)		Very (N = 2192)		aRR [a]	95% CI		Somewhat (N = 2029)		Slightly (N = 883)		Not at all (N = 217)	
	N	%	N	% [b]				N	% [b]	N	% [b]	N	% [b]
Conditions for which received counseling in the last 12 months [e]													
Depression	3075	56.6	1177	38.8	0.85	0.75	0.97	1215	40.0	526	17.3	119	3.9
PTSD	1922	35.4	779	41.1	1.11	1.00	1.24	704	37.2	339	17.9	73	3.9
Anxiety disorder	2109	38.8	812	39.0	0.97	0.87	1.08	839	40.3	357	17.1	74	3.6
Other mental health problem	1937	35.7	750	39.1	0.87	0.79	0.97	750	39.1	332	17.3	86	4.5
Alcohol/drug problems	327	6.0	119	36.6	0.93	0.77	1.12	119	36.6	69	21.2	18	5.5
Any ≥2 conditions	2775	51.1	1068	39.0	1.11	0.96	1.28	1092	39.8	480	17.5	101	3.7
None of the above	776	14.3	323	44.8	0.94	0.82	1.08	238	33.0	121	16.8	39	5.4
Counseling frequency in last 12 months													
>1 per week	299	5.7	148	50.7	1.57	1.34	1.85	99	33.9	40	13.7	5	1.7
1 per week	1768	33.4	797	45.4	1.25	1.11	1.41	649	37.0	267	15.2	42	2.4
2–3 times per month	1274	24.1	539	42.8	1.23	1.09	1.39	515	40.9	176	14.0	30	2.4
1 per month	880	16.6	331	38.0	1.12	0.97	1.29	355	40.7	148	17.0	38	4.4
<1 per month	1067	20.2	348	33.0	1.00	Reference			36.3	235	22.3	90	8.5
Received medication for a mental health problem in the last 12 months													
No	2335	43.0	1011	44.4	1.00	Reference		829	36.4	347	15.2	92	4.0
Yes	3094	57.0	1181	38.8	0.91	0.83	0.99	1200	39.4	536	17.6	125	4.1
Sought counseling prior to the last 12 months													
No	543	10.6	175	32.8	1.00	Reference		209	39.2	111	20.8	38	7.1
Yes	4601	89.4	1937	42.7	1.34	1.14	1.57	1718	37.9	717	15.8	162	3.6
Ever been without insurance in last 12 months													
No	4963	92.1	2018	41.5	1.00	Reference		1862	38.2	794	16.3	194	4.0
Yes	425	7.9	159	38.2	1.17	0.99	1.38	150	36.1	85	20.4	22	5.3
Unmet mental healthcare need in last 12 months													
No	4982	94.2	2090	42.7	1.00	Reference		1899	38.8	755	15.4	147	3.0
Yes	306	5.8	50	16.9	0.45	0.31	0.65	82	27.8	100	33.9	63	21.4
Previous unmet mental healthcare need [f]													
No	2935	68.9	1309	45.3	1.00	Reference		1082	37.4	416	14.4	84	2.9
Yes	1327	31.1	445	34.2	0.84	0.76	0.93	510	39.2	276	21.2	71	5.5

[a] Risk ratio represents the relative probability that perceived helpfulness – very helpful vs. all other categories (somewhat, slightly, and not at all). [b] Denominators exclude N = 108 missing responses for perceived helpfulness of therapy in last 12 months. [c] Evaluated among those not missing any PCL items across four Waves (N = 3569); persistent PTSD as measured by a score of ≥44 at all waves. [d] Non-persistent PTSD was defined as those who had PCL-17 scores ≥44 on at least one Wave (1–4), but not at all four Waves. [e] Respondents could select all that apply; thus, counts sum to greater than the total and percentages sum to greater than 100%. Each risk ratio represents the comparison between those who received counseling for each condition vs. not that condition (i.e., all other indications). [f] As assessed at Waves 2 and 3.

Those with persistent PTSD were less likely to rate their recent counseling as very helpful (aRR = 0.68, 95% CI: 0.58, 0.81), and more likely to report that it was "not at all" (5.4%) or slightly" (21.8%) helpful compared with those who never had PTSD (2.2% and 12.3%, respectively). Those who had non-persistent PTSD (i.e., intermittent, delayed, or recovered) were also less likely to rate their recent counseling as very helpful compared with those who never had PTSD (aRR = 0.76, 95% CI: 0.68, 0.83). Although similar frequencies of helpfulness were observed across the conditions for which people received counseling, in adjusted models, those who received counseling for depression (vs. all other indications) were less likely to rate their counseling as very helpful, whereas those who received counseling for PTSD (vs. all other indications) were more likely to rate their counseling as very helpful.

The frequency of counseling was positively associated with perceived helpfulness such that those who sought counseling more often reported it to be "very helpful" compared with those who went less often. Similarly, those who had received therapy prior to the last 12 months were more likely to report that their current counseling was very helpful compared with those who had never before received therapy (aRR = 1.34, 95% CI: 1.14, 1.57). Those who received medication for a mental health problem in the last 12 months were slightly less likely to report that their counseling was very helpful (aRR = 0.91, 95% CI: 0.83, 0.99) compared with those who did not receive medication, although this difference was small (38.8% vs. 44.4%, respectively) and not consistent among those who reported that it was somewhat helpful (39.4% vs. 36.4%, respectively). Finally, those who reported unmet mental healthcare needs in the last 12 months and previously were less likely to report that their therapy was very helpful compared to those who did not have unmet mental healthcare needs.

4. Discussion

In a large cohort of individuals exposed to the trauma of the WTC disaster, this study documented mental health treatment utilization up to 15 years after 9/11. Approximately one-third of Registry enrollees sought counseling at some time after 9/11. Counseling was sought consistently over time after 9/11 up to 15 years after, although the largest increase was observed within the first year after the disaster. Predictors of seeking counseling included race/ethnicity, age at 9/11, education level attained, exposure to the WTC attacks, other post-9/11 traumatic experiences, mental health symptomology, and pre-9/11 counseling. Whites, Hispanics, and those of other races, those who were children at the time of 9/11, and those with high levels of exposure to the WTC attacks sought counseling soonest after 9/11. Among those who sought counseling, several trends were identified across types of practitioners seen. For example, Blacks, Asians, and those with lower education and income were less likely to seek counseling from mental health specialists (e.g., psychologists) and more likely to seek counseling from general practitioners such as family doctors or religious advisors compared with their White and more highly educated counterparts. Finally, among those who sought recent counseling, most enrollees perceived their counseling to have been at least somewhat helpful. Women, Blacks, those aged ≥65 years, and those with very high WTC exposures were more likely to rate their recent counseling as very helpful. These predictors of counseling and time to counseling after 9/11, types of practitioners seen, and perceived helpfulness of recent counseling did not vary when the population was restricted to those with significant PTSD or depression symptoms.

One of the strongest predictors of seeking counseling after 9/11 was having sought counseling before 9/11. Another study among 9/11-exposed individuals reported that new uptake of mental healthcare was rare after 9/11 among those who were not already receiving care beforehand [9]. Although this study was conducted only six months after 9/11, whereas ours was conducted 15 years after 9/11, results were very similar. Stuber et al. reported that, among those who were already receiving mental health services before 9/11, 82.7% sought mental healthcare after 9/11, which is comparable to the 75.9% in our study. In addition, we found that those who sought counseling more often, as well as those who were previously connected to care, were more likely to rate their recent counseling as very helpful compared to those who went less frequently or had not sought care prior. This may indicate that those with established provider–patient relationships, or those who are accustomed to seeking counseling fare better than those just starting out [29]. Alternatively, those already connected to care and those who go often may be experiencing more symptom abatement and, thus, satisfaction compared with those who may have intermittent care that may not be satisfying their needs [30]. This correlation between symptom abatement and reports of perceived benefit is consistent with our observation that persistent PTSD was associated with a reduced degree of perceived helpfulness of recent therapy compared with those who never had PTSD.

Another strong predictor of seeking counseling after 9/11 was younger age at the time of the event. Specifically, those who were children at the time of 9/11 were the most likely to seek mental health treatment and sought treatment more quickly compared with those of older ages at 9/11. This may reflect counseling programs that were provided in schools [31,32], as well as parents worrying about children's potential needs after the disaster [6,33]. Given the vulnerable life stage of children who were exposed to 9/11 and the resulting psychological consequences that are thought to be of greater severity in this age group [34,35], this relatively greater degree of uptake is reassuring. However, in our study, the absolute proportions show a different perspective, with just over half of those aged 0–17 years at 9/11 having sought counseling at some time after 9/11. This represents an underutilization of the services that were available, especially in the aftermath of the events, both in this age group and in the overall population. In addition, we found that these young individuals were the least likely to rate any recent counseling as very helpful compared with older age groups. However, it should be noted that, for the majority of those who sought counseling in the 12 months before survey administration (i.e., recent counseling), the indication was likely not related to 9/11. However, we did not explicitly ask whether the counseling sought was to address 9/11-related trauma.

Consistent with other studies in post-disaster settings [12], this study documented an underutilization in counseling and mental health treatment. Despite several public health programs devoted to mental health, only about one-third of enrollees reported seeking counseling at some time in the 15 years after 9/11. This is similar to what was observed in the aftermath of Hurricane Katrina, although studied time frames were shorter [36]; however, even so, after initiation, drop-outs in treatment were common. In addition, we observed significant delays in seeking counseling across several strata. These types of delays in seeking treatment are common [37,38]. One major driver of utilization of care and delay in seeking it that was consistently documented is stigma [39,40]. Although we did not measure this, it was shown that certain populations are differentially more likely to be affected by stigma, including Blacks and Asians, males, and young people. Future studies in 9/11-exposed populations should explore race/ethnicity-specific barriers to care, including perceived stigma.

Another relevant issue for mental healthcare delivery in post-disaster settings is that natural reactions to disasters change over time [41]. The course of reactions is generally referred to as "threat" or "impact" (i.e., immediate), short-term, and long-term. These different phases present the need for different types of mental healthcare support. For example, in the aftermath of the Hanshin Awaji earthquake in 1995, depressive symptoms did not manifest in most of the affected population until weeks to months after the event [42]. This presents a very different need than the shock- and grief-related reactions that are more common in the "impact" phase [41]. Specifically, we reported a racial/ethnic disparity in receipt of counseling. Blacks and particularly Asians were the least likely to seek counseling after 9/11 compared with other racial and ethnic groups. It was repeatedly noted in the literature that Asian Americans are less likely to seek mental health treatment compared with other racial and ethnic groups, especially non-Hispanic Whites [43–49]. This is attributed to language barriers, deficiencies in cultural competence in the delivery of care, general lack of awareness of such service availability, and cultural differences in the conception of mental illness itself. These data have implications for improving the accessibility of culturally competent mental health services for Blacks and Asians.

This study benefited from several strengths. Firstly, this study provided long-term information on mental health treatment utilization after 9/11. Most published studies to date reported on mental health treatment utilization up to a maximum of two years post-disaster [15,17], whereas this study had data up to 15 years after 9/11. This is an important addition to the literature because we were able to document the degree of delays in treatment in a trauma-exposed population. However, it should be noted that, due to this long follow-up time, our examination of mental health treatment likely included visits related to 9/11, as well as utilization unrelated to the events of 9/11, and we were unable to discern between the two. Another attribute was that, although several studies were published on the topic of post-9/11 mental health service utilization, to our knowledge, this is the first that collected data on the type of practitioner sought. This type of information is important because we identified trends and disparities in care-seeking behavior across various demographics. These findings may inform future disaster response plans with regard to establishing more equitable care to all those potentially affected.

However, we also note this study's limitations. Firstly, the Wave 4 survey asked about age at first counseling, irrespective of 9/11. Thus, our analysis of time to counseling after 9/11 was limited to those who sought counseling for the first time after 9/11. This limited our ability to examine the determinants of time to counseling after 9/11 among those who had sought treatment before 9/11 as well. Secondly, despite the information we had over time on several mental health conditions and symptoms, we were not able to assess whether mental health treatment was associated with improvement in symptoms because we did not ask detailed questions over time on treatment initiation and continuation or types of therapy and specific medication use and duration of use. In order to answer this question, in addition to longitudinal data on mental health symptomology, an in-depth study would be necessary that asked about specific treatment modes, practitioner characteristics, duration of treatments, use of medications over time, and more. Thirdly, although we asked about the type of practitioner sought for counseling, it is possible that enrollees were not able to reliably report the specific type, especially more subtle distinctions such as psychologists vs. psychiatrists. However, we were able to observe differences and disparities across different providers. Fourthly, we did not collect data on specific mental health or neurodevelopmental conditions before 9/11. Having this data would have allowed us to explore whether these disorders conferred an additional risk of developing PTSD after 9/11 [50], and perhaps an increased likelihood of seeking treatment. Lastly, our study was limited to Registry enrollees who completed the Wave 4 survey, which was administered in 2015–2016. These enrollees represented just over half (51.6%) of those originally enrolled in 2003–2004. Therefore, selection bias is a concern due to the potential for selective participation across several strata. However, previous investigation of this issue showed that, although those with PTSD symptoms were slightly less likely to continue to participate in Registry surveys than those without, the degree of exposure to the WTC attacks was not associated with participation over time [51]. Furthermore, the Registry was not able to enroll all WTC-exposed individuals, which was estimated to be over 400,000, of which the Registry recruited more than 71,000 (17.4% enrollment rate) [52]. The enrollment rate was highest among rescue and recovery workers (33.5%) and lowest among passersby (12.0%). Unfortunately, however, we do not have information on those who did not enroll.

5. Conclusions

The WTC terrorist attacks exposed thousands, if not millions, of individuals in NYC to trauma, resulting in a significant mental health burden and subsequent need for services. Overall, approximately one-third of WTC-exposed individuals sought counseling up to 15 years post-9/11, which represents an underutilization that is consistent with other post-disaster literature. Those who were White or Hispanic, children at the time of 9/11, and had high levels of exposure to the WTC attacks were the most likely to seek counseling after 9/11 and had the shortest waiting times to seeking counseling. Among those who sought counseling, there was heterogeneity across several demographic strata in the types of practitioners seen, such as Blacks and Asians being less likely to seek counseling from mental health specialists compared with Whites. These results highlight the need for tailoring outreach to specific demographic subgroups in post-disaster settings. This study used data up to 15 years post-disaster to document mental health treatment utilization patterns, trends, and disparities that have implications for future preparedness plans and needs assessments.

Author Contributions: Conceptualization, M.H.J., C.N., L.J.P., and R.M.B.; formal analysis, M.H.J.; methodology, M.H.J., C.N., P.S., and R.M.B.; project administration, R.M.B.; supervision, R.M.B.; writing—original draft, M.H.J.; writing—review and editing, C.N., L.J.P., and R.M.B.

Acknowledgments: This publication was supported by Cooperative Agreement Numbers 2U50/OH009739 and 5U50/OH009739 from the National Institute for Occupational Safety and Health (NIOSH) of the Centers for Disease Control and Prevention (CDC); U50/ATU272750 from the Agency for Toxic Substances and Disease Registry (ATSDR), CDC, which included support from the National Center for Environmental Health, CDC; and by the New York City Department of Health and Mental Hygiene (NYC DOHMH). Its contents are solely the responsibility of the authors and do not necessarily represent the official views of NIOSH, CDC, or the Department of Health and Human Services.

Conflicts of Interest: The authors declare no conflicts of interest. The founding sponsors had no role in the design of the study; in the collection, analyses, or interpretation of data; in the writing of the manuscript, and in the decision to publish the results.

References

1.   Herman, D.; Felton, C.; Susser, E. Mental health needs in New York State following the September 11th attacks. *J. Urban Health* **2002**, *79*, 322–331. [CrossRef] [PubMed]

2.   Brackbill, R.M.; Hadler, J.L.; DiGrande, L.; Ekenga, C.C.; Farfel, M.R.; Friedman, S.; et al. Asthma and posttraumatic stress symptoms 5 to 6 years following exposure to the World Trade Center terrorist attack. *JAMA* **2009**, *302*, 502–516. [CrossRef] [PubMed]

3.   Galea, S.; Nandi, A.; Vlahov, D. The epidemiology of post-traumatic stress disorder after disasters. *Epidemiol. Rev.* **2005**, *27*, 78–91. [CrossRef] [PubMed]

4.   Neria, Y.; DiGrande, L.; Adams, B.G. Posttraumatic stress disorder following the September 11, 2001, terrorist attacks: A review of the literature among highly exposed populations. *Am. Psychol.* **2011**, *56*, 429. [CrossRef] [PubMed]

5.   Felton, C.J. Project liberty: A public health response to New Yorkers' mental health needs arising from the World Trade Center terrorist attacks. *J. Urban Health* **2002**, *79*, 429–433. [CrossRef] [PubMed]

6.   Fairbrother, G.; Stuber, J.; Galea, S.; Pfefferbaum, B.; Fleischman, A.R. Unmet need for counseling services by children in New York City after the September 11th attacks on the World Trade Center: Implications for pediatricians. *Pediatrics* **2004**, *113*, 1367–1374. [CrossRef]

7.   Dasaro, C.R.; Holden, W.L.; Berman, K.D.; Crane, M.A.; Kaplan, J.R.; Lucchini, R.G.; Luft, B.J.; Moline, J.M.; Teitelbaum, S.L.; Tirunagari, U.S.; et al. Cohort profile: World trade center health program general responder cohort. *Int. J. Epidemiol.* **2015**, *46*, e9. [CrossRef]

8.   Petrsoric, L.; Miller-Archie, S.A.; Welch, A.; Cone, J.; Farfel, M. Considerations for future disaster registries: Effectiveness of treatment referral outreach in addressing long-term unmet 9/11 disaster needs. *Disaster Prev. Manag. Int. J.* **2018**, *27*, 321–333. [CrossRef]

9.   Stuber, J.; Galea, S.; Boscarino, J.A.; Schlesinger, M. Was there unmet mental health need after the September 11, 2001 terrorist attacks? *Soc. Psychiatry Psychiatr. Epidemiol.* **2006**, *41*, 230–240. [CrossRef]

10.   Green, D.C.; Buehler, J.W.; Silk, B.J.; Thompson, N.J.; Schild, L.A.; Klein, M.; Berkelman, R.L. Trends in healthcare use in the New York City region following the Terrorist Attacks of 2001. *Biosecur. Bioterror. Biodef. Strategy Pract. Sci.* **2006**, *4*, 263–275. [CrossRef]

11.   Norris, F.H.; Friedman, M.J.; Watson, P.J. 60,000 disaster victims speak: Part II. Summary and implications of the disaster mental health research. *Psychiatry Interpers. Biol. Process.* **2002**, *65*, 240–260. [CrossRef]

12.   Rodriguez, J.J.; Kohn, R. Use of mental health services among disaster survivors. *Curr. Opin. Psychiatry* **2008**, *21*, 370–378. [CrossRef] [PubMed]

13.   Boscarino, J.A.; Adams, R.E.; Stuber, J.; Galea, S. Disparities in mental health treatment following the World Trade Center Disaster: Implications for mental health care and health services research. *J. Trauma. Stress* **2005**, *18*, 287–297. [CrossRef] [PubMed]

14.   Boscarino, J.A.; Galea, S.; Adams, R.E.; Ahern, J.; Resnick, H.; Vlahov, D. Mental health service and medication use in New York City after the September 11, 2001, terrorist attack. *Psychiatr. Serv.* **2004**, *55*, 274–283. [CrossRef] [PubMed]

15. Boscarino, J.A.; Adams, R.E.; Figley, C.R. Mental health service use 1-year after the World Trade Center disaster: Implications for mental health care. *Gen. Hosp. Psychiatry* **2004**, *26*, 346–358. [CrossRef] [PubMed]

16. Boscarino, J.A.; Galea, S.; Ahern, J.; Resnick, H.; Vlahov, D. Utilization of mental health services following the September 11th terrorist attacks in Manhattan, New York City. *Int. J. Emerg. Ment. Health* **2002**, *4*, 143–155. [PubMed]

17. Boscarino, J.A.; Adams, R.E.; Figley, C.R. Mental health service use after the World Trade Center disaster: Utilization trends and comparative effectiveness. *J. Nerv. Ment. Dis.* **2011**, *199*, 91. [CrossRef]

18. Farfel, M.; DiGrande, L.; Brackbill, R.; Prann, A.; Cone, J.; Friedman, S.; Walker, D.J.; Pezeshki, G.; Thomas, P.; Galea, S.; et al. An overview of 9/11 experiences and respiratory and mental health conditions among World Trade Center Health Registry enrollees. *J. Urban Health* **2008**, *85*, 880–909. [CrossRef]

19. Adams, R.E.; Boscarino, J.A. Stress and well-being in the aftermath of the World Trade Center attack: The continuing effects of a communitywide disaster. *J. Community Psychol.* **2005**, *33*, 175–190. [CrossRef]

20. Brackbill, R.M.; Stellman, S.D.; Perlman, S.E.; Walker, D.J.; Farfel, M.R. Mental health of those directly exposed to the World Trade Center disaster: Unmet mental health care need, mental health treatment service use, and quality of life. *Soc. Sci. Med.* **2013**, *81*, 110–114. [CrossRef]

21. Blanchard, E.B.; Jones-Alexander, J.; Buckley, T.C.; Forneris, C.A. Psychometric properties of the PTSD Checklist (PCL). *Behav. Res. Therapy* **1996**, *34*, 669–673. [CrossRef]

22. Ruggiero, K.J.; Del Ben, K.; Scotti, J.R.; Rabalais, A.E. Psychometric properties of the PTSD Checklist—Civilian version. *J. Trauma. Stress* **2003**, *16*, 495–502. [CrossRef] [PubMed]

23. Weathers, F.W.; Litz, B.T.; Herman, D.; Huska, J.; Keane, T. *The PTSD Checklist-Civilian Version (PCL-C)*; National Center for PTSD: Boston, MA, USA, 1994.

24. American Psychiatric Association. *Diagnostic and Statistical Manual of Mental Disorders: DSM-IV1994*; American Psychiatric Association: Washington, DC, USA, 2013.

25. McDonald, S.D.; Calhoun, P.S. The diagnostic accuracy of the PTSD checklist: A critical review. *Clin. Psychol. Rev.* **2010**, *30*, 976–987. [CrossRef] [PubMed]

26. Kroenke, K.; Strine, T.W.; Spitzer, R.L.; Williams, J.B.; Berry, J.T.; Mokdad, A.H. The PHQ-8 as a measure of current depression in the general population. *J. Affect. Disorders* **2009**, *114*, 163–173. [CrossRef] [PubMed]

27. Kroenke, K.; Spitzer, R.L. The PHQ-9: A new depression diagnostic and severity measure. *Psychiatr. Ann.* **2002**, *32*, 509–515. [CrossRef]

28. Kroenke, K.; Spitzer, R.L.; Williams, J.B. The PHQ-9: Validity of a brief depression severity measure. *J. Gen. Intern. Med.* **2001**, *16*, 606–613. [CrossRef] [PubMed]

29. Fuertes, J.N.; Mislowack, A.; Bennett, J.; Paul, L.; Gilbert, T.C.; Fontan, G.; Boylan, L.S. The physician–patient working alliance. *Patient Educ. Counsel.* **2007**, *66*, 29–36. [CrossRef]

30. Ankuta, G.Y.; Abeles, N. Client satisfaction, clinical significance, and meaningful change in psychotherapy. *Prof. Psychol. Res. Pract.* **1993**, *24*, 70. [CrossRef]

31. Stuber, J.; Fairbrother, G.; Galea, S.; Pfefferbaum, B.; Wilson-Genderson, M.; Vlahov, D. Determinants of counseling for children in Manhattan after the September 11 attacks. *Psychiatr. Serv.* **2002**, *53*, 815–822. [CrossRef]

32. Hoven, C.; Duarte, C.; Cohen, M.; Lucas, C.; Gregorian, N.; Rosen, C. *Effects of the World Trade Center Attack on NYC Public School Students*; New York City Board of Education: New York, NY, USA, 2002.

33. Janicke, D.M.; Finney, J.W.; Riley, A.W. Children's health care use a prospective investigation of factors related to care-seeking. *Med. Care* **2001**, *39*, 990–1001. [CrossRef]

34. Klein, T.P.; Devoe, E.R.; Miranda-Julian, C.; Linas, K. Young children's responses to September 11th: The New York City experience. *Infant Ment. Health J.* **2009**, *30*, 1–22. [CrossRef] [PubMed]

35. Davis, L.; Siegel, L.J. Posttraumatic stress disorder in children and adolescents: A review and analysis. *Clin. Child Fam. Psychol. Rev.* **2000**, *3*, 135–154. [CrossRef] [PubMed]

36. Wang, P.S.; Gruber, M.J.; Powers, R.E.; Schoenbaum, M.; Speier, A.H.; Wells, K.B.; Kessler, R.C. Mental health service use among Hurricane Katrina survivors in the eight months after the disaster. *Psychiatr. Serv.* **2007**, *58*, 1403–1411. [CrossRef] [PubMed]

37. Wang, P.S.; Berglund, P.A.; Olfson, M.; Kessler, R.C. Delays in initial treatment contact after first onset of a mental disorder. *Health Serv. Res.* **2004**, *39*, 393–416. [CrossRef] [PubMed]

38. Yousaf, O.; Grunfeld, E.A.; Hunter, M.S. A systematic review of the factors associated with delays in medical and psychological help-seeking among men. *Health Psychol. Rev.* **2015**, *9*, 264–276. [CrossRef] [PubMed]

39. Clement, S.; Schauman, O.; Graham, T.; Maggioni, F.; Evans-Lacko, S.; Bezborodovs, N.; et al. What is the impact of mental health-related stigma on help-seeking? A systematic review of quantitative and qualitative studies. *Psychol. Med.* **2015**, *45*, 11–27. [CrossRef] [PubMed]
40. Ward, E.C.; Wiltshire, J.C.; Detry, M.A.; Brown, R.L. African American men and women's attitude toward mental illness, perceptions of stigma, and preferred coping behaviors. *Nurs. Res.* **2013**, *62*, 185–194. [CrossRef] [PubMed]
41. Cohen, R.E. Mental health services for victims of disasters. *World Psychiatry* **2002**, *1*, 149. [PubMed]
42. Shinfuku, N. Disaster mental health: Lessons learned from the Hanshin Awaji earthquake. *World Psychiatry* **2002**, *1*, 158–159.
43. Sue, S.; Cheng, J.K.Y.; Saad, C.S.; Chu, J.P. Asian American mental health: A call to action. *Am. Psychol.* **2012**, *67*, 532. [CrossRef]
44. Kim, G.; Loi, C.X.A.; Chiriboga, D.A.; Jang, Y.; Parmelee, P.; Allen, R.S. Limited English proficiency as a barrier to mental health service use: A study of Latino and Asian immigrants with psychiatric disorders. *J. Psychiatr. Res.* **2011**, *45*, 104–110. [CrossRef] [PubMed]
45. McGuire, T.G.; Miranda, J. New evidence regarding racial and ethnic disparities in mental health: Policy implications. *Health Affairs* **2008**, *27*, 393–403. [CrossRef]
46. Alegría, M.; Chatterji, P.; Wells, K.; Cao, Z.; Chen, C.-n.; Takeuchi, D.; Jackson, J.; Meng, X.-L. Disparity in depression treatment among racial and ethnic minority populations in the United States. *Psychiatr. Serv.* **2008**, *59*, 1264–1272. [CrossRef]
47. Leong, F.T.; Lau, A.S. Barriers to providing effective mental health services to Asian Americans. *Ment. Health Serv. Res.* **2001**, *3*, 201–214. [CrossRef] [PubMed]
48. Kung, W.W.; Lu, P.-C. How symptom manifestations affect help seeking for mental health problems among Chinese Americans. *J. Nervous Ment. Dis.* **2008**, *196*, 46–54. [CrossRef] [PubMed]
49. Kung, W.W.; Liu, X.; Huang, D.; Kim, P.; Wang, X.; Yang, L.H. Factors related to the probable PTSD after the 9/11 World Trade Center attack among Asian Americans. *J. Urban Health* **2018**, *95*, 255–266. [CrossRef]
50. Dell'Osso, L.; Carpita, B.; Cremone, I.M.; Muti, D.; Diadema, E.; Barberi, F.M.; Massimetti, C.; Brondino, N.; Petrosino, B.; Politi, P.; et al. The mediating effect of trauma and stressor related symptoms and ruminations on the relationship between autistic traits and mood spectrum. *Psychiatry Res.* **2018**, in press. [CrossRef] [PubMed]
51. Yu, S.; Brackbill, R.M.; Stellman, S.D.; Ghuman, S.; Farfel, M.R. Evaluation of non-response bias in a cohort study of World Trade Center terrorist attack survivors. *BMC Res. Notes* **2015**, *8*, 42. [CrossRef]
52. Murphy, J.; Brackbill, R.M.; Thalji, L.; Dolan, M.; Pulliam, P.; Walker, D.J. Measuring and maximizing coverage in the World Trade Center Health Registry. *Stat. Med.* **2007**, *26*, 1688–1701. [CrossRef] [PubMed]

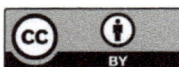

International Journal of
*Environmental Research
and Public Health*

MDPI

Article

Allergen Sensitization and Asthma Outcomes among World Trade Center Rescue and Recovery Workers

Belen Rojano [1], Erin West [1], Emily Ferdermann [1], Steven Markowitz [2], Denise Harrison [3], Laura Crowley [4], Paula Busse [5], Alex D. Federman [1] and Juan P. Wisnivesky [1,6,*]

[1] Division of General Internal Medicine, Department of Medicine, Icahn School of Medicine at Mount Sinai, New York, NY 10029, USA; belen.rojanobroz@mountsinai.org (B.R.); krystallyn@gmail.com (E.W.); emily.federmann@mountsinai.org (E.F.); alex.federman@mountsinai.org (A.D.F.)

[2] Barry Commoner Center for Health and the Environment, Queens College, City University of New York, Queens, New York, NY 11367, USA; steven.markowitz@qc.cuny.edu

[3] Department of Medicine, New York University School of Medicine, Bellevue Hospital Center, New York, NY 10016, USA; denise.harrison@nyulangone.org

[4] Division of Occupational and Environmental Medicine, Department of Environmental Medicine and Public Health, Icahn School of Medicine at Mount Sinai, New York, NY 10029, USA; laura.crowley@mssm.edu

[5] Division of Allergy and Immunology, Department of Medicine, Icahn School of Medicine at Mount Sinai, New York, NY 10029, USA; paula.busse@mssm.edu

[6] Division of Pulmonary, Critical Care, and Sleep Medicine, Department of Medicine, Icahn School of Medicine at Mount Sinai, New York, NY 10029, USA

* Correspondence: juan.wisnivesky@mssm.edu; Tel.: +1-212-8247567

Received: 15 January 2019; Accepted: 22 February 2019; Published: 1 March 2019

Abstract: A large number of World Trade Center (WTC) rescue and recovery workers are affected by asthma. While physical and mental health comorbidities have been associated with poor asthma control in this population, the potential role of allergen sensitization is unknown. This study examined the association of indoor sensitization and exposure as a risk factor for increased asthma morbidity in WTC workers. We used data from a prospective cohort of 331 WTC workers with asthma. Sensitization to indoor allergens was assessed by measurement of antigen-specific serum immunoglobulin E (IgE) levels. We used validated tools to evaluate the exposure to indoor allergens. Asthma morbidity outcomes included level of control (Asthma Control Questionnaire, ACQ), quality of life (Asthma Quality of Life Questionnaire, AQLQ) and acute resource utilization. The prevalence of sensitization to cat, dog, mouse, dust mite, cockroach, and mold allergens were 33%, 21%, 17%, 40%, 17%, and 17%, respectively. Unadjusted and regression analyses showed no significant relationship between sensitization and increased asthma morbidity ($p > 0.05$ for all comparisons), except for sensitization to Aspergillus Fumigatus, cat and mouse epithelium, which were associated with decreased morbidity.

Keywords: World Trade Center; indoor allergens sensitization; asthma quality of life; asthma control; asthma outcomes; mini asthma quality of life questionnaire; asthma morbidity; WTC-related asthma; immunoglobulin E; allergen exposure

---

1. Introduction

Multiple studies have documented high rates of asthma prevalence (approximately 30% cumulative incidence, 9 years after exposure) among World Trade Center (WTC) rescue and recovery workers [1,2]. Recent studies have also demonstrated that many WTC-exposed individuals suffer from substantial asthma morbidity, including poor disease control and a relatively high number of emergency room visits and hospitalizations [1]. The reasons for the poor outcomes observed among WTC workers are likely multifactorial and partially explained by an increased prevalence of comorbidities, such as gastroesophageal reflux (GERD) and chronic sinusitis, which are known to worsen asthma [1,3]. Similarly, post-traumatic stress disorder (PTSD), which has been described in up to 30% of WTC workers, is strongly associated with increased asthma morbidity [4].

Allergic sensitization is also associated with increased asthma morbidity, particularly in inner-city children [5,6]. Moreover, environmental remediation strategies to reduce indoor exposures have been shown to improve asthma control in this population [7,8]. The results of studies assessing the role of allergic sensitization in adult asthmatics are mixed [9–11]. Nonetheless, anti-immunoglobulin E (IgE) therapy is effective for antigen-sensitized patients and trigger avoidance is currently recommended as a major component of asthma self-management by the most recent national asthma guidelines [12]. The role sensitization and exposure to allergens on asthma outcomes in WTC workers has not been previously explored.

In this study, we determined the rates of sensitization to indoor allergens in a cohort of WTC workers with asthma, and assessed the relationship to asthma control and acute resource utilization.

2. Materials and Methods

2.1. Study Population

The study was conducted using data from a cohort of WTC workers with a physician diagnosis of asthma. Study participants were recruited between December 2012 and July 2016, from WTC workers who were followed by the Mount Sinai Hospital, North Shore-Long Island Jewish Health System/Queens College, and the New York University School of Medicine WTC Health Program. Criteria for recruitment into this program have been previously published [4,13] and include individuals who have volunteered or worked in the lower Manhattan, barge-loading piers or Staten Island landfill, and workers from the Port Authority Trans Hudson Corporation who were engaged in cleaning and personnel of the Office of the Chief Medical Examiner who processed human remains. Lower Manhattan residents, schoolchildren, building occupants, and passers-by were not included in this registry. Members of the Fire Department of the City of New York (FDNY) who are followed in a parallel program were also not included in the present study.

The current study was limited to patients with physician-diagnosed asthma who spoke English or Spanish and were ≥18 years of age at the time of enrollment. We excluded WTC workers with a prior diagnosis of chronic obstructive lung disease (COPD) and those who had history of >15 pack-years of smoking, due to the possibility of undiagnosed COPD. We also excluded workers with other chronic respiratory illnesses. Signed consent was obtained from all participants; the Institutional Review Boards of the Icahn School of Medicine at Mount Sinai, Queens College and New York University School of Medicine approved this study.

2.2. Study Variables

Study participants underwent an in-person standardized interview in English or Spanish to collect sociodemographic information and data regarding asthma history, including onset in relation to WTC exposure and medication regimen. We obtained information about physician diagnosis of GERD, allergic rhinitis, and chronic sinusitis, as well as other comorbidities. In order to diagnose the presence of mental health conditions (PTSD, panic disorder and depression) patients underwent a structured clinical psychiatric interview (SCID) [14]. According to criteria published in previous studies, participants were assigned to one of four different groups depending on the level of WTC exposure: Low, intermediate, high, and very high [1].

2.3. Allergic Sensitization and Exposure Assessments

Sensitization to indoor allergens was assessed using serum IgE levels in peripheral blood; a level >0.35 kU/L was considered indicative of sensitization [12,15]. The allergens included were, cat epithelium and dander, dog, mouse epithelium, house dust mites (*Dermatophagoides Farinae* and

Dermatophagoides Pteronyssinus), cockroaches (*Blatella Germanica* or *Periplaneta Americana*), and molds (*Alternaria Alternata* and *Aspergillus Fumigatus*). Serum IgE levels were determined using the Thermo Fisher Scientific Analyzer Phadia™ 1000® (Phadia AB, Uppsala, Sweden). Home environmental exposures were ascertained using survey questions previously validated against findings from home inspections [16–18]. The survey included questions about the presence of pets at home, visible molds, mildew, wet spots, and/or cockroaches. In addition, study participants were asked about the presence of dust at home, home cleaning behaviors, and if the participants kept windows closed during the allergy seasons.

2.4. Outcomes

We used the Asthma Control Questionnaire (ACQ) to assess the level of asthma control [19]. The ACQ is a validated tool available in English and Spanish and has been extensively used in clinical practice and research [20]. Higher ACQ scores indicate worse asthma control and a change of >0.5 units is considered clinically significant [19]. The impact of allergic sensitization on quality of life was assessed with the Mini Asthma Quality of Life Questionnaire (AQLQ) [21]. This validated tool includes 15 questions in four domains (symptoms, environment, emotions and activities) and has good reliability and responsiveness [21,22]. A higher score on the AQLQ indicates better quality of life related to asthma [21]. We also collected information about asthma-related resource utilization (visits to emergency department, hospitalizations, use of oral corticosteroids) in the previous year.

2.5. Statistical Analysis

The means with standard deviations and percentages with 95% confidence intervals (CI) were used to describe the baseline characteristics of the study participants. We used the *t*-test to compare ACQ and AQLQ scores of WTC workers sensitized versus those not sensitized to each specific indoor allergen. The chi-square test was used to compare acute resource utilization according to sensitization status. The adjusted association between sensitization status, ACQ, and AQLQ scores over time was assessed using linear regression to control for sociodemographic characteristics, asthma history, asthma onset in relation to 9/11 exposure, asthma regimen, WTC exposure level, and comorbidities. The potential relationship of acute resource utilization with sensitization to each allergen was evaluated using logistic regression analysis.

Power calculations showed that a total of approximately 220 patients were required for the study to have 80% power to detect a clinically significance difference of $\geq$0.5 units in ACQ and AQLQ scores among patients sensitized versus not sensitized to each indoor allergen. All statistical tests were performed with SAS statistical software (SAS Institute, Cary, NC, USA) using 2-tailed tests.

3. Results

3.1. Participant Characteristics

Overall, 373 WTC workers with asthma were enrolled in the study; of these, 42 lacked results for specific IgE and were excluded from these analyses. The mean (SD) age of study participants was 52.7 (8) years; 73% were male; 35% white, 13% Black, and 43% Hispanic (Table 1). Most WTC workers (72%) reported asthma onset after WTC exposure and 66% were prescribed an asthma controller medication. Among the cohort, the frequency of patients with well-controlled, uncontrolled, and very poorly controlled asthma was 27%, 26%, and 47%, respectively; almost half (49%) reported poor quality of life. In terms of resource utilization, 20% of WTC workers had a hospitalization or an ER visit related to their asthma in the previous 12 months, and 27% had received an oral corticosteroid burst for an exacerbation.

Table 1. Baseline characteristics of World Trade Center rescue and recovery workers with asthma.

Characteristic	Value
Age, years, mean (SD)	52.7 (8)
Male, No. (%)	240 (73)
Race/Ethnicity, No. (%)	
White	115 (35)
Black	44 (13)
Hispanic	142 (43)
Other	28 (8)
Refused/Unknown	2 (1)
Education, No. (%)	
Did not graduate high school	30 (9)
High School or GED	52 (16)
Some College	135 (41)
College Graduate or More Advanced Degree	114 (34)
Monthly Income < $3,000, No. (%)	183 (55)
Occupation, No. (%)	
Employed Full Time	141 (43)
Employed Part Time	35 (10)
Unemployed	19 (6)
On Disability	40 (12)
Retired	72 (22)
Not Working/Student/Other	24 (7)
Smoking Status No. (%)	
Current/former Smoker	101 (31)
Never Smoked	220 (66)
Refused/Unknown	10 (3)
WTC Exposure No. (%)	
Low	51 (15)
Intermediate	138 (42)
High	116 (35)
Very High	26 (8)
Asthma Onset Post 9/11, No. (%)	242 (72)
Hospitalization/Emergency Room Visit for Asthma in the Past Year, No. (%)	64 (20)
Oral Corticosteroid Use in Past 12 Months No. (%)	88 (27)
Asthma Control Level, No. (%)	
Well Controlled	91 (27)
Uncontrolled	86 (26)
Very Poorly Controlled	154 (47)
Asthma-related Quality of Life, No. (%)	
Good	172 (52)
Poor	159 (48)
On Asthma Controller Medication, No. (%)	218 (66)
Comorbidities No. (%)	
Gastric Esophageal Reflux Disorder	222 (67)
Sinusitis	207 (63)
Major Depression	88 (27)
Posttraumatic Stress Disorder	81 (24)

SD: standard deviation. No.: Number. WTC: World Trade Center.

Overall, 56% (95% CI: 51–62%) of WTC workers were sensitized to at least one indoor allergen (Table 2). The frequency of sensitization to cat, dog, mouse epithelium, *Dermatophagoides Farinae*, *Dermatophagoides Pteronyssines*, cockroach, *Alternaria Tenuis*, and *Aspergillus Fumigatus* was 33% (95% CI: 28–38%), 21% (95% CI: 17–26%), 17% (95% CI: 13–22%), 34% (95% CI: 30–40%), 32% (95% CI: 26–37%), 17% (95% CI: 13–21%), 11% (95% CI: 7–14%), and 10% (95% CI: 6–15%), respectively. Overall, 50% of participants had cats, dogs, or birds at home, 17% reported presence of mice/rats at home, 24% had observed cockroaches, 20% observed wet spots, 25% had mold/mildew at their home, and only 34% kept windows closed during the allergy season.

Table 2. Sensitization and exposure to indoor allergens among World Trade Center rescue and recovery workers with asthma.

Allergen	Number	Percentage (95% CI)
At least One Indoor Allergens	186	56 (51–62)
Cat Dander	110	33 (28–38)
Dog Dander	63	21 (17–26)
Mouse Epithelium	57	17 (13–22)
Dermatophagoides Farinae	115	34 (29–40)
Dermatophagoides Pteronyssines	105	32 (26–37)
Cockroach	57	17 (13–21)
Alternaria Tenuis	35	11 (7–14)
Aspergillus Fumigatus	20	10 (6–15)
Home Exposures		
Cats, dogs or birds living in home	165	50 (44–55)
Mice or rats	58	17 (13–22)
Cockroaches	79	24 (19–29)
Wet spots on walls, wallpaper, ceilings or carpets	68	20 (16–25)
Mold or mildew growing on surfaces	83	25 (20–30)
Keeps windows closed during allergen season	110	34 (29–40)

CI: confidence interval.

3.2. Unadjusted Associations between Sensitization and Asthma Morbidity

Unadjusted analyses showed no significant association between sensitization to most indoor allergen and ACQ and AQLQ scores ($p > 0.05$ for all comparisons) (Table 3). Only sensitization to Aspergillus Fumigatus (mean difference: -0.63; 95% CI: -1.17 to -0.09) was associated with a lower ACQ score. Similarly, sensitization to at least one allergen (mean difference: 0.29; 95% CI: 0.01 to 0.56), and sensitization to cat allergens (mean difference: 0.36; 95% CI: 0.08 to 0.65) were associated with higher AQLQ scores. In addition, the use of oral corticosteroids and acute resource utilization were not significantly associated with sensitization status to most allergens ($p > 0.05$ for all comparisons). However, sensitization to mouse epithelium (OR: 0.39; 95% CI: 0.18–0.86) was associated with a decreased use of oral corticoids in the year before enrollment. We also found that acute asthma-related resource utilization was lower in patients sensitized to at least one allergen (OR: 0.54; 95% CI: 0.29–0.99). Unadjusted analyses also showed no significant interaction between allergen sensitization and WTC exposure category ($p > 0.05$ for all comparisons), suggesting the effect of sensitization was not different according to the level of exposure at the WTC site.

Table 3. Unadjusted associations between sensitization to indoor allergens and asthma morbidity in World Trade Center rescue and recovery workers.

Exposure	Mean ACQ Difference, 95% CI	Mean AQLQ Difference, 95% CI	OCS Use OR, 95% CI	Resource Utilization OR, 95% CI
At Least One Allergen	−0.15 (−0.40, 0.09)	0.29 (0.01, 0.56) *	1.24 (0.75, 2.06)	0.54 (0.29, 0.99)
Cat Dander	−0.14 (−0.40, 0.11)	0.36 (0.08, 0.65) *	1.51 (0.91, 2.52)	0.66 (0.33, 1.31)
Dog Dander	0.04 (−0.28, 0.35)	0.21 (−0.15, 0.56)	0.83 (0.43, 1.60)	0.58 (0.23, 1.45)
Mouse Epithelium	0.12 (−0.21, 0.44)	0.04 (−0.32, 0.40)	0.39 (0.18, 0.86) *	0.62 (0.25, 1.54)
Dermatophagoides Farinae	0.03 (−0.23, 0.28)	0.10 (−0.18, 0.39)	1.06 (0.63, 1.77)	0.71 (0.36, 1.38)
Dermatophagoides Pteronyssines	−0.11 (−0.38, 0.15)	0.14 (−0.15, 0.44)	0.76 (0.44, 1.32)	0.75 (0.38, 1.48)
Cockroach	−0.04 (−0.37, 0.29)	0.01 (−0.35, 0.37)	0.91 (0.47, 1.77)	0.50 (0.19, 1.33)
Alternaria Tenuis	−0.33 (−0.73, 0.06)	0.39 (−0.06, 0.83)	0.55 (0.22, 1.38)	0.32 (0.07, 1.36)
Aspergillus Fumigatus	−0.63 (−1.17, −0.09) *	0.53 (−0.05, 1.12)	0.56 (0.18, 1.77)	0.29 (0.04, 2.25)

CI: confidence interval; OR: odds ratio; OCS: oral corticosteroids, ACQ: Asthma Control Questionnaire, AQLQ: Asthma Quality of Life Questionnaire. * Statistically significant at a <0.05 level.

3.3. Adjusted Associations between Indoor Sensitization and Asthma Control

Adjusted analyses also showed no statistically significant association between the sensitization to most allergens and ACQ and AQLQ scores, use of oral steroids, and previous utilization of health care services ($p > 0.05$ for all comparisons) (Table 4). However, sensitization to at least one indoor allergen (mean difference: 0.27; 95% CI: 0.03 to 0.50) or Dermatophagoides Pteronyssines (mean difference: 0.29; 95% CI: 0.03 to 0.55) were significantly associated with higher AQLQ scores. Finally, sensitization to at least one allergen (OR: 0.41; 95% CI: 0.20–0.85), and cockroach (OR: 0.27; 95% CI: 0.08–0.91) were significantly associated with lower rates of acute asthma-related resource utilization.

Table 4. Adjusted associations between sensitization to indoor allergens and asthma morbidity in World Trade Center rescue and recovery workers.

Exposure	Mean ACQ Difference, 95% CI	Mean AQLQ Difference, 95% CI	OCS Use OR and 95% CI	Utilization OR and 95% CI
At least One Allergen	−0.19 (−0.43, 0.04)	0.27 (0.03, 0.50) *	1.16 (0.65, 2.07)	0.41 (0.20, 0.85) *
Cat Dander	−0.09 (−0.34, 0.16)	0.17 (−0.09, 0.43)	1.46 (0.80, 2.66)	0.47 (0.21, 1.06)
Dog Dander	−0.06 (−0.37, 0.24)	0.29 (−0.02, 0.61)	0.77 (0.37, 1.62)	0.45 (0.16, 1.27)
Mouse Epithelium	0.20 (−0.11, 0.50)	−0.08 (−0.39, 0.24)	0.42 (0.17, 1.02)	0.41 (0.13, 1.31)
Dermatophagoides Farinae	0.02 (−0.23, 0.27)	0.06 (−0.19, 0.31)	1.10 (0.60, 2.00)	0.48 (0.21, 1.08)
Dermatophagoides Pteronyssines	−0.24 (−0.49, 0.01)	0.29 (0.03, 0.55) *	0.77 (0.40, 1.46)	0.56 (0.24, 1.31)
Cockroach	−0.29 (−0.61, 0.03)	0.30 (−0.03, 0.63)	0.81 (0.36, 1.80)	0.27 (0.08, 0.91) *
Alternaria Tenuis	−0.10 (−0.48, 0.28)	0.09 (−0.30, 0.48)	0.49 (0.17, 1.38)	0.31 (0.06, 1.60)
Aspergillus Fumigatus	−0.42 (−0.94, 0.10)	0.46 (−0.08, 0.99)	0.42 (0.10, 1.69)	0.44 (0.05, 4.14)

CI: confidence interval; OR: odds ratio; OCS: oral corticosteroids, ACQ: Asthma Control Questionnaire, AQLQ: Asthma Quality of Life Questionnaire. * Statistically significant at a <0.05 level.

4. Discussion

Asthma is a common WTC-related condition that is frequently poorly controlled and associated with substantial healthcare resource utilization [1]. In this study, we found that a large percentage of WTC workers are sensitized to common indoor allergens, similarly to the general population [23]. However, sensitization to most of the indoor allergens evaluated was not significantly associated with increased asthma morbidity or acute resource utilization, even among WTC workers exposed to these allergens. These results suggest that efforts to better control WTC-related asthma should focus on other established risk factors, such as other medical co-morbidities, PTSD, or low adherence to controller medication, and other effective self-management behaviors [1,2,4].

There is strong epidemiologic evidence linking allergen sensitization to increased asthma morbidity in inner-city children [5,6,24,25]. Moreover, the effectiveness of home-based environmental remediation and multi-trigger interventions in decreasing allergen exposure and reducing asthma morbidity is well-established [26,27]. Several studies have also evaluated the potential impact of allergic sensitization on asthma outcomes in adults. Specific allergens, in particular cockroach [5] and *Alternaria* [28], have been associated with more severe asthma; asthma deaths have been linked to high fungal spore counts in the environment [29]. Similarly, a study of 140 inner-city women with asthma showed a statistically significant association between increased asthma morbidity and exposure to cats among sensitized patients [30]. A study of elderly inner-city asthmatics showed that patients with high levels of cockroach-specific IgE had worse disease control and more severe airflow obstruction [10]. Similarly, a study of 5845 adults with asthma showed higher exacerbation rates in those sensitized to cat or dogs that had these pets at home [31]. Conversely, a study of 245 inner-city adults with persistent asthma showed no significant relationship between indoor allergen sensitization and asthma outcomes [9]. The European Respiratory Health Survey showed no association between the levels of cat allergen and/or sensitization status with asthma symptoms [32]. Our study extends these findings by showing a lack of association between sensitization and asthma morbidity in WTC workers.

Several factors may explain our findings. WTC-related asthma may be associated with a higher prevalence of airway neutrophilia [33]. Asthma is characterized by airway inflammation [34], characterized by an eosinophil-dominated pattern, especially in patients who have allergen-induced symptoms and an underlying T2 inflammatory profile. However, asthma is a heterogeneous disease and there is increased evidence that other mechanisms, such as a neutrophil-mediated inflammation, less often associated with atopy, could lead to enhanced bronchial reactivity and airflow obstruction in some patients [35]. Th-17 cells appear to play a key role in the pathophysiology of neutrophilic asthma, a disease often associated with worse control and resistance to inhaled corticosteroids [34,36–43]. Thus, if a larger proportion of WTC workers have neutrophil predominant asthma, it is expected that sensitization plays a decreased role in the underlying pathophysiology of this asthma phenotype, and hence its control. Further understanding about the most common patterns of airway inflammation in WTC workers with asthma is important for personalizing their management.

Many WTC workers have physical and/or mental health comorbidities known to increase asthma morbidity. These include GERD, chronic sinusitis, and rhinitis, as well as, PTSD, and major depression [1,3,4]. Thus, these conditions may be more important determinants of the level of asthma control in WTC workers, rather than the potential impact of allergic sensitization. While prior studies have showed that there is a strong negative impact of allergic sensitization among inner-city children with asthma, our cohort was limited to adults, who spent less time at home and therefore are less exposed to the home indoor environment [44].

Given the relatively high rate of allergen sensitization in our population of WTC workers with asthma, avoidance of environmental triggers could still contribute to improved control in some of these patients, particularly those with features of eosinophilic disease. However, our findings suggest that healthcare providers should also focus on other important asthma triggers in this population, such as other medical comorbidities and occupational exposures.

Our study has some limitations that should be mentioned. Our data were collected between 11 and 15 years of the WTC exposure, and therefore our findings represent a narrow window in time. Despite enrolling a relatively large number of WTC workers, our cohort did not represent all populations exposed to WTC disaster, such as firefighters, local residents, and passersby. Thus, our results may not be generalizable to these groups. Our study did not include a non-WTC asthma control group to assess for potential differences in the role and the impact of allergen sensitization. WTC rescue and recovery workers are a unique population given their exposures at the WTC site, range of occupations and associated exposures prior and after 9/11, healthy worker effect, and a high prevalence of physical and mental health comorbidities, many of which (e.g., GERD and PTSD) are associated with worse asthma control. Thus, it is very difficult to identify a control group to perform robust comparisons of the relationship between allergic sensitization and asthma morbidity in WTC versus no-WTC populations. However, in a prior study of non-WTC asthma patients recruited from the same institution [9], we found similar rates of sensitization to cats (41%), mouse epithelium (14%), dust mites (43%), molds (21%) than those reported in our WTC workers cohort. The prevalence of sensitization to cockroach was higher in the non-WTC asthma cohort (60% vs. 17%) that could be related to higher levels of cockroach exposure in this inner-city population and may explain some of the differences in our results. In this non-WTC population, adjusted analyses showed that allergy to cockroach, dust mites, cat, mouse, or molds were not associated with increased resource utilization or worse asthma outcomes. Some exceptions were the presence of dust mite sensitization that was related to increased use of oral steroids in the year before enrollment, mouse sensitization that was related with an increased number of hospitalizations, and cat sensitization that showed decreased number to ED visits during the follow up period. Similarly, our adjusted analyses showed significant associations between sensitization to some allergens (*Dermatophagoides Pteronyssines* and cockroach) with markers of decreased asthma morbidity. We used objective measures of allergen sensitization and validated cut-offs, however, we did not collect home samples to assess the actual levels of environmental exposure. Although self-reported measures may be subject to bias, we used validated items that have been correlated to direct home environmental assessments [16,21,22]. Similarly, we used validated instruments to assess asthma control and quality of life in study participants. We did not evaluate IgE sensitization to outdoor allergens, as they play a limited role in asthma exacerbations [45]. We found that sensitization to some allergens was associated with improved asthma control. However, these relationships were inconsistent across different asthma outcomes for specific allergens, and thus, more likely related to random sampling. Conversely, our study was not powered to find small differences in asthma control and quality of life among sensitized WTC workers; however, our sample was sufficient for identifying clinically meaningful differences in these outcomes. Finally, we did not assess the potential impact of outdoor allergens on asthma morbidity levels of WTC workers.

5. Conclusions

In summary, we found no significant associations between indoor allergen sensitization and exposure to asthma morbidity in WTC workers. Given the high rates of the absence of asthma control and decreased quality of life in this population, our findings can guide providers in their management strategies for WTC workers with asthma.

Author Contributions: Conceptualization, J.P.W.; methodology and investigation, J.P.W., S.M., D.H., L.C., P.B., and A.D.F.; project administration, J.P.W. and E.F.; data curation, E.W., E.F., J.P.W., and B.R.; formal analysis, E.W., B.R., and J.P.W.; writing—original draft preparation, B.R., E.W., E.F.; writing—review and editing, J.P.W., S.M., D.H., L.C., P.B., and A.D.F.; visualization, B.R., E.W., E.F., and J.P.W.; supervision, J.P.W.; funding acquisition, J.P.W.

Funding: This study was funded by the National Institute for Occupational Safety and Health (U01OH010405).

Acknowledgments: This study was supported by CDC/NIOSH grant U01OH010405. Data were provided by the General Responder Data Center at Mount Sinai (CDC/NIOSH contract 200-2017-93325). Rojano was supported by a Research Fellowship from the Fundación Alfonso Martín Escudero.

Conflicts of Interest: Wisnivesky has received a consultant honorarium from Merck, Astra Zeneca, and Quintiles, and research grants from Sanofi and Quorum. Busse received a grant and honorarium from Shire and honorarium from Behring, Pharming, Pearl Therapeutics, Biocryst, CVS Health, and GSK. The other authors have no conflict of interest to report.

References

1. Jordan, H.T.; Stellman, S.D.; Reibman, J.; Farfel, M.R.; Brackbill, R.M.; Friedman, S.M.; Li, J.; Cone, J.E. Factors associated with poor control of 9/11-related asthma 10–11 years after the 2001 World Trade Center terrorist attacks. *J. Asthma Off. J. Assoc. Care Asthma* **2015**, *52*, 630–637. [CrossRef] [PubMed]

2. Wisnivesky, J.P.; Teitelbaum, S.L.; Todd, A.C.; Boffetta, P.; Crane, M.; Crowley, L.; de la Hoz, R.E.; Dellenbaugh, C.; Harrison, D.; Herbert, R.; et al. Persistence of multiple illnesses in World Trade Center rescue and recovery workers: A cohort study. *Lancet* **2011**, *378*, 888–897. [CrossRef]

3. Li, J.; Brackbill, R.M.; Stellman, S.D.; Farfel, M.R.; Miller-Archie, S.A.; Friedman, S.; Walker, D.J.; Thorpe, L.E.; Cone, J. Gastroesophageal reflux symptoms and comorbid asthma and posttraumatic stress disorder following the 9/11 terrorist attacks on World Trade Center in New York City. *Am. J. Gastroenterol.* **2011**, *106*, 1933–1941. [CrossRef] [PubMed]

4. Mindlis, I.; Morales-Raveendran, E.; Goodman, E.; Xu, K.; Vila-Castelar, C.; Keller, K.; Crawford, G.; James, S.; Katz, C.L.; Crowley, L.E.; et al. Post-traumatic stress disorder dimensions and asthma morbidity in World Trade Center rescue and recovery workers. *J. Asthma Off. J. Assoc. Care Asthma* **2017**, *54*, 723–731. [CrossRef] [PubMed]

5. Rosenstreich, D.L.; Eggleston, P.; Kattan, M.; Baker, D.; Slavin, R.G.; Gergen, P.; Mitchell, H.; McNiff-Mortimer, K.; Lynn, H.; Ownby, D.; et al. The role of cockroach allergy and exposure to cockroach allergen in causing morbidity among inner-city children with asthma. *N. Engl. J. Med.* **1997**, *336*, 1356–1363. [CrossRef] [PubMed]

6. Sporik, R.; Holgate, S.T.; Platts-Mills, T.A.; Cogswell, J.J. Exposure to house-dust mite allergen (Der p I) and the development of asthma in childhood. A prospective study. *N. Engl. J. Med.* **1990**, *323*, 502–507. [CrossRef] [PubMed]

7. Crain, E.F.; Walter, M.; O'Connor, G.T.; Mitchell, H.; Gruchalla, R.S.; Kattan, M.; Malindzak, G.S.; Enright, P.; Evans, R., 3rd; Morgan, W.; et al. Home and allergic characteristics of children with asthma in seven U.S. urban communities and design of an environmental intervention: The Inner-City Asthma Study. *Environ. Health Perspect.* **2002**, *110*, 939–945. [CrossRef] [PubMed]

8. Carter, M.C.; Perzanowski, M.S.; Raymond, A.; Platts-Mills, T.A. Home intervention in the treatment of asthma among inner-city children. *J. Allergy Clin. Immunol.* **2001**, *108*, 732–737. [CrossRef] [PubMed]

9. Wisnivesky, J.P.; Sampson, H.; Berns, S.; Kattan, M.; Halm, E.A. Lack of association between indoor allergen sensitization and asthma morbidity in inner-city adults. *J. Allergy Clin. Immunol.* **2007**, *120*, 113–120. [CrossRef] [PubMed]

10. Rogers, L.; Cassino, C.; Berger, K.I.; Goldring, R.M.; Norman, R.G.; Klugh, T.; Reibman, J. Asthma in the elderly: Cockroach sensitization and severity of airway obstruction in elderly nonsmokers. *Chest* **2002**, *122*, 1580–1586. [CrossRef] [PubMed]

11. Kanchongkittiphon, W.; Mendell, M.J.; Gaffin, J.M.; Wang, G.; Phipatanakul, W. Indoor environmental exposures and exacerbation of asthma: An update to the 2000 review by the Institute of Medicine. *Environ. Health Perspect.* **2015**, *123*, 6–20. [CrossRef] [PubMed]

12. Platts-Mills, T.A.; Vervloet, D.; Thomas, W.R.; Aalberse, R.C.; Chapman, M.D. Indoor allergens and asthma: Report of the Third International Workshop. *J. Allergy Clin. Immunol.* **1997**, *100*, S2–S24. [CrossRef]

13. Brackbill, R.M.; Hadler, J.L.; DiGrande, L.; Ekenga, C.C.; Farfel, M.R.; Friedman, S.; Perlman, S.E.; Stellman, S.D.; Walker, D.J.; Wu, D.; et al. Asthma and posttraumatic stress symptoms 5 to 6 years following exposure to the World Trade Center terrorist attack. *Jama* **2009**, *302*, 502–516. [CrossRef] [PubMed]

14. First, M.B.; Williams, J.B.; Spitzer, R.L.; Gibbon, M. *Structured Clinical Interview for DSM-IV-TR Axis I Disorders, Clinical Trials Version (SCID-CT)*; Biometrics Research, New York State Psychiatric Institute: New York, NY, USA, 2007.

15. Pastorello, E.A.; Incorvaia, C.; Ortolani, C.; Bonini, S.; Canonica, G.W.; Romagnani, S.; Tursi, A.; Zanussi, C. Studies on the relationship between the level of specific IgE antibodies and the clinical expression of allergy: I. Definition of levels distinguishing patients with symptomatic from patients with asymptomatic allergy to common aeroallergens. *J. Allergy Clin. Immunol.* **1995**, *96*, 580–587. [CrossRef]

16. Dales, R.E.; Schweitzer, I.; Bartlett, S.; Raizenne, M.; Burnett, R. Indoor Air Quality and Health: Reproducibility of Respiratory Symptoms and Reported Home Dampness and Molds using a Self-Administered Questionnaire. *Indoor Air* **1994**, *4*, 2–7. [CrossRef]

17. Dales, R.E.; Zwanenburg, H.; Burnett, R.; Franklin, C.A. Respiratory health effects of home dampness and molds among Canadian children. *Am. J. Epidemiol.* **1991**, *134*, 196–203. [CrossRef] [PubMed]

18. Halm, E.A.; Mora, P.; Leventhal, H. No symptoms, no asthma: The acute episodic disease belief is associated with poor self-management among inner-city adults with persistent asthma. *Chest* **2006**, *129*, 573–580. [CrossRef] [PubMed]

19. Juniper, E.F.; Bousquet, J.; Abetz, L.; Bateman, E.D. Identifying 'well-controlled' and 'not well-controlled' asthma using the Asthma Control Questionnaire. *Respir. Med.* **2006**, *100*, 616–621. [CrossRef] [PubMed]

20. Nathan, R.A.; Sorkness, C.A.; Kosinski, M.; Schatz, M.; Li, J.T.; Marcus, P.; Murray, J.J.; Pendergraft, T.B. Development of the asthma control test: A survey for assessing asthma control. *J. Allergy Clin. Immunol.* **2004**, *113*, 59–65. [CrossRef] [PubMed]

21. Juniper, E.F.; Guyatt, G.H.; Cox, F.M.; Ferrie, P.J.; King, D.R. Development and validation of the Mini Asthma Quality of Life Questionnaire. *Eur. Respir. J.* **1999**, *14*, 32–38. [CrossRef] [PubMed]

22. Sanjuas, C.; Alonso, J.; Sanchis, J.; Casan, P.; Broquetas, J.M.; Ferrie, P.J.; Juniper, E.F.; Anto, J.M. The quality-of-life questionnaire with asthma patients: The Spanish version of the Asthma Quality of Life Questionnaire. *Archivos de Bronconeumologia* **1995**, *31*, 219–226. [PubMed]

23. Busse, P.J.; Cohn, R.D.; Salo, P.M.; Zeldin, D.C. Characteristics of allergic sensitization among asthmatic adults older than 55 years: Results from the National Health and Nutrition Examination Survey, 2005–2006. *Ann. Allergy Asthma Immunol. Off. Publ. Am. Coll. Allergy Asthma Immunol.* **2013**, *110*, 247–252. [CrossRef] [PubMed]

24. Bacharier, L.B.; Dawson, C.; Bloomberg, G.R.; Bender, B.; Wilson, L.; Strunk, R.C. Hospitalization for asthma: Atopic, pulmonary function, and psychological correlates among participants in the Childhood Asthma Management Program. *Pediatrics* **2003**, *112*, e85–e92. [CrossRef] [PubMed]

25. Vargas, P.A.; Simpson, P.M.; Gary Wheeler, J.; Goel, R.; Feild, C.R.; Tilford, J.M.; Jones, S.M. Characteristics of children with asthma who are enrolled in a Head Start program. *J. Allergy Clin. Immunol.* **2004**, *114*, 499–504. [CrossRef] [PubMed]

26. Rabito, F.A.; Carlson, J.C.; He, H.; Werthmann, D.; Schal, C. A single intervention for cockroach control reduces cockroach exposure and asthma morbidity in children. *J. Allergy Clin. Immunol.* **2017**, *140*, 565–570. [CrossRef] [PubMed]

27. Reddy, A.L.; Gomez, M.; Dixon, S.L. An Evaluation of a State-Funded Healthy Homes Intervention on Asthma Outcomes in Adults and Children. *J. Public Health Manag. Pract. JPHMP* **2017**, *23*, 219–228. [CrossRef] [PubMed]

28. O'Hollaren, M.T.; Yunginger, J.W.; Offord, K.P.; Somers, M.J.; O'Connell, E.J.; Ballard, D.J.; Sachs, M.I. Exposure to an aeroallergen as a possible precipitating factor in respiratory arrest in young patients with asthma. *N. Engl. J. Med.* **1991**, *324*, 359–363. [CrossRef] [PubMed]

29. Targonski, P.V.; Persky, V.W.; Ramekrishnan, V. Effect of environmental molds on risk of death from asthma during the pollen season. *J. Allergy Clin. Immunol.* **1995**, *95*, 955–961. [CrossRef]

30. Lewis, S.A.; Weiss, S.T.; Platts-Mills, T.A.; Burge, H.; Gold, D.R. The role of indoor allergen sensitization and exposure in causing morbidity in women with asthma. *Am. J. Respir. Crit. Care Med.* **2002**, *165*, 961–966. [CrossRef] [PubMed]

31. Gergen, P.J.; Mitchell, H.E.; Calatroni, A.; Sever, M.L.; Cohn, R.D.; Salo, P.M.; Thorne, P.S.; Zeldin, D.C. Sensitization and Exposure to Pets: The Effect on Asthma Morbidity in the US Population. *J. Allergy Clin. Immunol. Pract.* **2018**, *6*, 101–107. [CrossRef] [PubMed]

32. Chen, C.M.; Thiering, E.; Zock, J.P.; Villani, S.; Olivieri, M.; Modig, L.; Jarvis, D.; Norback, D.; Verlato, G.; Heinrich, J. Is there a threshold concentration of cat allergen exposure on respiratory symptoms in adults? *PLoS ONE* **2015**, *10*, e0127457. [CrossRef] [PubMed]

33. Weiden, M.D.; Kwon, S.; Caraher, E.; Berger, K.I.; Reibman, J.; Rom, W.N.; Prezant, D.J.; Nolan, A. Biomarkers of World Trade Center Particulate Matter Exposure: Physiology of distal airway and blood biomarkers that predict FEV(1) decline. *Semin. Respir. Crit. Care Med.* **2015**, *36*, 323–333. [CrossRef] [PubMed]

34. Fahy, J.V. Eosinophilic and neutrophilic inflammation in asthma: Insights from clinical studies. *Proc. Am. Thorac. Soc.* **2009**, *6*, 256–259. [CrossRef] [PubMed]

35. Bogaert, P.; Naessens, T.; De Koker, S.; Hennuy, B.; Hacha, J.; Smet, M.; Cataldo, D.; Di Valentin, E.; Piette, J.; Tournoy, K.G.; et al. Inflammatory signatures for eosinophilic vs. neutrophilic allergic pulmonary inflammation reveal critical regulatory checkpoints. *Am. J. Physiol. Lung Cell. Mol. Physiol.* **2011**, *300*, L679–L690. [CrossRef] [PubMed]

36. Douwes, J.; Gibson, P.; Pekkanen, J.; Pearce, N. Non-eosinophilic asthma: Importance and possible mechanisms. *Thorax* **2002**, *57*, 643–648. [CrossRef] [PubMed]

37. Al-Ramli, W.; Prefontaine, D.; Chouiali, F.; Martin, J.G.; Olivenstein, R.; Lemiere, C.; Hamid, Q. T(H)17-associated cytokines (IL-17A and IL-17F) in severe asthma. *J. Allergy Clin. Immunol.* **2009**, *123*, 1185–1187. [CrossRef] [PubMed]

38. Barnes, P.J. Immunology of asthma and chronic obstructive pulmonary disease. *Nat. Rev. Immunol.* **2008**, *8*, 183–192. [CrossRef] [PubMed]

39. Bullens, D.M.; Truyen, E.; Coteur, L.; Dilissen, E.; Hellings, P.W.; Dupont, L.J.; Ceuppens, J.L. IL-17 mRNA in sputum of asthmatic patients: Linking T cell driven inflammation and granulocytic influx? *Respir. Res.* **2006**, *7*, 135. [CrossRef] [PubMed]

40. Hashimoto, T.; Akiyama, K.; Kobayashi, N.; Mori, A. Comparison of IL-17 production by helper T cells among atopic and nonatopic asthmatics and control subjects. *Int. Arch. Allergy Immunol.* **2005**, *137* (Suppl. 1), 51–54. [CrossRef] [PubMed]

41. Cundall, M.; Sun, Y.; Miranda, C.; Trudeau, J.B.; Barnes, S.; Wenzel, S.E. Neutrophil-derived matrix metalloproteinase-9 is increased in severe asthma and poorly inhibited by glucocorticoids. *J. Allergy Clin. Immunol.* **2003**, *112*, 1064–1071. [CrossRef] [PubMed]

42. Levy, B.D.; De Sanctis, G.T.; Devchand, P.R.; Kim, E.; Ackerman, K.; Schmidt, B.A.; Szczeklik, W.; Drazen, J.M.; Serhan, C.N. Multi-pronged inhibition of airway hyper-responsiveness and inflammation by lipoxin A(4). *Nat. Med.* **2002**, *8*, 1018–1023. [CrossRef] [PubMed]

43. Ordonez, C.L.; Shaughnessy, T.E.; Matthay, M.A.; Fahy, J.V. Increased neutrophil numbers and IL-8 levels in airway secretions in acute severe asthma: Clinical and biologic significance. *Am. J. Respir. Crit. Care Med.* **2000**, *161*, 1185–1190. [CrossRef] [PubMed]

44. Holgate, S.T.; Polosa, R. The mechanisms, diagnosis, and management of severe asthma in adults. *Lancet* **2006**, *368*, 780–793. [CrossRef]

45. Nelson, H.S. The importance of allergens in the development of asthma and the persistence of symptoms. *J. Allergy Clin. Immunol.* **2000**, *105*, S628–S632. [CrossRef] [PubMed]

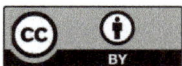

International Journal of
*Environmental Research
and Public Health*

MDPI

Article

9/11 Residential Exposures: The Impact of World Trade Center Dust on Respiratory Outcomes of Lower Manhattan Residents

Vinicius C. Antao [1,2], L. Lászlo Pallos [1], Shannon L. Graham [1], Youn K. Shim [1], James H. Sapp [1], Brian Lewis [1], Steven Bullard [1], Howard E. Alper [3], James E. Cone [3], Mark R. Farfel [3] and Robert M. Brackbill [3,*]

[1] Division of Toxicology and Human Health Sciences, Agency for Toxic Substances and Disease Registries, 4770 Buford Highway NE, Mail Stop F-58, Atlanta, GA 30341, USA; antaov@hss.edu (V.C.A.); Laszlo.Pallos@cdc.HHS.gov (L.L.P.); buu9@cdc.gov (S.L.G.); yak3@cdc.gov (Y.K.S.); ozs1@cdc.gov (J.H.S.); bkl9@cdc.gov (B.L.); asz3@cdc.gov (S.B.)

[2] Center for the Advancement of Value in Musculoskeletal Care, Hospital for Special Surgery, 535 East 70th Street, New York, NY 10021, USA

[3] Department of Health and Mental Hygiene, World Trade Center Health Registry, 125 Worth St, New York, NY 10013, USA; halper@health.nyc.gov (H.E.A.); jcone@health.nyc.gov (J.E.C.); mfarfel@health.nyc.gov (M.R.F.)

* Correspondence: rbrackbi@health.nyc.gov; Tel.: +1-(646)-632-6609; Fax: +1-(646)-632-5175

Received: 4 February 2019; Accepted: 28 February 2019; Published: 5 March 2019

Abstract: Thousands of lower Manhattan residents sustained damage to their homes following the collapse of the Twin Towers on 11 September 2001. Respiratory outcomes have been reported in this population. We sought to describe patterns of home damage and cleaning practices in lower Manhattan and their impacts on respiratory outcomes among World Trade Center Health Registry (WTCHR) respondents. Data were derived from WTCHR Wave 1 (W1) (9/2003–11/2004) and Wave 2 (W2) (11/2006–12/2007) surveys. Outcomes of interest were respiratory symptoms (shortness of breath (SoB), wheezing, persistent chronic cough, upper respiratory symptoms (URS)) first occurring or worsening after 9/11 W1 and still present at W2 and respiratory diseases (asthma and chronic obstructive pulmonary disease (COPD)) first diagnosed after 9/11 W1 and present at W2. We performed descriptive statistics, multivariate logistic regression and geospatial analyses, controlling for demographics and other exposure variables. A total of 6447 residents were included. Mean age on 9/11 was 45.1 years (±15.1 years), 42% were male, 45% had ever smoked cigarettes, and 44% reported some or intense dust cloud exposure on 9/11. The presence of debris was associated with chronic cough (adjusted OR (aOR) = 1.56, CI: 1.12–2.17), and upper respiratory symptoms (aOR = 1.56, CI: 1.24–1.95). A heavy coating of dust was associated with increased shortness of breath (aOR = 1.65, CI: 1.24–2.18), wheezing (aOR = 1.43, CI: 1.03–1.97), and chronic cough (aOR = 1.59, CI: 1.09–2.28). Dusting or sweeping without water was the cleaning behavior associated with the largest number of respiratory outcomes, such as shortness of breath, wheezing, and URS. Lower Manhattan residents who suffered home damage following the 9/11 attacks were more likely to report respiratory symptoms and diseases compared to those who did not report home damage.

Keywords: WTC attack; respiratory symptoms; lower Manhattan residents; cleaning practices

1. Introduction

The terrorist attacks in New York City on 11 September 2001 (9/11) led to the destruction of the World Trade Center (WTC) Twin Towers and six other adjacent buildings. The collapse of the two towers released a massive cloud of dust and debris that damaged surrounding buildings within and around the WTC complex, a 16-acre area that was subsequently called Ground Zero [1]. The plume of dust reached an altitude of 1500 meters and, depending on meteorological conditions, extended to lower Manhattan and the New York and New Jersey metropolitan areas. More than 100,000 μm per cubic meter of particles were estimated to be present in the air during the first few minutes after the collapse of each building [2].

The contents of settled WTC dust have been extensively analyzed and were characterized as a mixture of cement dust, glass fibers, asbestos, lead, polycyclic aromatic hydrocarbons, polychlorinated biphenyls, organochlorine pesticides, and polychlorinated furans and dioxins [1,3–5]. Indoor dust was primarily comprised of inhalable particles (<53 μm). In contrast, most outdoor dust was primarily comprised of larger particles [6].

Approximately 25,000 lower Manhattan residents were physically and emotionally affected by this disaster [7]. Two months after the attacks, air quality and surface dust were among the main concerns of lower Manhattan residents [7]. Most WTC-related residential exposures were caused by re-suspension of settled indoor dust [2] during cleaning efforts or in poorly cleaned environments. This is a large motivator for our analyses of cleaning practices.

A number of studies demonstrated the deleterious health effects of household exposures in the context of the WTC attacks. Most of them were relatively small case-control studies [8–11]. Increased asthma prevalence was previously reported among WTC Health Registry (WTCHR) enrollees who experienced a heavy layer of dust in their homes [12]. Acute and chronic exposures were also associated with lower respiratory symptoms among WTCHR participants [13]. However, prior studies, specifically Lin et al. [8] and Maslow [13], had limited samples of residents (n = 1317; n = 479, respectively). Maslow [13] did not evaluate associations between exposures and specific respiratory symptoms. Although Lin et al. [8] did assess lower and upper respiratory symptoms, they did not include diagnosed conditions such as asthma or chronic obstructive pulmonary disease.

With a large sample of residents in lower Manhattan and a comprehensive set of outcomes, the present study describes patterns of home damage and cleaning practices, as a surrogate for household exposures since measures of exposure in homes is limited. We initially looked at geospatial relationships between Ground Zero location and exposure and health outcomes. We then conducted multivariate logistic regression analyses to find potential associations between those variables among a large sample of WTCHR respondents.

2. Methods

The WTCHR monitors the health of people exposed to the 9/11 WTC disaster through periodic health surveys and is housed within the New York City Department of Health and Mental Hygiene (NYCDHMH). The WTCHR is the largest effort in the United States to monitor health after a disaster of this kind and includes data on 68,444 adults, including lower Manhattan residents, rescue and recovery workers, and building occupants and passers-by. More details on the WTCHR can be found elsewhere [14] and online at https://www1.nyc.gov/site/911health/about/wtc-health-registry.page.

For this report, data were derived from WTCHR Wave 1 (W1) survey (baseline), collected between 9/2003 and 11/2004, and Wave 2 (W2) survey (first follow-up), collected between 11/2006 and 12/2007. We included W1 and W2 participants 18 years and older, whose primary residence on September 11th was located in lower Manhattan, south of Canal Street. Residents who performed rescue and recovery work were excluded from this analysis.

The Centers for Disease Control and Prevention (CDC) and NYCDHMH institutional review boards approved the Registry protocols. A Federal Certificate of Confidentiality was obtained, as was verbal informed consent.

2.1. Environmental and Household Exposures

In the W1 Survey, respondents were asked if they were outdoors after the towers' collapse and to report their location when they first encountered the dust cloud (closest cross street intersection, closest landmark, or closest subway stop) [14]. The W2 survey information was used to categorize dust exposures into "intense", "some", and "none". The "intense" dust exposure was defined as having been in the dust cloud on 9/11 and reporting at least one of five experiences: being unable to see more than a few feet; having difficulty walking or finding one's way; trouble finding shelter; being covered with dust; or not being able to hear. The "some" category consisted of those who had reported being in the dust and debris cloud at Wave 1 but who did not experience intense exposure and "none" were those who reported no dust cloud exposure at all. These categories of exposure to the dust cloud (1 = none, 2 = some, or 3 = intense) were combined with reported location at the time of first encounter with the dust cloud (reported at W1) to produce Figure 1 for the geospatial analysis.

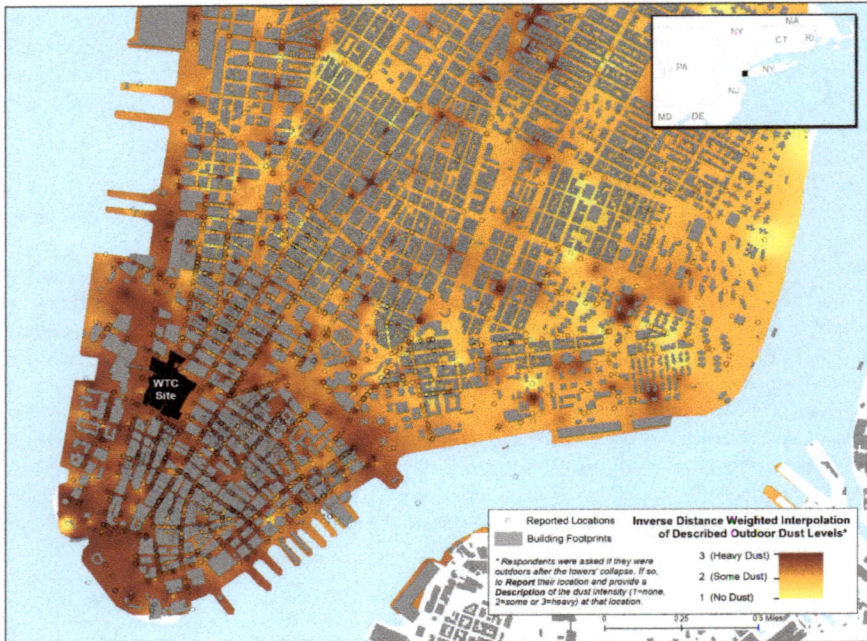

Figure 1. Inverse distance weighted (IDW) interpolation of reported levels of dust cloud intensity (1 = none, 2 = some or 3 = intense) among World Trade Center (WTC) Health Registry respondents (n = 23,466) (Wave 1 survey, 9/2003–11/2004).

Wave 2 also included detailed questions about conditions inside the homes after 9/11 as well as cleaning practices and replacing of household items. WTCHR participants were asked about the presence of "a fine coating of dust on surfaces", "a heavy coating of dust on surfaces (so thick one couldn't see what was underneath)", "broken window(s)", "damage to home or furnishings", and "debris from the disaster". In addition, enrollees answered whether or not they had personally "cleaned ventilation ducts", "cleaned with a damp cloth or wet mop or wet sponge", "used a vacuum (with or without a high-efficiency particulate air or HEPA filter)", and "dusted or swept without water." Moreover, enrollees were inquired whether or not they replaced "carpet or rugs", "furniture (replaced or re-upholstered)", "drapes, blinds or curtains", and "air conditioners" as a result of the 9/11 events.

2.2. Health Outcomes

Outcomes of interest were self-reported respiratory symptoms and self-reported physician diagnoses of respiratory diseases, asked at both W1 and W2 surveys. Symptoms included shortness of breath, wheezing, persistent chronic cough, and upper respiratory symptoms, first occurring or worsening after 9/11 and present at W2. Respiratory diseases comprised asthma or reactive airways dysfunction syndrome (RADS) and chronic obstructive pulmonary disease (COPD), first diagnosed after 9/11 and present at W2.

2.3. Geospatial Analyses

Initially, to explore potential geospatial relationships between Ground Zero location and exposures and health outcomes, we mapped exposures and health outcomes of WTCHR resident enrollees in lower Manhattan using ArcGIS version 10.2 (ESRI, Redlands, CA, USA). These variables were mapped at the census tract level of geography using 2000 Census tract boundaries. For this part of the analysis, "yes" responses for any of the health outcomes variables were summed per census tracts (Boolean OR, not arithmetic sum). Similarly, exposure variables (fine coating of dust on surfaces, heavy coating of dust on surfaces, broken windows, damage to home or furnishings, and debris from the disaster was present) were also grouped and categorized as "yes" or "no" and mapped by census tract totals. The number of enrollees within each census tract was used as the denominator of the proportions represented on the maps. In addition, point values of dust cloud exposure were modeled using inverse distance weighted (IDW) interpolation to create a surface representation of the dust levels throughout lower Manhattan. IDW uses measured values (point locations) to predict values for unmeasured surrounding areas.

2.4. Statistical Analyses

We examined demographic characteristics, household exposures resulting from the 9/11 attacks, and cleaning practices among the study population using descriptive statistics (means, standard deviations, and proportions). We also calculated the prevalence (%) of self-reported respiratory symptoms and respiratory diseases. The relationship between cleaning practices and conditions inside the homes after 9/11 was assessed using multivariate logistic regression analyses adjusted for age, race, education, income, sex. Analyses were also controlled for "priority group", a stratification of registrants into higher and lower priority groups for the purposes of targeting and outreach, which to a degree reflects a resident's distance from the WTC site. Priority group 1 included residents as of 9/11 at addresses located south of Chamber Street; Group 2 included residents located on or north of Chamber but south of Canal Street; a third resident group, Group 0, was defined upon recognition of the inclusion of respondents living on or north of Canal in zip codes overlapping the Canal boundary or in other NYC boroughs. Also, the analyses were controlled for any exposure outside, to the dust cloud.

Each of the cleaning practices (dusted or swept without water; cleaned with damp cloth, sponge, or mop; used a vacuum to clean; and cleaned ventilation ducts) was modeled using logistic regression. Based on medical considerations and plausibility of real relationships being present, the list of all variables was narrowed to 17 potential explanatory variables for cleaning practices using 'purposive' or *a priori* selection. The predictors or covariates included five home exposures (fine coating of dust, heavy coating of dust, broken windows, damage in the home or furnishings, presence of debris in the home). The covariates also included four replacement behaviors (replaced AC, carpets, drapes, furniture). Lastly, each model contained terms for eight confounders, as listed in Section 3.2 (Table 3).

The cleaning practices themselves, other than the cleaning behavior specified outcome, are also modeled as predictors. These other cleaning practices were conditioned on the presence of dust in the home. For example, "cleaned ventilation ducts" was modelled including the other three cleaning practices as predictors (i.e., dusted or swept without water; used a vacuum to clean; and cleaned with damp cloth, sponge, or mop). The covariate cleaning practices were considered only if reported in conjunction with the presence of either fine or heavy dust (e.g., vacuum and fine or heavy dust had to be "yes" for the derived covariate "vacuum" to be "yes"). We fitted the four logistic models with all 17 variables included. Adjusted odds ratios (aOR), and their 95% confidence intervals (95% CI), for each cleaning method are provided in Section 3.2 (Table 3).

Each health outcome variable was modelled in a similar way. Based on medical considerations and likelihood of real relationships being present, the list of all covariates was narrowed to 21 explanatory variables for health outcomes (again, 'purposive' or *a priori* selection). Each of the six health outcomes was modeled using logistic regression with covariates as follows:

(a) Five demographic variables (age at 9/11, race, sex, education, and income);
(b) Resident priority group, indicating degree of registrant recruitment by area (partially a surrogate for location relative to the WTC site);
(c) Dust cloud exposure category (intense, some, none);
(d) Ever having smoked (at least 100 cigarettes in a lifetime);
(e) Five variables of exposures in the home (broken windows, debris in the home, fine dust, heavy dust, and damage in the home);
(f) Four variables containing data on behavior regarding replacement of various major items in the home (having replaced air-conditioning, carpeting, drapes, and furniture); and
(g) Four variables for the presence of cleaning practices, which are conditioned on the presence of dust in the home.

Again, the covariate cleaning practices were considered only if reported in conjunction with the presence of either fine or heavy dust (e.g., vacuum and fine or heavy dust had to be "yes" for the derived covariate "vacuum" to be "yes"). Smoking status was queried as "Have (you) smoked at least 100 cigarettes in (your) entire life?" Adjusted odds ratios (aOR), and their 95% confidence intervals (95% CI), for each health outcome were computed for all variables in the model including demographic, exposure, and cleaning practices. All analyses were performed using SAS version 9.3 (SAS Institute Inc, Cary, NC, USA).

3. Results

A total of 6447 lower Manhattan residents were included in this study. Table 1 shows their demographic characteristics. Mean age on 9/11 was 45.1 years (±15.1 years). Around 42% were male and 67% had completed college or post-graduate work. Forty-five percent had ever smoked cigarettes and 44% reported some or intense dust cloud exposure on 9/11.

Table 1. Demographic characteristics of 6447 Lower Manhattan residents enrolled in the World Trade Center (WTC) Health Registry.

Characteristic	N	%
Age on 9/11/2001 (yrs, mean ± SD)	45.1 ± 15.1	-
Sex (male)	2688	41.7
Race		
White	4281	66.4
Black	325	5
Hispanic	579	9
Asian	1061	16.5
Other/Unknown	201	3.1
Education *		
<High school	504	7.9
High school	738	11.5
Some college	893	14
College +	4265	66.6

Table 1. *Cont.*

Characteristic	N	%
Income level		
Less than 25K	1322	20.9
25 to <50K	1181	18.6
50 to <75K	836	13.2
75 to <100K	1801	28.4
100K or more	1197	18.9
Ever smoking *	2903	45.4
Dust cloud exposure on 9/11 *		
None	3446	56.3
Some	1196	19.5
Intense	1479	24.2

* Percentages do not reflect total N due to missing values.

3.1. Geospatial Representation of Exposures and Symptoms

Figures 1–3, respectively, display the geospatial distributions of self-reported outdoor location at the time of first encountering the dust cloud by intensity of exposure, indoor dust and damage to residences, and any reported respiratory symptoms up to 6 years after the 9/11 attacks. Figures 1 and 2 show more frequent reports of higher indoor and outdoor exposures on edges of lower Manhattan, especially the western side along the Hudson River. Over 50% of WTCHR enrollees residing in census tracts in both the lower western and eastern sides of Manhattan reported having dust or debris in the home. The proportion reporting indoor home exposure declined rapidly further north and east up to the Registry Canal Street boundary for residents. The distribution of respiratory symptoms depicted in the Figure 3 map overlaps in large part with the distribution of reported residential exposures. The percentage of enrollees by census tract who reported any respiratory symptom ranged from less than 1% furthest North and East approaching Canal Street to 50% or more of enrollee respondents who lived in census tracts along the Hudson River adjacent to the WTC site.

3.2. Home Damage and Cleaning Practices

Table 2 shows the types of home damage and household cleaning practices of WTCHR lower Manhattan residents. The majority of residents reported a fine coating of dust on interior surfaces, while 17% had a heavy coating of dust, enough to make it impossible to see what was underneath. Only 6% had broken windows and less than 15% reported damage to home or furnishings. Presence of debris was reported by 12% of the respondents. Cleaning practices varied greatly: more than half of participants reported cleaning with a damp cloth, sponge, or mop, whereas 23% reported dusting or sweeping without water. Around 20% of participants replaced carpets, furniture, or drapes, blinds, and curtains. Almost one third replaced air conditioners (individually, or the building).

Table 2. Self-reported household exposures resulting from the 9/11 attacks, cleaning practices, and other characteristics among 6447 Lower Manhattan residents enrolled in the World Trade Center (WTC) Health Registry.

Characteristics	N *	%
Fine coating of dust	3974/6241	63.7
Heavy coating of dust	1067/6251	17.1
Broken windows	368/6256	5.9
Damage to home or furnishings	927/6250	14.8
Presence of debris	759/6256	12.1
Cleaned ventilation ducts	1061/5931	17.9
Cleaned with damp cloth, sponge, or mop	3307/5919	55.9
Used a vacuum to clean	2687/5934	45.3
Dusted or swept without water	1263/5407	23.4
Replaced carpet or rugs	1201/6090	19.7
Replaced furniture	1304/6090	21.4
Replaced drapes, blinds, or curtains	1232/6090	20.2
Replaced air conditioners	1896/6090	31.1

* Changes in denominators are due to non-response.

Figure 2 shows that the majority of respondents reporting any type of home damage were located near the WTC site.

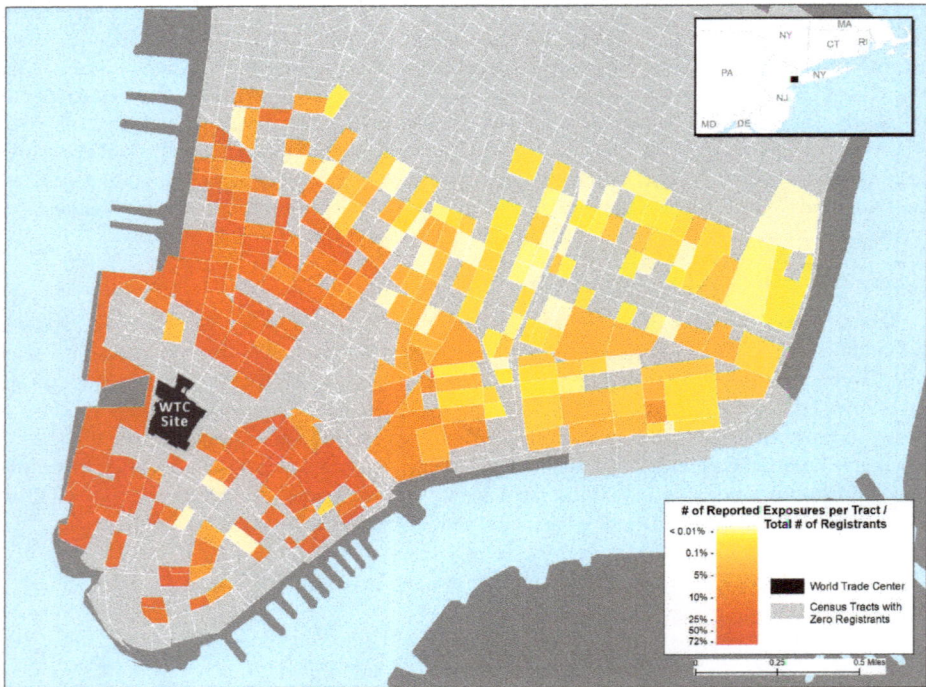

Figure 2. Proportion of World Trade Center (WTC) Health Registry participants reporting any fine coating of dust on surfaces, heavy coating of dust on surfaces, broken window (s), damage to home or furnishings, or debris in their Lower Manhattan residences (n = 6348) (Wave 2 survey, 11/2006–12/2007).

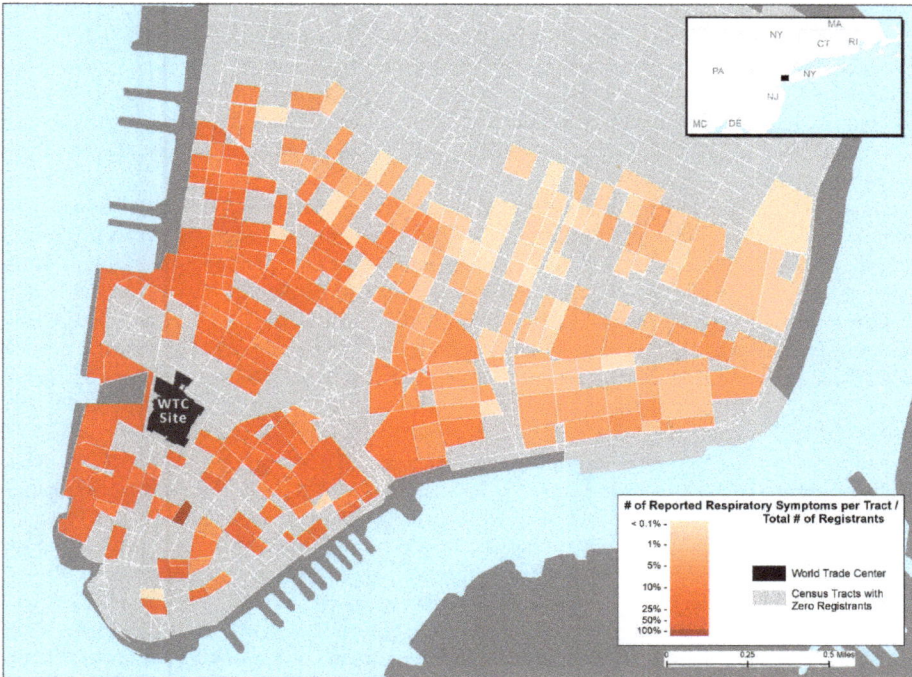

Figure 3. Proportion of World Trade Center (WTC) Health Registry participants reporting any respiratory outcome (shortness of breath, wheezing, chronic cough, upper respiratory symptoms, asthma/reactive airways dysfunction syndrome, chronic obstructive pulmonary disease) (n = 6348) (Wave 2 survey, 11/2006–12/2007).

Table 3 shows that those who dusted or swept without water were more likely to report the presence of debris (aOR = 1.31; 95% Confidence Interval (CI) 1.06–1.61) as to other reported exposures.

Table 3. Associations between cleaning practices and home exposures among 6,447 Lower Manhattan residents enrolled in the World Trade Center (WTC) Health Registry.

Exposure/Cleaning Practices	Adjusted Odds Ratio (95% Confidence Interval) *			
	Dusted or Swept without Water	Cleaned with Damp Cloth, Sponge, or Mop	Used a Vacuum to Clean	Cleaned Ventilation Ducts
Fine coating of dust	0.99 (0.82, 1.20)	**1.85 (1.59, 2.14)**	**0.63 (0.53, 0.74)**	**0.38 (0.27, 0.52)**
Heavy coating of dust	1.03 (0.82, 1.29)	1.08 (0.88, 1.33)	**0.64 (0.52, 0.79)**	**0.59 (0.42, 0.83)**
Broken windows	1.24 (0.86, 1.79)	**0.69 (0.48, 0.99)**	0.97 (0.67, 1.39)	0.95 (0.57, 1.59)
Damage to home or furnishings	0.92 (0.73, 1.14)	0.90 (0.72, 1.12)	**1.25 (1.01, 1.54)**	**1.34 (1.01, 1.79)**
Presence of debris	**1.31 (1.06, 1.61)**	1.07 (0.87, 1.33)	1.20 (0.98, 1.48)	1.16 (0.87, 1.53)
Dusted or swept without water	-	**1.50 (1.26, 1.79)**	**1.76 (1.50, 2.07)**	**1.76 (1.43, 2.18)**
Cleaned with damp cloth, sponge, or mop	**1.47 (1.23, 1.74)**	-	**4.59 (3.95, 5.34)**	**3.92 (2.94, 5.23)**
Used a vacuum to clean	**1.73 (1.48, 2.03)**	**4.71 (4.04, 5.50)**	-	**1.95 (1.56, 2.43)**
Cleaned ventilation ducts	**1.74 (1.41, 2.15)**	**5.28 (3.72, 7.50)**	**2.08 (1.65, 2.62)**	-

* Each model has terms for eight confounders: models are adjusted for any effect due to age at 9/11, education, income level, race, sex, smoking status, and dust cloud exposure and resident priority group. - = not in the particular logistic model. Each column gives a distinct logistic model fit, with the column heading being the dependent (response) cleaning practice variable. (Statistically significant adjusted odds ratios in bold).

Using a damp cloth, sponge, or mop was also associated with reporting a fine coating of dust (aOR = 1.85; 95% CI 1.59–2.14). In contrast, those who used water for cleaning were less likely to report broken windows. Lower Manhattan residents who reported using a vacuum to clean, as well as those who reported cleaning ventilation ducts, were less likely to report a fine or a heavy coating of dust, but more likely to report damage to home or furnishings, Table 3). Cleaning practices were also associated with each other, with cleaning with damp cloth, sponge, or mop having the strongest association with using a vacuum to clean (aOR = 4.71; 95% CI 4.04–5.50) and cleaning ventilation ducts (aOR = 5.28; 95% CI 3.72–7.50). These results were expected, yet including these terms made for more thorough modeling.

Prevalence of respiratory outcomes was as follows: shortness of breath (16.1 %), wheezing (10.7%), chronic cough (6.8%), upper respiratory symptoms (60.8%), asthma or reactive airways dysfunction syndrome (RADS) (7.9%), and chronic obstructive pulmonary disease (COPD) (5.4%) (Table 4). A total of 68% of lower Manhattan residents reporting any respiratory outcome were located within 0.5 miles from Ground Zero (Figure 3). Table 5 shows odds ratios and 95% confidence intervals for respiratory outcomes in relation to several characteristics of home damage and cleaning practices. (See explanatory comments given previously, as Tables 3 and 5 have the same layout). Those who reported a heavy coating of dust had 65% (95% CI 1.24–2.18), 43% (95% CI 1.03–1.97) and 59% (95% CI 1.09–2.28) higher odds of reporting shortness of breath, wheezing, or chronic cough, respectively. Residents who reported damage to home or furnishings had a 33% (95% CI 1.01–1.75) increased odds of reporting shortness of breath and 36% (95% CI 1.06–1.74) increased odds of reporting upper respiratory symptoms. Presence of debris was associated with chronic cough (aOR = 1.56; CI 1.12–2.17) and upper respiratory symptoms (aOR = 1.56; CI 1.24–1.95). Lower Manhattan residents who reported replacing air conditioners had higher odds of reporting upper respiratory symptoms (aOR = 1.32; CI 1.14–1.54). Replacing carpets was associated with increased COPD (aOR = 1.49; CI 1.03–2.16), while replacing drapes was associates with increased shortness of breath (aOR = 1.31; CI 1.03–1.65). Dusting or sweeping without water was the cleaning behavior associated with the largest number (three) of respiratory outcomes. Residents who did that had higher odds of reporting shortness of breath (aOR = 1.37; 95% CI 1.11–1.69), wheezing (aOR = 1.49; CI 1.17–1.90), and upper respiratory symptoms (aOR = 1.28; CI 1.08–1.53). Cleaning with a damp cloth, sponge, or mop and cleaning ventilation ducts were also associated with some respiratory outcomes including URS for damp cloth (aOR = 1.40; 95% CI 1.18–1.64) and wheezing and cough with ventilation duct cleaning (aOR = 1.48; 95% CI 1.08–2.01 and aOR = 1.94; 95% CI 1.38–2.73, respectively).

Table 4. Prevalence of self-reported post-9/11, respiratory symptoms and respiratory diseases present at Wave 2 (W2) (11/2006–12/2007) surveys among 6447 Lower Manhattan residents enrolled in the World Trade Center (WTC) Health Registry.

Symptom/Disease	N *	%
Shortness of breath	983/6126	16.1
Wheezing	668/6234	10.7
Chronic cough	439/6415	6.8
Upper respiratory symptoms	3761/6,190	60.8
Asthma/RADS [†]	434/5466	7.9
Chronic obstructive pulmonary disease	320/5931	5.4

* Changes in denominators are due to non-response. [†] RADS = Reactive airways dysfunction syndrome.

Table 5. Post-9/11 respiratory symptoms or diseases present at W2 in relation to home exposures and cleaning practices among 6447 Lower Manhattan residents enrolled in the World Trade Center (WTC) Health Registry.

Exposure/Cleaning Practices	Adjusted Odds Ratios (95% Confidence Interval) * for Each Respiratory Condition					
	Shortness of Breath	Wheezing	Chronic Cough	URS **	Asthma/RADS †	COPD ‡
Light coating of dust	1.25 (0.98–1.59)	1.10 (0.84, 1.45)	1.06 (0.77, 1.47)	1.11 (0.93, 1.31)	1.01 (0.74, 1.39)	1.19 (0.84, 1.70)
Broken Windows	0.95 (0.60, 1.50)	1.46 (0.91, 2.36)	0.88 (0.68, 1.62)	0.98 (0.66, 1.44)	1.16 (0.63, 2.12)	1.01 (0.51, 1.99)
Heavy coating of dust	**1.65 (1.24, 2.18)**	**1.43 (1.03, 1.97)**	**1.59 (1.09, 2.28)**	1.08 (0.87, 1.35)	1.21 (0.82, 1.79)	1.35 (0.89, 2.05)
Damage to home or furnishings	**1.33 (1.01, 1.75)**	1.31 (0.96–1.81)	0.82 (0.56, 1.19)	**1.36 (1.06, 1.74)**	1.11 (0.74, 1.65)	1.11 (0.73, 1.68)
Presence of debris	1.62 (0.97, 1.64)	1.19 (0.88, 1.61)	**1.56 (1.12, 2.17)**	**1.56 (1.24, 1.95)**	0.92 (0.63, 1.35)	0.94 (0.63, 1.40)
Replaced air conditioner	1.06 (0.87, 1.28)	1.08 (0.87, 1.34)	1.24 (0.96, 1.60)	**1.32 (1.14, 1.54)**	0.91 (0.69, 1.19)	1.31 (0.99, 1.74)
Replaced carpets	0.90 (0.70, 1.17)	1.05 (0.78, 1.41)	1.07 (0.76, 1.50)	1.03 (0.83, 1.28)	1.21 (0.85, 1.73)	1.49 (1.03, 2.16)
Replaced drapes	**1.31 (1.03, 1.65)**	0.98 (0.75, 1.29)	1.02 (0.74, 1.40)	1.11 (0.90, 1.36)	0.99 (0.71, 1.39)	0.96 (0.67, 1.38)
Replaced furniture	1.24 (0.97, 1.59)	1.13 (0.85, 1.51)	1.24 (0.89, 1.73)	1.14 (0.93, 1.40)	1.40 (0.99, 1.96)	0.89 (0.62, 1.29)
Dusted or swept without water	**1.37 (1.11, 1.69)**	**1.49 (1.17, 1.90)**	1.21 (0.91, 1.61)	**1.28 (1.08, 1.53)**	**1.35 (1.00, 1.81)**	1.16 (0.85, 1.61)
Cleaned with damp cloth, sponge, mop	1.15 (0.92, 1.43)	1.01 (0.79, 1.30)	1.05 (0.78, 1.41)	**1.40 (1.18, 1.64)**	0.91 (0.67, 1.22)	0.96 (0.69, 1.32)
Cleaned ventilation ducts	1.23 (0.93, 1.64)	**1.48 (1.08, 2.01)**	**1.94 (1.38, 2.73)**	1.18 (0.92, 1.53)	1.23 (0.82, 1.82)	1.30 (0.86, 1.96)
Vacuumed	0.96 (0.78, 1.19)	1.06 (0.84, 1.34)	0.95 (0.71, 1.25)	1.01 (0.86, 1.19)	0.99 (0.75, 1.33)	0.94 (0.69, 1.29)

* Each model has terms for eight confounders: models are adjusted for any effect due to age at 9/11, education, income level, race, sex, smoking status, and dust cloud exposure and resident priority group. ** URS = Upper respiratory symptoms. † RADS = Reactive airways dysfunction syndrome. ‡ COPD = Chronic obstructive pulmonary disease. Each column gives a separate logistic model fit, with the column heading being the dependent (response) health outcome variable. (Statistically significant adjusted odds ratios in bold).

4. Discussion

This is the largest study to evaluate respiratory outcomes among lower Manhattan residents who reported household exposures as a result of the 9/11 terrorist attacks. Our findings are consistent with increased respiratory symptoms and diseases, which are associated with several levels of home damage and different cleaning practices, and corroborate other studies in similar populations [8–11,13] or subset of the WTCHR resident population [13].

The explosion and collapse of buildings and subsequent fires at Ground Zero produced a large plume of dust and smoke that released particles and gases into the air. Characterization of both outdoor and indoor dust samples identified asbestos, glass fibers, lead, and polycyclic aromatic hydrocarbons (PAHs), among numerous other contaminants [1,4,5]. In fact, indoor samples contained more inhalable dust particles than did outdoor dust [6]. Our data show that the majority of lower Manhattan residents in the WTCHR may have been exposed to airborne contaminants because of some type of home damage following the 9/11 attacks. The presence of dust was the most common problem, but more severe damage, such as broken windows and furniture, were also reported. A case-control study comparing lower and upper Manhattan residents found that 30.7% of residents in the affected region reported some physical damage to their homes and 86.4% reported dust [8]. As expected, our geospatial analysis demonstrates that a higher proportion of WTCHR participants reporting any home damage were located in the vicinity of Ground Zero.

As a result of the presence of dust, debris, and other damage, lower Manhattan residents personally cleaned their homes using a variety of methods. Lin et al. reported that 74.3% of residents in the affected area personally cleaned their homes [8]. The majority of residents participating in the present study reported using wet cleaning practices, such as using a damp cloth, sponge, or mop, which are likely to minimize suspension of dust and have been recommended by the Environmental Protection Agency (EPA) in that context [3,15]. However, many residents reported dusting or sweeping without water and even cleaning ventilation ducts by themselves. These practices were associated with the presence of debris and may have resulted in excessive dust exposure. In addition, numerous residents reported that household items, such as carpets, furniture, curtains, and air conditioners were replaced, which may have been associated with more severe damage to their homes. Among other measures, the EPA designed and implemented a Residential Dust Cleanup Program in 2002, to ensure that lower Manhattan residents were protected from potential WTC-related exposures [16].

Upper respiratory symptoms were the most common health outcomes reported by lower Manhattan residents in the WTCHR. This finding is consistent with other WTC studies among residents [10] and rescue and recovery workers [17–19]. According to Lin et al., residents living within 1.5 km of the WTC site experienced a 200 percent increase of at least one persistent upper respiratory symptom compared to controls in the Upper West Side of Manhattan [10]. Our study also demonstrates high rates of persistent shortness of breath, wheezing, and chronic cough among lower Manhattan residents. These findings are in line with those of Lin et al., who reported that increased rates of lower respiratory symptoms persisted among lower Manhattan residents two and four years after the 9/11 attacks [9]. Moreover, most residents reporting any persistent respiratory symptoms in our study were located within a 0.5-mile radius of Ground Zero. Lin et al. also described an apparent trend when comparing residents below and not below Canal St.: the former had stronger associations between location and both any new-onset and persistent new-onset respiratory symptoms [9]. Reibman et al. also reported that four times as many lower Manhattan residents presented wheezing compared to a control population. In addition, three times as many residents reported cough and shortness of breath [11].

Our results demonstrate an association between respiratory health outcomes and numerous types of home damage and cleaning practices. In particular, the presence of a heavy coating of dust was associated with shortness of breath, wheezing and cough and the presence of debris with chronic cough and upper respiratory symptoms. Lin et al. reported that upper respiratory symptoms were associated with both dust and physical damage to home, with statistically significant cumulative incidence ratios (CIRs) ranging from 1.27 to 1.71. In addition, the association between lower respiratory symptoms and exposures yielded CIRs between 1.31 and 1.44 [8]. In our study, the use of dry cleaning practices, such as dusting or sweeping without water, was associated with shortness of breath, wheezing, and upper respiratory symptoms. In contrast, only one health outcome was associated with cleaning with a damp cloth, sponge, or mop. It is not clear if the cleaning practice with water provided some protective effects by limiting re-suspension of dust, since in our analysis the cleaning practices with and without water were not mutually exclusive. Both practices were also associated with other methods of cleaning. Furthermore, cleaning practice with water was significantly associated with fine coating of dust (OR = 1.85; 95% CI, 1.59–2.14) versus cleaning practice without water was not (OR = 0.99; 95% CI, 0.82–1.20). Nevertheless, Lin et al. did not find statistically significant associations between self-cleaning of homes and lower respiratory symptoms at 2- and 4-year follow ups of lower Manhattan residents (N = 136 and 69 participants, respectively) [9].

A strength of this study is the ability to demonstrate persistent health outcomes in a large sample of lower Manhattan residents exposed in their homes to airborne contaminants resulting from the 9/11 terrorist attacks. Our analyses controlled for potential confounders, such as the intensity of exposure to the cloud of dust and debris, smoking, and priority group or area of recruitment, which may serve as a surrogate for location in lower Manhattan.

However, this study is subject to several limitations. Self-selection bias may affect our results. Lower Manhattan residents who developed respiratory symptoms and diseases after 9/11/2001 may have been more likely to enroll in the WTC registry than asymptomatic persons. Medical records were not obtained which might have been used to verify reported conditions. In addition, smoking was defined as ever/never, without taking into account pack-years. Also, there was essentially no ability to validate the reported exposures quantitatively, because environmental sampling was not conducted. Nonetheless, it is unlikely that differences between respondents and non-respondents and misclassification of disease status would have an influence on the intensity of home damage reporting and selection of cleaning practices. Recall bias is also a limitation since questionnaires for W2 were applied over 5 years after the event of interest. In an attempt to account for this aspect, we verified responses on W1 and W2 for consistency. In addition, information on time to return home and use of respiratory protection while cleaning was not available. It is possible that severely damaged home inhabitants took longer to return to their homes or did so only after renovations, which potentially reduced dust exposures. Similarly, residents may have used different degrees of respiratory protection while cleaning surfaces. These factors would have *reduced* the apparent effect of the reported home damage on respiratory health outcomes.

5. Conclusions

This analysis demonstrates that lower Manhattan residents who suffered home damage following the 9/11 attacks are more likely to report respiratory symptoms and diseases in the WTCHR. It also highlights the specific kinds of damage or other specific exposure events, such as cleaning practices, which are statistically related to such increased symptoms and diseases. These health outcomes persisted for at least 5–6 years after the event, which may have translated into lower quality of life.

Author Contributions: Conceptualization, V.C.A., R.M.B., M.R.F., L.L.P., S.L.G., J.E.C.; Formal analysis, L.L.P., B.L., H.E.A.; Methodology, V.C.A., L.L.P., S.L.G., H.E.A., Y.K.S., S.B., J.H.S.; Project Administration, V.C.A., M.R.F., R.M.B., J.E.C.; Writing, V.C.A., J.H.S., L.L.P., Y.K.S., R.M.B.; Reviewing and editing, V.C.A., L.L.P., J.H.S., Y.K.S., J.E.C., M.R.F., H.E.A., R.M.B.

Funding: This study was supported by Cooperative Agreement U50/ATU272750 from the Agency for Toxic Substances and Disease Registry (ATSDR) and the Centers for Disease Control and Prevention (CDC), which included support from the National Center for Environmental Health and by Cooperative Agreement U50/OH009739 from the National Institute for Occupational Safety and Health (NIOSH) and the New York City Department of Health and Mental Hygiene. The findings and conclusions in this report are those of the authors and do not necessarily represent the views of the ATSDR or CDC/NIOSH.

Conflicts of Interest: The authors declare they have no competing financial interests.

References

1. Lioy, P.J.; Weisel, C.P.; Millette, J.R.; Eisenreich, S.; Vallero, D.; Offenberg, J.; Buckley, B.; Turpin, B.; Zhong, M.; Cohen, M.D.; et al. Characterization of the dust/smoke aerosol that settled east of the World Trade Center (WTC) in lower Manhattan after the collapse of the WTC 11 September 2001. *Environ. Health Perspect.* **2002**, *110*, 703–714. [CrossRef] [PubMed]

2. Lioy, P.J.; Georgopoulos, P. The anatomy of the exposures that occurred around the World Trade Center site: 9/11 and beyond. *Ann. N. Y. Acad. Sci.* **2006**, *1076*, 54–79. [CrossRef] [PubMed]

3. Centers for Disease Control and Prevention. Prevention, Potential exposures to airborne and settled surface dust in residential areas of lower Manhattan following the collapse of the World Trade Center—New York City, November 4–December 11, 2001. *MMWR Morb. Mortal Wkly. Rep.* **2003**, *52*, 131–136.

4. Lorber, M.; Gibb, H.; Grant, L.; Pinto, J.; Pleil, J.; Cleverly, D. Assessment of inhalation exposures and potential health risks to the general population that resulted from the collapse of the World Trade Center towers. *Risk Anal.* **2007**, *27*, 1203–1221. [CrossRef] [PubMed]

5. Offenberg, J.H.; Eisenreich, S.J.; Gigliotti, C.L.; Chen, L.C.; Xiong, J.Q.; Quan, C.; Lou, X.; Zhong, M.; Gorczynski, J.; Yiin, L.M.; et al. Persistent organic pollutants in dusts that settled indoors in lower Manhattan after September 11, 2001. *J. Expo. Anal. Environ. Epidemiol.* **2004**, *14*, 164–172. [CrossRef] [PubMed]

6. Yiin, L.M.; Millette, J.R.; Vette, A.; Ilacqua, V.; Quan, C.; Gorczynski, J.; Kendall, M.; Chen, L.C.; Weisel, C.P.; Buckley, B.; et al. Comparisons of the dust/smoke particulate that settled inside the surrounding buildings and outside on the streets of southern New York City after the collapse of the World Trade Center, September 11, 2001. *J. Air Waste Manag. Assoc.* **2004**, *54*, 515–528. [CrossRef] [PubMed]

7. Centers for Disease Control and Prevention. Community needs assessment of lower Manhattan residents following the World Trade Center attacks—Manhattan, New York City, 2001. *MMWR Morb. Mortal. Wkly. Rep.* **2002**, *51*, 10–13.

8. Lin, S.; Jones, R.; Reibman, J.; Bowers, J.; Fitzgerald, E.F.; Hwang, S.A. Reported respiratory symptoms and adverse home conditions after 9/11 among residents living near the World Trade Center. *J. Asthma* **2007**, *44*, 325–332. [CrossRef] [PubMed]

9. Lin, S.; Jones, R.; Reibman, J.; Morse, D.; Hwang, S.A. Lower respiratory symptoms among residents living near the World Trade Center, two and four years after 9/11. *Int. J. Occup. Environ. Health* **2010**, *16*, 44–52. [CrossRef] [PubMed]

10. Lin, S.; Reibman, J.; Bowers, J.A.; Hwang, S.A.; Hoerning, A.; Gomez, M.I.; Fitzgerald, E.F. Upper respiratory symptoms and other health effects among residents living near the World Trade Center site after September 11, 2001. *Am. J. Epidemiol.* **2005**, *162*, 499–507. [CrossRef] [PubMed]

11. Reibman, J.; Lin, S.; Hwang, S.A.; Gulati, M.; Bowers, J.A.; Rogers, L.; Berger, K.I.; Hoerning, A.; Gomez, M.; Fitzgerald, E.F. The World Trade Center residents' respiratory health study: New-onset respiratory symptoms and pulmonary function. *Environ. Health Perspect.* **2005**, *113*, 406–411. [CrossRef] [PubMed]

12. Brackbill, R.M.; Hadler, J.L.; DiGrande, L.; Ekenga, C.C.; Farfel, M.R.; Friedman, S.; Perlman, S.E.; Stellman, S.D.; Walker, D.J.; Wu, D.; et al. Asthma and posttraumatic stress symptoms 5 to 6 years following exposure to the World Trade Center terrorist attack. *JAMA* **2009**, *302*, 502–516. [CrossRef] [PubMed]

13. Maslow, C.B.; Friedman, S.M.; Pillai, P.S.; Reibman, J.; Berger, K.I.; Goldring, R.; Stellman, S.D.; Farfel, M. Chronic and acute exposures to the world trade center disaster and lower respiratory symptoms: Area residents and workers. *Am. J. Public Health* **2012**, *102*, 1186–1194. [CrossRef] [PubMed]

14. Farfel, M.; DiGrande, L.; Brackbill, R.; Prann, A.; Cone, J.; Friedman, S.; Walker, D.J.; Pezeshki, G.; Thomas, P.; Galea, S.; et al. An overview of 9/11 experiences and respiratory and mental health conditions among World Trade Center Health Registry enrollees. *J. Urban Health* **2008**, *85*, 880–909. [CrossRef] [PubMed]

15. Environmental Protection Agency. Interim Final WTC Residential Confirmation Study. In 2003. Available online: http://www.epa.gov/wtc/reports/confirmation_cleaning_study.pdf (accessed on 18 December 2014).

16. Environmental Protection Agency. World Trade Center Residential Dust Cleanup Program. Final Report. In 2005. Available online: http://permanent.access.gpo.gov/gpo41622/residential-dust-cleanup-final-report.pdf (accessed on 28 January 2016).

17. Antao, V.C.; Pallos, L.L.; Shim, Y.K.; Sapp, J.H., 2nd; Brackbill, R.M.; Cone, J.E.; Stellman, S.D.; Farfel, M.R. Respiratory protective equipment, mask use, and respiratory outcomes among World Trade Center rescue and recovery workers. *Am. J. Ind. Med.* **2011**, *54*, 897–905. [CrossRef] [PubMed]

18. De la Hoz, R.E.; Shohet, M.R.; Chasan, R.; Bienenfeld, L.A.; Afilaka, A.A.; Levin, S.M.; Herbert, R. Occupational toxicant inhalation injury: The World Trade Center (WTC) experience. *Int. Arch. Occup. Environ. Health* **2008**, *81*, 479–485. [CrossRef] [PubMed]

19. Herbert, R.; Moline, J.; Skloot, G.; Metzger, K.; Baron, S.; Luft, B.; Markowitz, S.; Udasin, I.; Harrison, D.; Stein, D.; et al. The World Trade Center disaster and the health of workers: Five-year assessment of a unique medical screening program. *Environ. Health Perspect.* **2006**, *114*, 1853–1858. [CrossRef] [PubMed]

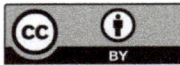

International Journal of
Environmental Research and Public Health

MDPI

Article

Sarcoid-Like Granulomatous Disease: Pathologic Case Series in World Trade Center Dust Exposed Rescue and Recovery Workers

Vasanthi R. Sunil [1,*,†], Jared Radbel [2,†], Sabiha Hussain [2], Kinal N. Vayas [1], Jessica Cervelli [1], Malik Deen [2], Howard Kipen [3], Iris Udasin [3], Robert Laumbach [3], Jag Sunderram [2], Jeffrey D. Laskin [3] and Debra L. Laskin [1]

[1]   Ernest Mario School of Pharmacy, Rutgers University, Piscataway, NJ 08854, USA;
     kinalv5@pharmacy.rutgers.edu (K.N.V.); j.cervelli@pharmacy.rutgers.edu (J.C.);
     laskin@eohsi.rutgers.edu (D.L.L.)
[2]   Robert Wood Johnson Medical School, Rutgers University, New Brunswick, NJ 08901, USA;
     jr1106@rwjms.rutgers.edu (J.R.); sabiha.hussain@rutgers.edu (S.H.); malik.deen@rutgers.edu (M.D.);
     sunderja@rwjms.rutgers.edu (J.S.)
[3]   School of Public Health, Rutgers University, Piscataway, NJ 08854, USA; kipen@eohsi.rutgers.edu (H.K.);
     iu22@eohsi.rutgers.edu (I.U.); laumbach@eohsi.rutgers.edu (R.L.); jlaskin@eohsi.rutgers.edu (J.D.L.)
*   Correspondence: sunilva@pharmacy.rutgers.edu; Tel.: +1-848-445-6190; Fax: +1-732-445-0119
†   The authors contributed equally to this work.

Received: 23 January 2019; Accepted: 26 February 2019; Published: 6 March 2019

Abstract: Sarcoid-like granulomatous diseases (SGD) have been previously identified in cohorts of World Trade Center (WTC) dust-exposed individuals. In the present studies, we analyzed lung and/or lymph node biopsies from patients referred to our clinic with suspected WTC dust-induced lung disease to evaluate potential pathophysiologic mechanisms. Histologic sections of lung and/or lymph node samples were analyzed for markers of injury, oxidative stress, inflammation, fibrosis, and epigenetic modifications. Out of seven patients examined, we diagnosed four with SGD and two with pulmonary fibrosis; one was diagnosed later with SGD at another medical facility. Patients with SGD were predominantly white, obese men, who were less than 50 years old and never smoked. Cytochrome b5, cytokeratin 17, heme oxygenase-1, lipocalin-2, inducible nitric oxide synthase, cyclooxygenase 2, tumor necrosis factor α, ADP-ribosylation factor-like GTPase 11, mannose receptor-1, galectin-3, transforming growth factor β, histone-3 and methylated histone-3 were identified in lung and lymph nodes at varying levels in all samples examined. Three of the biopsy samples with granulomas displayed peri-granulomatous fibrosis. These findings are important and suggest the potential of WTC dust-induced fibrotic sarcoid. It is likely that patient demographics and/or genetic factors influence the response to WTC dust injury and that these contribute to different pathological outcomes.

Keywords: WTC; fibrotic sarcoid; injury; inflammation; fibrosis

---

1. Introduction

Following the collapse of the World Trade Center (WTC) towers on 11 September, 2001, toxic dust was suspended in the air of lower Manhattan and Brooklyn. Over time, rescue and recovery workers exposed to WTC dust developed various respiratory diseases involving both the airways (asthma-like airway hyper-reactivity, bronchiolitis), and less commonly, the lung parenchyma (eosinophilic pneumonia, fibrosis, sarcoid-like granulomatous disease) [1,2]. Most notable is sarcoid-like granulomatous disease (SGD), which has been diagnosed at relatively high rates in cohorts of firefighters and rescue workers who have been followed since 2001 [3]. This condition is distinct from frank sarcoidosis which is a diagnosis of exclusion, once other known causes of granulomatous disease have been ruled out. It may be that WTC dust-induced SGD is a unique pathology, with potential for specific therapeutic interventions.

Although WTC dust has been extensively characterized [4], little is known about the pathophysiologic mechanisms underlying the development of SGD and other lung pathologies. Studies in rodents have reported increased expression of genes associated with inflammation and oxidative stress in the lung following WTC dust exposure [5,6]. However, in these studies, granulomatous inflammation was not observed, making determination of the pathogenesis of WTC dust-induced SGD in humans, problematic.

In this report, we describe the pathologic findings in seven patients exposed to WTC dust who presented with ambiguous clinical pulmonary diagnoses. In all of the patients, we identified markers of injury, oxidative stress, inflammation, and epigenetic changes in lung and/or lymph nodes. Based on pathologic findings, five of the patients demonstrated evidence of SGD and three of these had peri-granulomatous fibrosis. These findings are important as they suggest the possibility of development of fibrosis in patients with WTC dust-induced SGD. This may lead to changes in clinical outcomes and treatment strategies.

2. Methods

2.1. Patients

Investigators at the Environmental and Occupational Health Sciences Institute (EOHSI) of Rutgers University are part of a New York/New Jersey consortium that has been following a cohort of rescue and recovery workers exposed to dust and other materials at the WTC site. These individuals included rescue, recovery, debris-cleanup, law enforcement, and related support service workers, and volunteers in lower Manhattan (south of Canal St.), the Staten Island Landfill, and/or the barge loading piers, who worked on-site for at least 4 h/day between 11 and 14 September, 2001, for at least 24 h during September 2001, or for at least 80 h total time between September and December 2001 [7]. From among approximately 2000 patients followed at EOHSI, 7 were referred for biopsy between 2007 and 2011, if a final pulmonary diagnosis despite symptom review and full evaluation including pulmonary function testing (PFT) and computerized tomography (CT) scan interpretation required tissue analysis. Patient demographics were collected, including WTC dust exposure levels as described by Wisnivesky et al. [2]. Lung and/or mediastinal lymph node specimens were obtained for both histopathologic evaluation and immunohistochemical staining. All subjects gave informed consent for inclusion before they participated in the study. The study was conducted in accord with the Declaration of Helsinki, and the protocol was approved by the Ethics Committee of the Rutgers Institutional Review Board.

2.2. Pulmonary Function Testing (PFT)

PFTs were performed using NSpire Health pulmonary functioning testing devices (NSpire Health, Longmont, CO, USA), that were calibrated in the Rutgers University Robert Wood Johnson Medical School Pulmonary Function Laboratory. Test results were interpreted according to American Thoracic Society guidelines and results collected for each patient [8].

2.3. CT Scans

Tidal breathing CT was performed from lung apex to lung base without the use of intravenous contrast material. All results were interpreted by board-certified radiologists.

2.4. Sample Collection, Histology and Immunohistochemistry

We collected lung samples by transbronchial biopsy (TBB) from 3 patients, and by video-assisted thoracoscopy (VATS) from 2 patients. Three patients had mediastinal lymph node biopsies obtained via mediastinoscopy (Med). Samples were fixed in 3% paraformaldehyde for 4 h and then transferred to 50% ethanol. Histological sections (4 μm) were prepared and stained with hematoxylin and eosin (H and E) or Masson's trichrome stain. Tissues were analyzed by a board-certified pulmonary pathologist (M. Deen) for the extent of inflammation, including macrophage and neutrophil localization, alterations in alveolar epithelial barriers, fibrin deposition, edema, granuloma formation, and fibrosis. Representative images were acquired at high resolution (magnification 60×) using an Olympus VS120 Virtual Microscopy System, scanned and viewed using OlyVIA version 2.6 software (Olympus Life Sciences, Center Valley, PA, USA).

For immunohistochemistry, tissue sections were deparaffinized with xylene (4 min, ×2) followed by decreasing concentrations of ethanol (100%–50%) and finally, water. After antigen retrieval using citrate buffer (10.2 mM sodium citrate, 0.05% Tween 20, pH 6.0) and quenching of endogenous peroxidase with 3% H_2O_2 for 10–30 min, sections were incubated for 1–4 h at room temperature with 5–100% goat serum to block nonspecific binding. This was followed by overnight incubation at 4 °C with rabbit IgG or rabbit polyclonal anti-cytochrome b5 (1:250, Abcam, Cambridge, MA, USA), anti-cytokeratin 17 (1:1000, Abcam), anti-heme oxygenase (HO)-1 (1:650, Enzo Life Sciences, Farmingdale, NY, USA), anti-lipocalin (Lcn)-2 (1:250, Abcam), anti-inducible nitric oxide synthase (iNOS) (1:500, Abcam), anti-cyclooxygenase (COX)-2 (1:100, Abcam), anti-tumor necrosis factor (TNF)α (1:50, Abcam), anti-ADP-ribosylation factor-like GTPase (ARL)11 (1:100, Bioss Antibodies, Woburn, MA, USA), anti-mannose receptor (MR)-1 (1:500, Abcam), anti-galectin (Gal)-3 (1:400, R&D Systems, Minneapolis, MN, USA), anti-transforming growth factor (TGF)β (1:50, Abcam), anti-histone H3 (1:50, Cell Signaling, Danvers, MA, USA), or anti-mono-methyl histone H3K4 (1:100, Cell Signaling) antibodies. Sections were then incubated with biotinylated secondary antibody (Vector Labs, Burlingame, CA, USA) for 30 min at room temperature. Binding was visualized using a DAB (3,3′ diaminobenzidine) peroxidase substrate kit (Vector Labs). Sections of lung and/or lymph nodes from all 7 subjects were analyzed for each antibody.

3. Results

3.1. Patient Demographics and Diagnoses

Patient demographics are presented in Table 1. The patients were predominantly male (100%), white (non-Hispanic; 100%), and former smokers (57%). Based on pathological findings (see below), patients were divided into two groups; those with SGD (*n* = 5) and those with other pathology (*n* = 2). Of the patients with SGD, 100% were white males, overweight or obese (BMI = 25–29 (20%); BMI ≥ 30 (80%)), 80% were <50 years old (mean age 43.5), and 60% never smoked (Table 1). Four of the five patients with SGD had an intermediate WTC dust exposure level, and one had a high level of exposure [2]. The two non-SGD patients had high WTC dust exposure levels (Table 1). The clinical, radiographic and pathologic characteristics of patients undergoing biopsy are presented in Table 2. The reasons for biopsy in patients with SGD (patients #1–5) were mediastinal/hilar adenopathy and pulmonary nodules (Table 2). Other patients displayed a mix of lymphadenopathy, fibrosis, nodules, and emphysema. Of patients with SGD, patients #1 and #2 had normal pulmonary function, while patients #3 and #4 displayed restrictive physiology and patient #5 had mixed obstruction and restriction (Table 3). The two patients without SGD (#6 and #7) had restrictive physiology (Table 3).

3.2. Pathological Results

Biopsy samples from three of the seven patients (patients #1, #3 and #4) showed well-formed non-caseating granulomas in lymph nodes suggesting SGD; patient #2 exhibited scant, poorly formed granuloma in the lung (Table 2 and Figure 1). In two of the patients (#3 and #4), only lymph nodes were biopsied; in one patient (#2), only lung parenchyma was biopsied. In patient #1, both lymph nodes and lung were biopsied, and both tissue types exhibited non-caseating granulomas (Figure 1). Masson's trichrome staining of tissues revealed the presence of well-formed granulomas and evidence of peri-granulomatous fibrosis in lymph nodes of patients #1, #3 and #4 (Figure 2). Of the other three patients without granulomatous changes (#5–#7), pathological diagnoses in the lung included mild fibrosis, bronchial inflammation and acute and chronic lung injury (Table 2 and Figure 1). Patient #5 was diagnosed later with SGD at another medical facility after obtaining additional tissue via VATS.

Table 1. Demographic characteristics of patients undergoing biopsy.

Characteristics	Total Number (%)	SGD Number (%)	Other Diseases Number (%)
Gender			
Male	7 (100)	5 (100)	2 (100)
Female	0 (0)	0 (0)	0 (100)
Age			
<50	4 (57)	4 (80)	(0)
50–59	1 (14)	1 (20)	0 (0)
60–69	2 (29)	0 (0)	2 (100)
Race/Ethnicity			
White (non-Hispanic)	7 (100)	5 (100)	2 (100)
Black (non-Hispanic)	0 (0)	0 (0)	0 (0)
Hispanic	0 (0)	0 (0)	0 (0)
Smoking Status			
Current	0 (0)	0 (0)	0 (0)
Past	4 (57)	2 (40)	2 (100)
Never	3 (43)	3 (60)	0 (0)
BMI (kg/m^2)			
< 25	0 (0)	0 (0)	0 (0)
25–29	3 (43)	1 (20)	2 (100)
30–39	4 (57)	4 (80)	0 (0)
WTC Exposure Category [2]			
Very High	0 (0)	0 (0)	0 (0)
High	3 (43)	1 (20)	2 (100)
Intermediate	4 (57)	4 (80)	0 (0)
Low	0 (0)	0 (0)	0 (0)

Abbreviations: SGD, sarcoid-like granulomatous disease; BMI, body mass index; WTC, World Trade Center.

Table 2. Clinical, radiographic and pathologic presentation of patients.

PT#	Reason for Referral	CT Impression	Biopsy	Lung Pathology	Lymph Node Pathology	Diagnosis
1	Lung nodules, mediastinal LAD	Mediastinal LAD, ground glass, sub-centimeter peripheral nodules, very mild fibrotic changes	VATS and Med	Bilateral upper lobe: Non-caseating granulomas with surrounding fibrosis Right upper and lower lobe: Scant, poorly formed granulomas	Non-caseating granulomas with surrounding fibrosis	SGD
2	Chronic cough and dyspnea	Multiple nodules	VATS	NC	NC	SGD
3	Hilar and mediastinal LAD and chronic bronchitis	Hilar and mediastinal LAD, apical pleural thickening	Med	NC	Non-caseating granulomas with surrounding fibrosis	SGD
4	Hilar LAD	Mediastinal and hilar LAD with bilateral pleural-based nodules	Med	NC	Non-caseating granuloma with surrounding fibrosis	SGD
5	Dyspnea and fatigue	Pulmonary nodules with mediastinal LAD	TBB	Right lower lobe: Focal areas of lung injury. (proteinaceous exudate with fibrin deposit)	NC	SGD (Diagnosed later at another medical facility)
6	Cough, dyspnea	Punctate calcified granulomas in lower lobes, bronchiectasis, mild intralobular septal thickening, scattered ground glass, mediastinal LAD	TBB	Left lower lobe: Focal interstitial fibrosis	NC	Pulmonary fibrosis and adenocarcinoma of the lung
7	Cough, dyspnea	Centrilobular emphysema, interstitial fibrosis. No adenopathy	TBB	Right upper lobe Unremarkable.	NC	Pulmonary fibrosis

Abbreviations: PT#, patient number; CT, computerized tomography; LAD, lymphadenopathy; VATS, video-assisted thoracoscopy; Med, mediastinoscopy; TBB, trans-bronchial biopsy; SGD, sarcoid-like granulomatous disease; NC, sample not collected.

Table 3. Pulmonary function test findings in patients undergoing biopsy.

PT#	Spirometry			Lung Volumes		DLCO (%)	Impression
	FEV$_1$ (%)	FVC (%)	FEV$_1$/FVC (%)	VC (%)	TLC (%)		
1	98	100	97	98	93	103	WNL
2	100	104	96	103	109	104	WNL
3	88	84	104	81	82	85	Mild RTLD
4	98	94	104	83	73	69	Mild RILD
5	42	58	72	51	62	69	Severe Mixed OLD & RILD
6	98	87	112	80	78	57	Mild RILD
7	80	77	104	80	77	86	Mild RTLD

Abbreviations: PT#: patient number; FEV$_1$: forced expiratory volume in 1 s; FVC: forced vital capacity; VC: vital capacity; TLC: total lung capacity; DLCO: diffusing capacity for carbon monoxide; WNL: within normal limits; RTLD: restrictive thoracic lung disease; RILD: restrictive interstitial lung disease; OLD: obstructive lung disease. Bolded values were below normal confidence intervals.

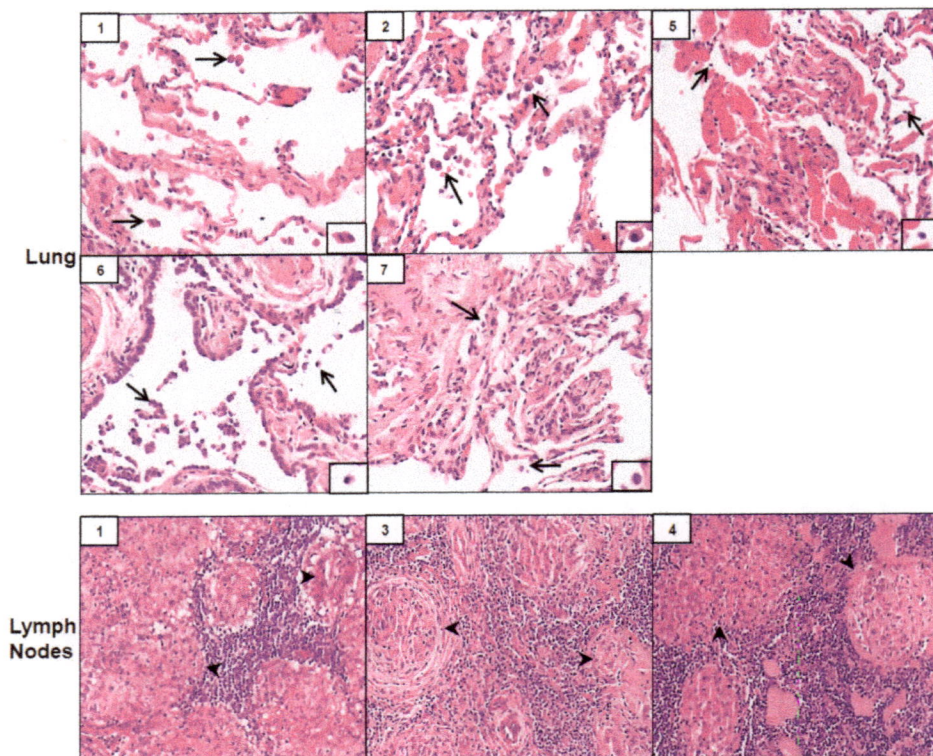

Figure 1. Histology of lung and lymph nodes. Biopsies of lung (top and middle panels) and lymph nodes (bottom panels), collected from World Trade Center (WTC) rescue and recovery workers, were sectioned and stained with Hematoxylin and Eosin (H&E). Inset, patient number. Magnification, 20×; arrows, alveolar macrophages; arrowheads, lymphocytes.

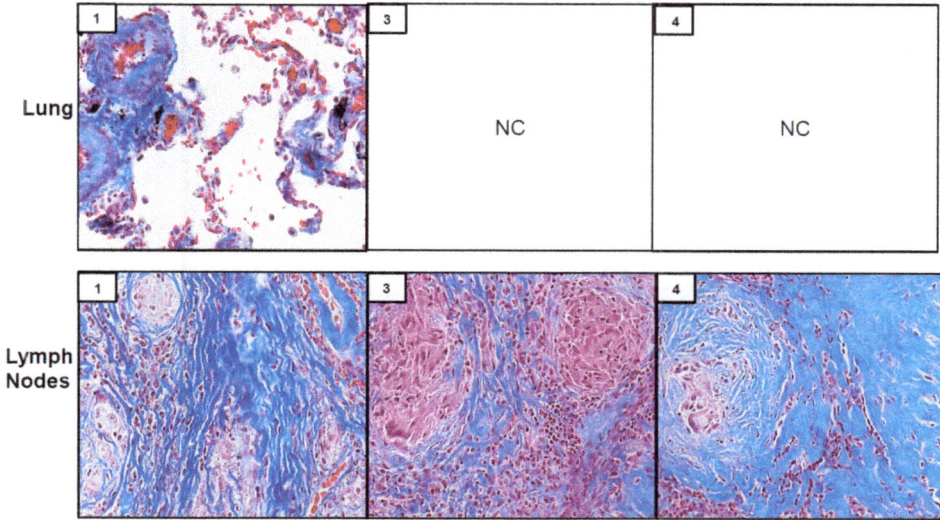

Figure 2. Trichrome staining of lung and lymph nodes. Biopsies of lung (top panel) and lymph nodes (bottom panels), collected from WTC rescue and recovery workers were sectioned and stained with Masson's trichrome. Inset, patient number; NC, tissue not collected. Magnification, 13.2×.

3.3. Expression of Markers of Injury, Oxidative Stress, Inflammation, Fibrosis, and Epigenetic Changes

Analysis of tissue sections by immunohistochemistry revealed the presence of cytochrome b5 and cytokeratin 17, markers of injury in lung (patients #1, # 2, #5, #6 and #7) and lymph nodes (patients #1, #3 and #4) (Figure 3). Whereas cytochrome b5 expression was uniformly distributed throughout the lung, including alveolar macrophages and epithelial cells, cytokeratin 17 was more prominent in alveolar macrophages. However, the intensity of expression of both of these markers varied between patients. Markers of oxidative stress including HO-1 and Lcn-2 were upregulated in alveolar macrophages and lymph node biopsies from all patients (Figure 4). As observed with cytochrome b5 and cytokeratin 17, the intensity of expression varied between patients. We also noted upregulation of the proinflammatory proteins iNOS, COX-2, TNFα, and ARL11 to varying degrees in alveolar macrophages and lymph nodes in all patient samples examined (Figures 5 and 6). Anti-inflammatory/pro-fibrotic markers of macrophage activation, including MR-1, the galactoside-binding lectin, Gal-3, and TGFβ were also upregulated (Figures 7 and 8). Additionally, histone H3 and methylated (K4) histone H3K4, epigenetic markers of inflammation/fibrosis were identified in lung and lymph nodes with varying intensities in all patient samples examined (Figure 9).

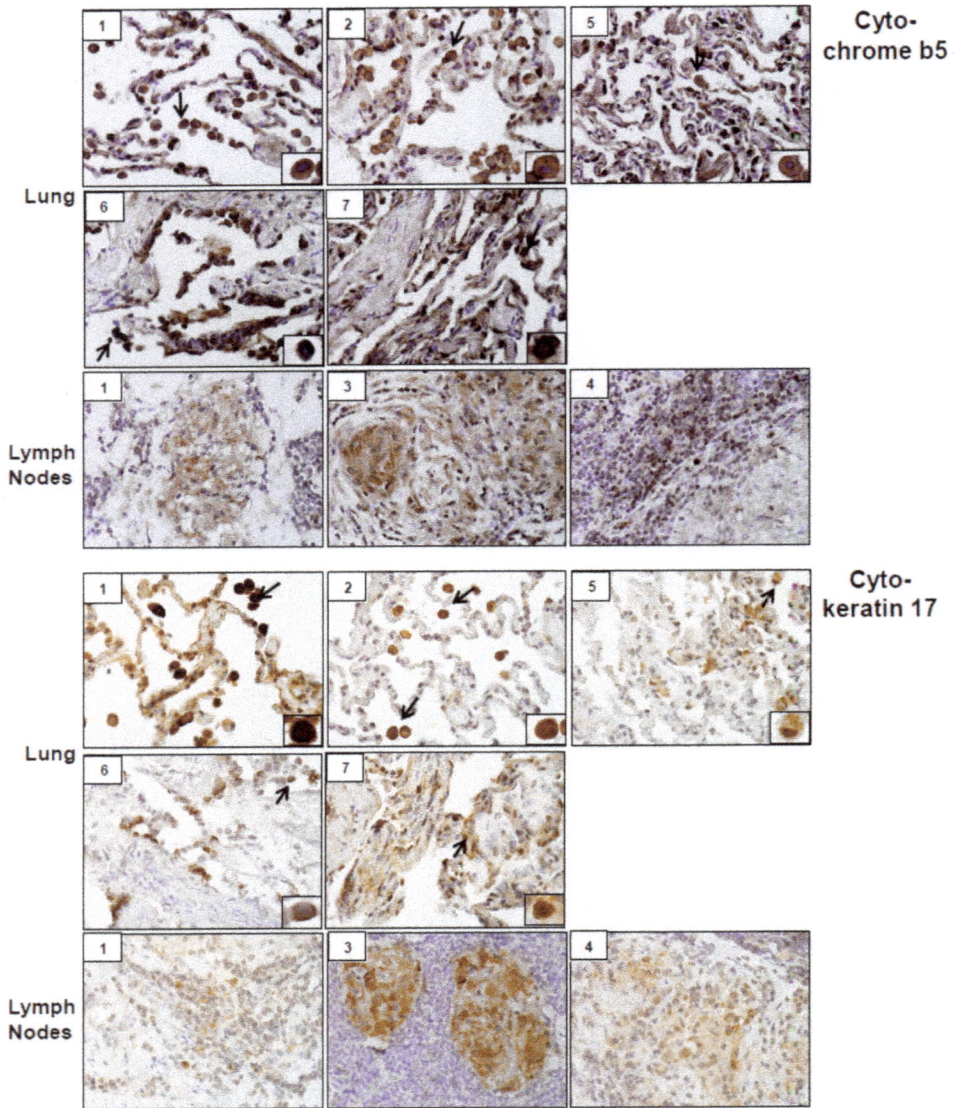

Figure 3. Cytochrome b5 and cytokeratin 17 expression in lung and/or lymph nodes collected from WTC rescue and recovery workers. Sections were immunostained with antibody to cytochrome b5 or cytokeratin 17. Binding was visualized using a 3,3′ diaminobenzidine (DAB) peroxidase substrate kit. One representative section from each patient is shown. Inset, patient number. Magnification, 60×; arrows, alveolar macrophages.

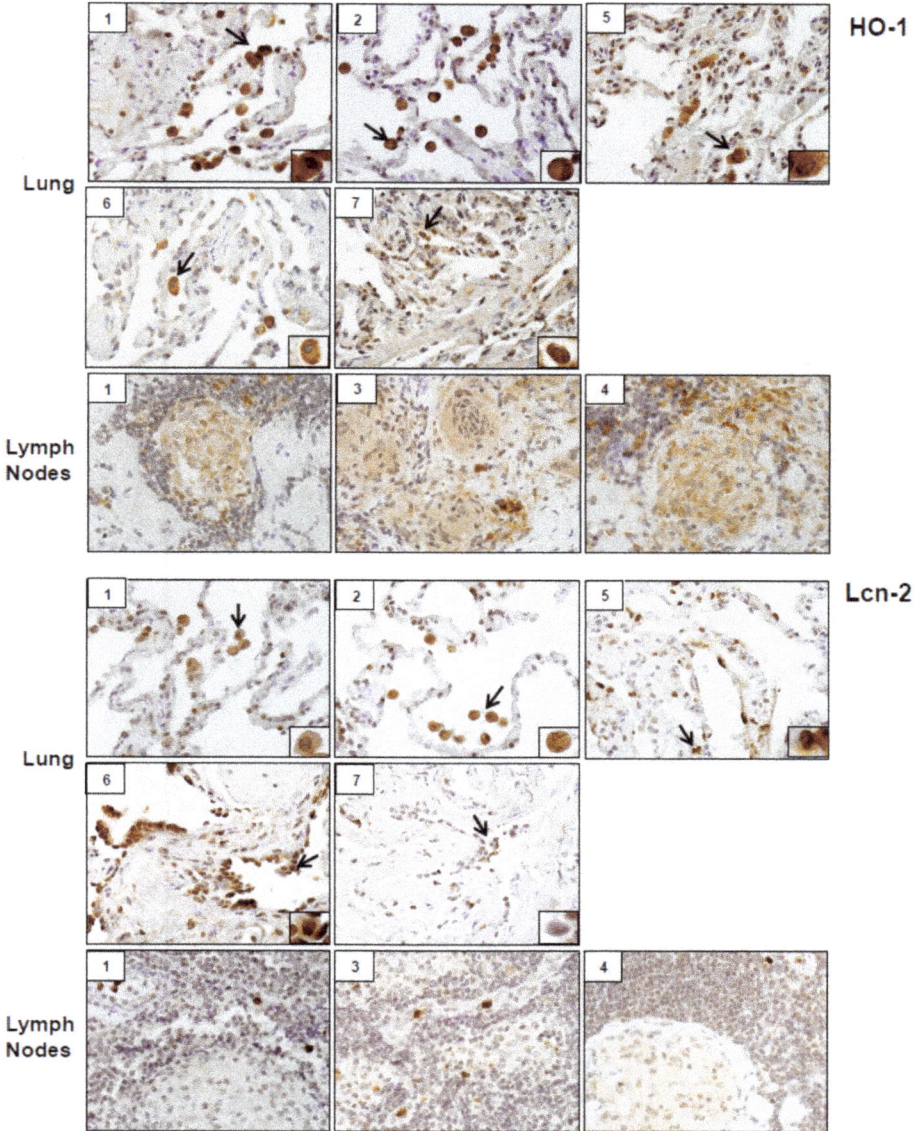

Figure 4. Hemeoxygenase (HO)-1 and Lipocalin (Lcn)-2 expression in lung and/or lymph nodes collected from WTC rescue and recovery workers. Sections were immunostained with antibody to HO-1 or Lcn-2. Binding was visualized using a DAB peroxidase substrate kit. One representative section from each patient is shown. Inset, patient number. Magnification, 60×; arrows, alveolar macrophages.

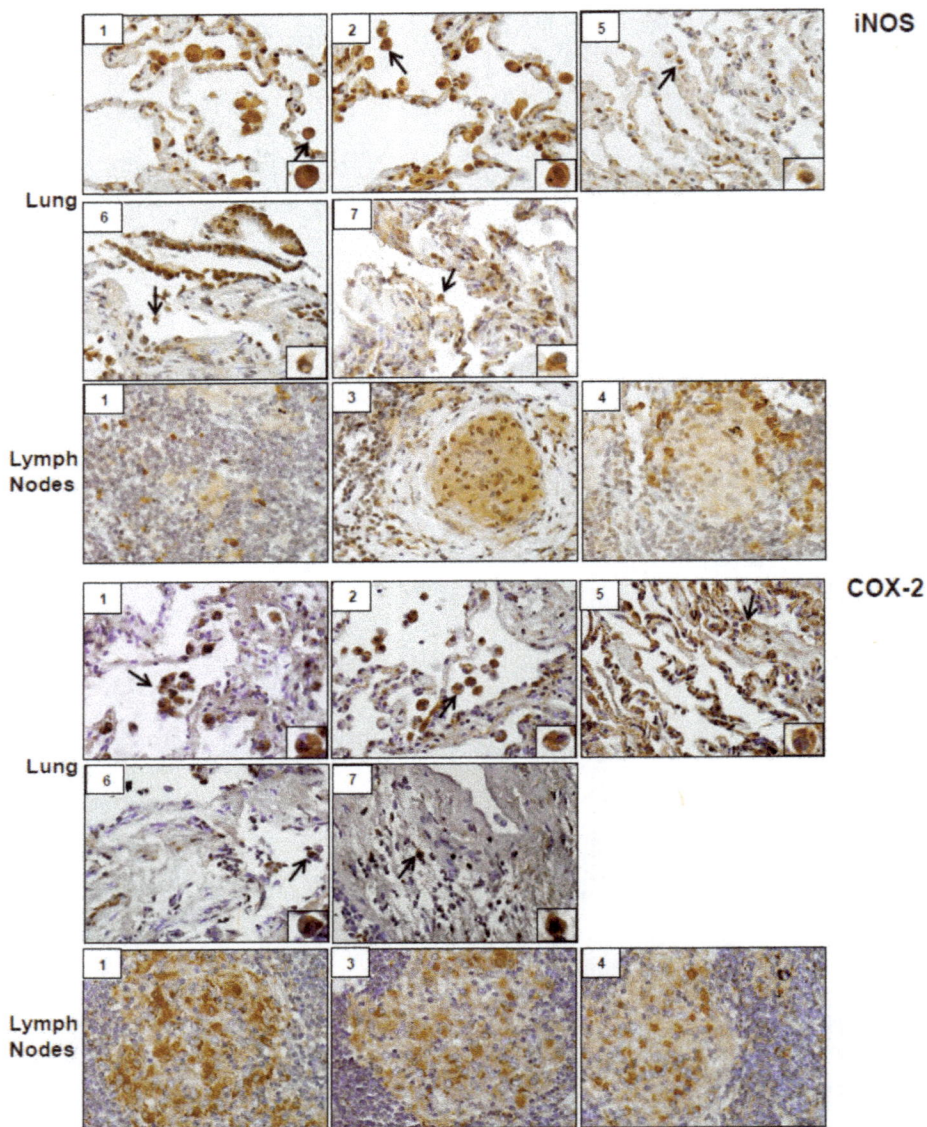

Figure 5. Inducible nitric oxide synthase (iNOS) and Cyclooxygenase (COX)-2 expression in lung and/or lymph nodes collected from WTC rescue and recovery workers. Sections were immunostained with antibody to iNOS or COX-2. Binding was visualized using a DAB peroxidase substrate kit. One representative section from each patient is shown. Inset, patient number. Magnification, 60×; arrows, alveolar macrophages.

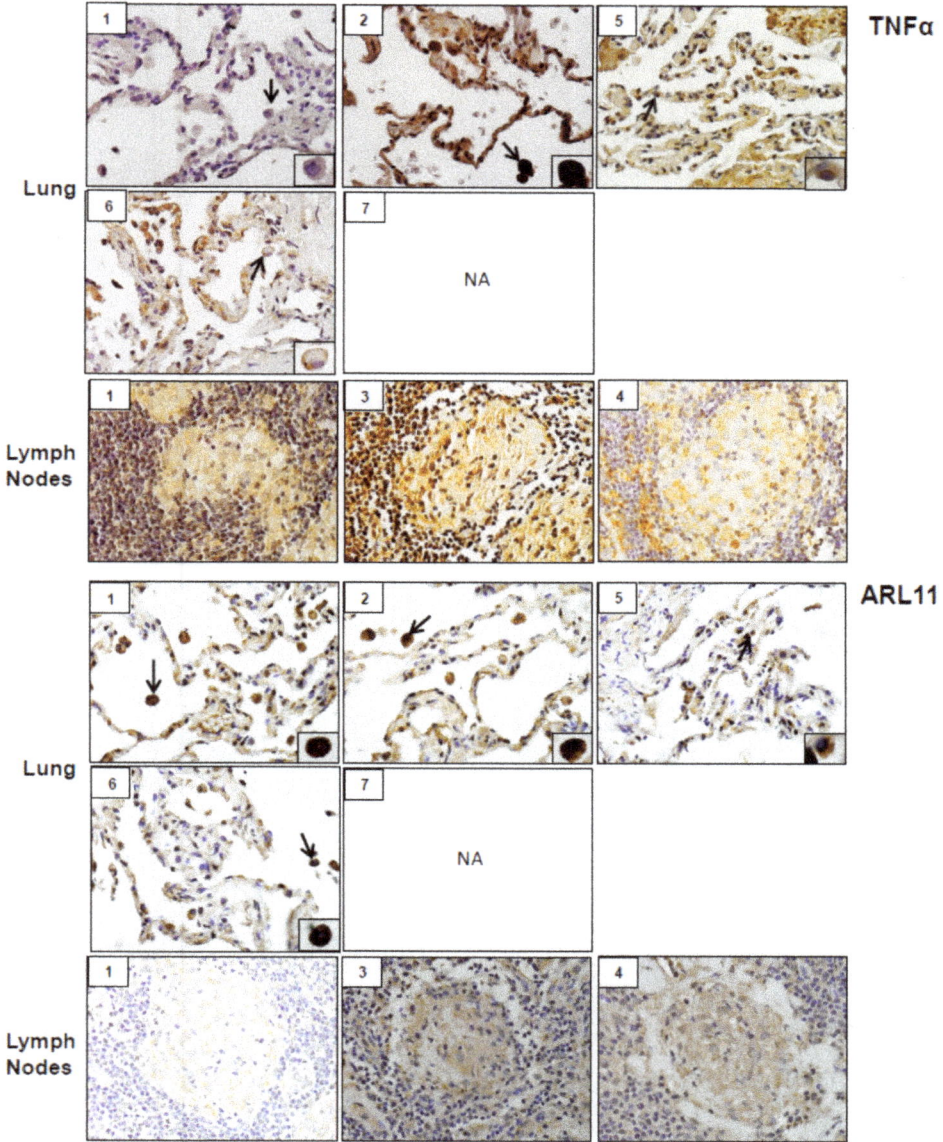

Figure 6. Tumor necrosis factor (TNF)α and ADP-ribosylation factor-like GTPase (ARL)11 expression in lung and/or lymph nodes collected from WTC rescue and recovery workers. Sections were immunostained with antibody to TNFα or ARL11. Binding was visualized using a DAB peroxidase substrate kit. One representative section from each patient is shown. Inset, patient number; NA, tissue not available. Magnification, 60×; arrows, alveolar macrophages.

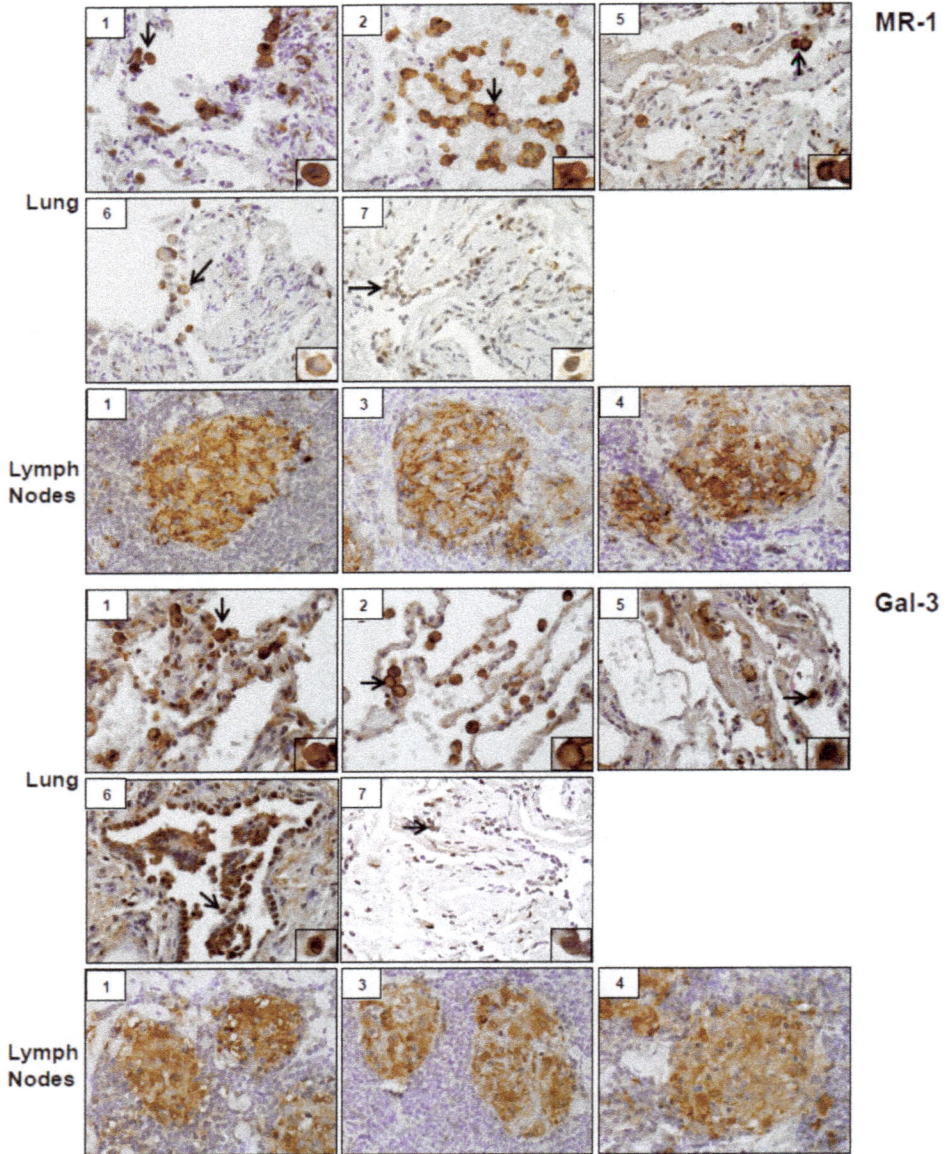

Figure 7. Mannose receptor (MR)-1 and Galectin (Gal)-3 expression in lung and/or lymph nodes collected from WTC rescue and recovery workers. Sections were immunostained with antibody to MR-1 or Gal-3. Binding was visualized using a DAB peroxidase substrate kit. One representative section from each patient is shown. Inset, patient number. Magnification, 60×; arrows, alveolar macrophages.

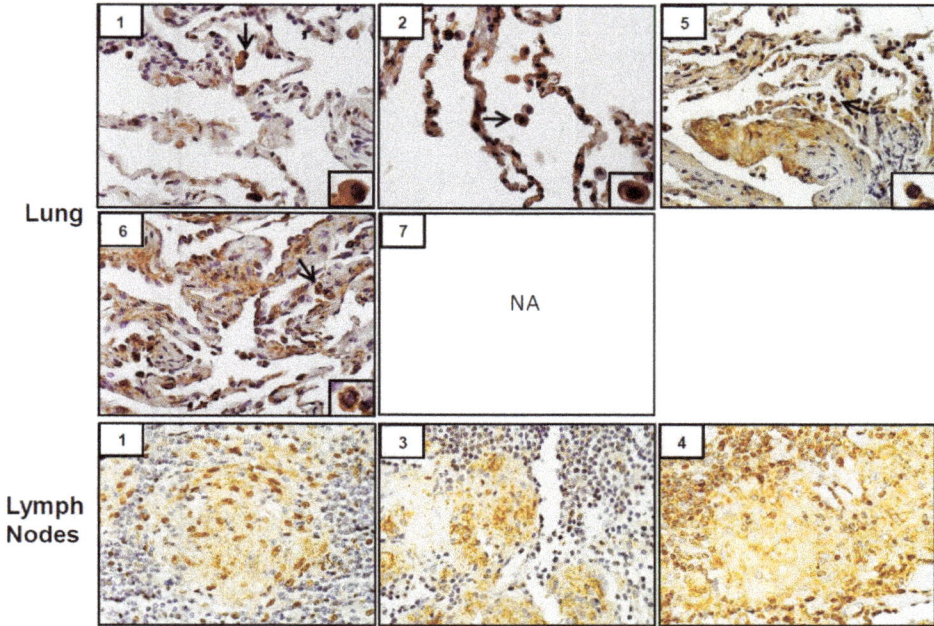

Figure 8. Transforming growth factor (TGF)β expression in lung and/or lymph nodes collected from WTC rescue and recovery workers. Sections were immunostained with antibody to TGFβ. Binding was visualized using a DAB peroxidase substrate kit. One representative section from each patient is shown. Inset, patient number; NA, tissue not available. Magnification, 60×; arrows, alveolar macrophages.

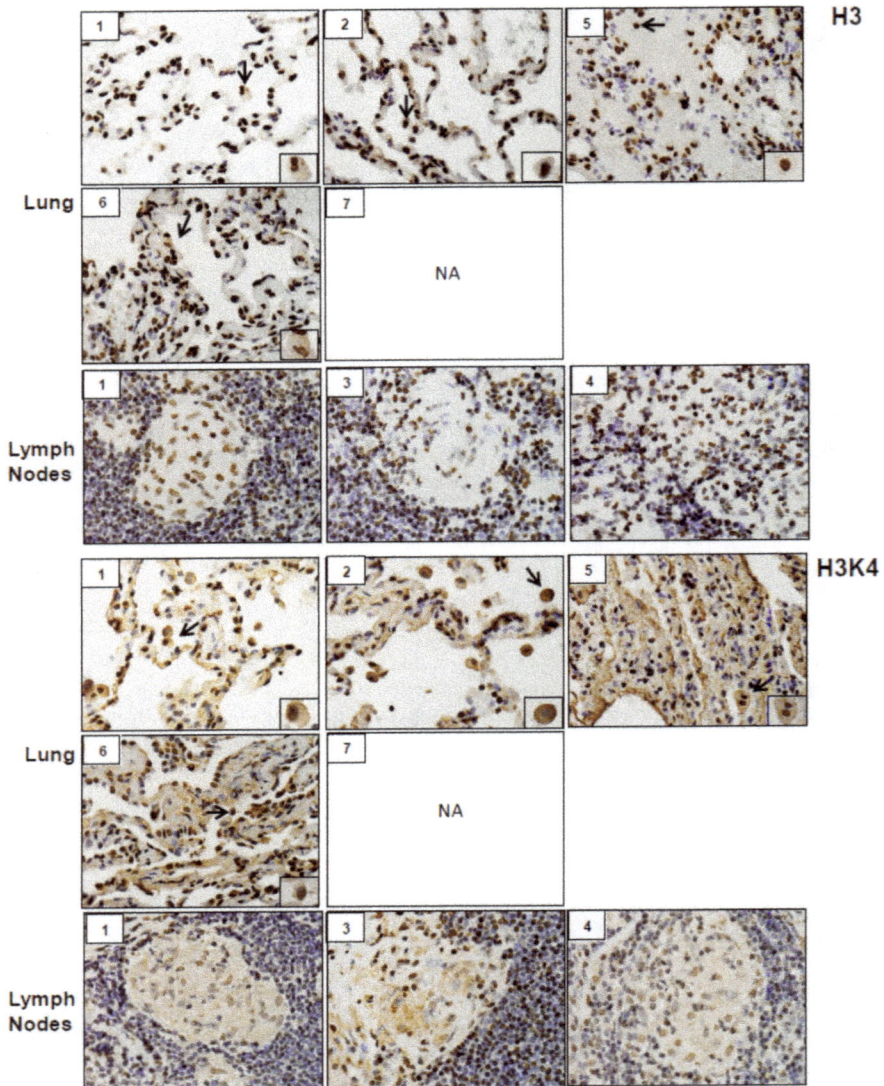

Figure 9. Histone H3 and methylated (K4) histone H3K4 expression in lung and/or lymph nodes collected from WTC rescue and recovery workers. Sections were immunostained with antibody to H3 or H3K4. Binding was visualized using a DAB peroxidase substrate kit. One representative section from each patient is shown. Inset, patient number; NA, tissue not available. Magnification, 60×; arrows, alveolar macrophages.

4. Discussion

The present studies report that five of the seven patients referred to our clinic for diagnostic evaluation exhibited SGD, as evidenced by non-caseating granulomas in lung and/or lymph nodes. SGD has previously been described among a subset of WTC rescue and recovery workers [9,10]. Mechanisms underlying the development of this disease remain unknown [11–15]. Non-caseating granuloma formation is a type of foreign body reaction which involves trapping of remnants of foreign materials that cannot be degraded and/or destroyed by macrophages [16]. The appearance of non-caseating granulomas in WTC dust-exposed patients is in line with findings that WTC dust contained organic and inorganic particles which have been implicated in the development of granulomatous pulmonary disease [17].

Inflammation and oxidative stress are common responses to inhalation of particles and fibers including silica and asbestos, components of WTC dust, and they are thought to be involved in pulmonary disease pathogenesis [18–20]. As a first step in elucidating WTC dust-induced SGD mechanisms, we analyzed the expression of markers of oxidative stress, inflammation, and injury in lung and/or lymph nodes of WTC dust-exposed patients followed in our clinic. Lung and/or lymph node samples from all patients examined stained positively for markers of pro-inflammatory M1 macrophages including iNOS, COX-2, TNFα and ARL11 [21–23]. iNOS and COX-2 mediate the production of reactive nitrogen species and proinflammatory eicosanoids, respectively. These mediators are known to contribute to M1 macrophage activation and lung injury induced by diverse toxicants, and they may play a similar role in the pathogenic response to WTC dust [21]. In this regard, COX-2 has been reported to be upregulated by silica, a component of WTC dust, in rodents, cultured fibroblasts, and in sarcoid granulomas [4,18,24–26]. ARL11 has recently been identified as a regulator of proinflammatory macrophage activation and TNFα release [22,27]. TNFα has been implicated in lung injury induced by silica [26], suggesting a potential mechanism of disease pathogenesis following WTC dust exposure.

Previous studies showed that WTC dust induces oxidative stress [5,6]. Consistent with these reports, tissue samples from all patients examined were found to stain positively for the oxidative stress markers, HO-1 and Lcn-2. In addition to their anti-oxidant activity, these proteins promote anti-inflammatory responses. Macrophage Lcn-2 has previously been shown to reduce granulomatous inflammation in mycobacterial pulmonary infections [28]. Upregulation of HO-1 and Lcn-2 in granulomas of WTC dust-exposed patients may reflect a compensatory attempt to limit inflammation and granuloma progression. Increases in proinflammatory macrophage mediators and oxidative stress were associated with lung damage as evidenced by upregulation of cytochrome b5 and cytokeratin 17 in macrophages and epithelial cells. Similar increases in these proteins have been reported in acute lung injury induced by inhaled ozone and *S. aureus* enterotoxin [23,29,30].

The activity of proinflammatory/cytotoxic M1 macrophages is balanced by anti-inflammatory/pro-fibrotic M2 macrophages, which downregulate inflammation and initiate wound repair. However, when overactivated, M2 macrophages promote fibrosis [21]. Findings that macrophages in histologic sections of WTC dust-exposed patients stained positively for MR-1 and Gal-3 suggest M2 macrophage activation [31]. This is in accord with findings that Gal-3 promotes M2 polarization of macrophages and contributes to lung fibrosis [32,33].

Coordinate with the presence of M2 macrophages, we found that tissue samples stained positively for the pro-fibrotic protein TGF β. Of note, patients with well-formed granulomas (#1, #3 and #4) also exhibited peri-granulomatous fibrosis, as evidenced by trichrome staining. Fibrotic sarcoidosis is characterized pathologically as fibrotic destruction at sites of prior granulomatous inflammation [34]. The granulomas are thought to function as a nidus for the development of fibrosis that can encompass larger areas of the respiratory tract, resulting in collagen deposition in broncho-vascular tracts and interlobular septae, cystic distortion and honeycombing of the lung [35,36]. It remains to be determined if peri-granulomatous fibrosis in our series is an early indicator of progressive fibrotic disease in patients with WTC dust-induced SGD. The most recent follow up of a large WTC dust-exposed firefighter cohort with SGD did not report clinical evidence of fibrotic disease [13]. Our pathological series suggests that fibrosis may develop in these patients with time. This is important as the development of fibrosis in sarcoidosis represents a significant change in the clinical course that is associated with increased morbidity and mortality [34,35].

It is important to note that expression of inflammatory proteins was observed in all patients exposed to WTC dust, regardless of the presence of granulomas. As we did not have controls to assess for comparison, a causal link has not been established. It is likely that specific patient demographics, such as smoking, obesity, age, and/or genetic/epigenetic factors influence the immune response to WTC dust injury, contributing to different pathological outcomes. In this regard, our patients with SGD were predominantly non-smokers, obese and <50 years of age at diagnosis. This is similar to the demographic profile of larger cohorts of New York City firefighters and first responders exposed to WTC dust [3,13]. Evidence suggests that sarcoidosis is more likely to develop in young, obese, non-smokers [37,38]. These factors are known to affect the adaptive immune response by inducing T-cell differentiation towards a Th1 phenotype [39–42]. This may contribute to the development of WTC dust-induced SGD. Lung and lymph node biopsies in our cohort, also stained positively for histone H3 and H3K4, suggesting the possibility that epigenetic factors may also contribute to SGD.

All five patients with SGD had intermediate/high exposure to WTC dust. Previous studies demonstrated a strong correlation between WTC dust exposure levels and the development of lung disease with very high exposure levels causing the most disease [2]. Our studies suggest that intermediate levels of WTC dust exposure may be a sufficient risk factor for developing SGD with fibrosis. It is also possible that heterogeneity in WTC dust, such as composition (silica, metal) and particle size, affect the pathologic response [36]. These possibilities require further investigation.

Limitations

In this case series studies, we are limited in any inferences we can make about associations, since our sample size was small and non-random, and we did not have case-matched controls.

5. Conclusions

In summary, our studies demonstrate the presence of SGD in five of seven patients exposed to intermediate/high levels of WTC dust. Lung and/or lymph nodes exhibited signs of oxidative stress, inflammation, tissue damage, and fibrosis. This was associated with upregulation of proinflammatory and pro-fibrotic markers and epigenetic alterations. Our observations of peri-granulomatous fibrosis in some of the patients with SGD are novel. Further studies are required to elucidate the precise mechanisms underlying this pathology in subsets of WTC dust-exposed patients.

Author Contributions: Conceptualization, V.R.S., H.K. and D.L.L.; data curation, S.H.; formal analysis, V.R.S. and J.R.; funding acquisition, H.K., I.U. and D.L.L.; investigation, V.R.S. and D.L.L.; methodology, V.R.S., K.N.V., J.C. and M.D.; project administration, D.L.L.; resources, D.L.L.; supervision, V.R.S. and D.L.L.; writing—original draft, V.R.S. and J.R.; writing—review and editing, S.H., H.K., I.U., R.L., J.S., J.D.L. and D.L.L.

Funding: This work was supported by the National Institutes of Health [grant numbers: ES005022, ES004738, and AR055073], and the National Institute for Occupational Safety and Health [grant number: U100H008239].

Conflicts of Interest: The authors declare no conflict of interest.

References

1. Guidotti, T.L.; Prezant, D.; de la Hoz, R.E.; Miller, A. The evolving spectrum of pulmonary disease in responders to the World Trade Center tragedy. *Am. J. Ind. Med.* **2011**, *54*, 649–660. [CrossRef] [PubMed]
2. Wisnivesky, J.P.; Teitelbaum, S.L.; Todd, A.C.; Boffetta, P.; Crane, M.; Crowley, L.; de la Hoz, R.E.; Dellenbaugh, C.; Harrison, D.; Herbert, R.; et al. Persistence of multiple illnesses in World Trade Center rescue and recovery workers: A cohort study. *Lancet* **2011**, *378*, 888–897. [CrossRef]
3. Webber, M.P.; Yip, J.; Zeig-Owens, R.; Moir, W.; Ungprasert, P.; Crowson, C.S.; Hall, C.B.; Jaber, N.; Weiden, M.D.; Matteson, E.L.; et al. Post-9/11 sarcoidosis in WTC-exposed firefighters and emergency medical service workers. *Respir. Med.* **2017**, *132*, 232–237. [CrossRef] [PubMed]
4. Lioy, P.J.; Weisel, C.P.; Millette, J.R.; Eisenreich, S.; Vallero, D.; Offenberg, J.; Buckley, B.; Turpin, B.; Zhong, M.; Cohen, M.D.; et al. Characterization of the dust/smoke aerosol that settled east of the World Trade Center (WTC) in lower Manhattan after the collapse of the WTC 11 September 2001. *Environ. Health Perspect.* **2002**, *110*, 703–714. [CrossRef] [PubMed]

5.   Cohen, M.D.; Vaughan, J.M.; Garrett, B.; Prophete, C.; Horton, L.; Sisco, M.; Kodavanti, U.P.; Ward, W.O.; Peltier, R.E.; Zelikoff, J.; et al. Acute high-level exposure to WTC particles alters expression of genes associated with oxidative stress and immune function in the lung. *J. Immunotoxicol.* **2015**, *12*, 140–153. [CrossRef] [PubMed]

6.   Sunil, V.R.; Vayas, K.N.; Fang, M.; Zarbl, H.; Massa, C.; Gow, A.J.; Cervelli, J.A.; Kipen, H.; Laumbach, R.J.; Lioy, P.J.; et al. World Trade Center (WTC) dust exposure in mice is associated with inflammation, oxidative stress and epigenetic changes in the lung. *Exp. Mol. Pathol.* **2017**, *102*, 50–58. [CrossRef] [PubMed]

7.   Herbert, R.; Moline, J.; Skloot, G.; Metzger, K.; Baron, S.; Luft, B.; Markowitz, S.; Udasin, I.; Harrison, D.; Stein, D.; et al. The World Trade Center disaster and the health of workers: Five-year assessment of a unique medical screening program. *Environ. Health Perspect.* **2006**, *114*, 1853–1858. [CrossRef] [PubMed]

8.   Miller, M.R.; Hankinson, J.; Brusasco, V.; Burgos, F.; Casaburi, R.; Coates, A.; Crapo, R.; Enright, P.; van der Grinten, C.P.; Gustafsson, P.; et al. Standardisation of spirometry. *Eur. Respir. J.* **2005**, *26*, 319–338. [CrossRef] [PubMed]

9.   Crowley, L.E.; Herbert, R.; Moline, J.M.; Wallenstein, S.; Shukla, G.; Schechter, C.; Skloot, G.S.; Udasin, I.; Luft, B.J.; Harrison, D.; et al. "Sarcoid like" granulomatous pulmonary disease in World Trade Center disaster responders. *Am. J. Ind. Med.* **2011**, *54*, 175–184. [CrossRef] [PubMed]

10.   Izbicki, G.; Chavko, R.; Banauch, G.I.; Weiden, M.D.; Berger, K.I.; Aldrich, T.K.; Hall, C.; Kelly, K.J.; Prezant, D.J. World Trade Center "sarcoid-like" granulomatous pulmonary disease in New York City Fire Department rescue workers. *Chest* **2007**, *131*, 1414–1423. [CrossRef] [PubMed]

11.   Chen, E.S.; Song, Z.; Willett, M.H.; Heine, S.; Yung, R.C.; Liu, M.C.; Groshong, S.D.; Zhang, Y.; Tuder, R.M.; Moller, D.R. Serum amyloid A regulates granulomatous inflammation in sarcoidosis through Toll-like receptor-2. *Am. J. Respir. Crit. Care Med.* **2010**, *181*, 360–373. [CrossRef] [PubMed]

12.   Facco, M.; Cabrelle, A.; Calabrese, F.; Teramo, A.; Cinetto, F.; Carraro, S.; Martini, V.; Calzetti, F.; Tamassia, N.; Cassatella, M.A.; et al. TL1A/DR3 axis involvement in the inflammatory cytokine network during pulmonary sarcoidosis. *Clin. Mol. Allergy* **2015**, *13*, 16. [CrossRef] [PubMed]

13.   Hena, K.M.; Yip, J.; Jaber, N.; Goldfarb, D.; Fullam, K.; Cleven, K.; Moir, W.; Zeig-Owens, R.; Webber, M.P.; Spevack, D.M.; et al. Clinical Course of Sarcoidosis in World Trade Center-Exposed Firefighters. *Chest* **2018**, *153*, 114–123. [CrossRef] [PubMed]

14.   Schnerch, J.; Prasse, A.; Vlachakis, D.; Schuchardt, K.L.; Pechkovsky, D.V.; Goldmann, T.; Gaede, K.I.; Muller-Quernheim, J.; Zissel, G. Functional Toll-Like Receptor 9 Expression and CXCR3 Ligand Release in Pulmonary Sarcoidosis. *Am. J. Respir. Cell Mol. Biol.* **2016**, *55*, 749–757. [CrossRef] [PubMed]

15.   Wiken, M.; Idali, F.; Al Hayja, M.A.; Grunewald, J.; Eklund, A.; Wahlstrom, J. No evidence of altered alveolar macrophage polarization, but reduced expression of TLR2, in bronchoalveolar lavage cells in sarcoidosis. *Respir. Res.* **2010**, *11*, 121. [CrossRef] [PubMed]

16.   Valeyre, D.; Prasse, A.; Nunes, H.; Uzunhan, Y.; Brillet, P.Y.; Muller-Quernheim, J. Sarcoidosis. *Lancet* **2014**, *383*, 1155–1167. [CrossRef]

17.   Safirstein, B.H.; Klukowicz, A.; Miller, R.; Teirstein, A. Granulomatous pneumonitis following exposure to the World Trade Center collapse. *Chest* **2003**, *123*, 301–304. [CrossRef] [PubMed]

18.   Fubini, B.; Hubbard, A. Reactive oxygen species (ROS) and reactive nitrogen species (RNS) generation by silica in inflammation and fibrosis. *Free Radic. Biol. Med.* **2003**, *34*, 1507–1516. [CrossRef]

19.   Rimal, B.; Greenberg, A.K.; Rom, W.N. Basic pathogenetic mechanisms in silicosis: Current understanding. *Curr. Opin. Pulm. Med.* **2005**, *11*, 169–173. [CrossRef] [PubMed]

20.   Valavanidis, A.; Vlachogianni, T.; Fiotakis, K.; Loridas, S. Pulmonary Oxidative Stress, Inflammation and Cancer: Respirable Particulate Matter, Fibrous Dusts and Ozone as Major Causes of Lung Carcinogenesis through Reactive Oxygen Species Mechanisms. *Int. J. Environ. Res. Public Health* **2013**, *10*, 3886–3907. [CrossRef] [PubMed]

21.   Laskin, D.L.; Sunil, V.R.; Gardner, C.R.; Laskin, J.D. Macrophages and tissue injury: Agents of defense or destruction? *Ann. Rev. Pharmacol. Toxicol.* **2011**, *51*, 267–288. [CrossRef] [PubMed]

22.   Platko, K.; Lebeau, P.; Austin, R.C. MAPping the kinase landscape of macrophage activation. *J. Biol. Chem.* **2018**, *293*, 9910–9911. [CrossRef] [PubMed]

23.   Sunil, V.R.; Francis, M.; Vayas, K.N.; Cervelli, J.A.; Choi, H.; Laskin, J.D.; Laskin, D.L. Regulation of ozone-induced lung inflammation and injury by the beta-galactoside-binding lectin galectin-3. *Toxicol. Appl. Pharmacol.* **2015**, *284*, 236–245. [CrossRef] [PubMed]

24. Choi, J.K.; Lee, S.G.; Lee, J.Y.; Nam, H.Y.; Lee, W.K.; Lee, K.H.; Kim, H.J.; Lim, Y. Silica induces human cyclooxygenase-2 gene expression through the NF-kappaB signaling pathway. *J. Environ. Pathol. Toxicol. Oncol.* **2005**, *24*, 163–174. [CrossRef] [PubMed]

25. Christophi, G.P.; Caza, T.; Curtiss, C.; Gumber, D.; Massa, P.T.; Landas, S.K. Gene expression profiles in granuloma tissue reveal novel diagnostic markers in sarcoidosis. *Exp. Mol. Pathol.* **2014**, *96*, 393–399. [CrossRef] [PubMed]

26. Kawasaki, H. A mechanistic review of silica-induced inhalation toxicity. *Inhal. Toxicol.* **2015**, *27*, 363–377. [CrossRef] [PubMed]

27. Arya, S.B.; Kumar, G.; Kaur, H.; Kaur, A.; Tuli, A. ARL11 regulates lipopolysaccharide-stimulated macrophage activation by promoting mitogen-activated protein kinase (MAPK) signaling. *J. Biol. Chem.* **2018**, *293*, 9892–9909. [CrossRef] [PubMed]

28. Guglani, L.; Gopal, R.; Rangel-Moreno, J.; Junecko, B.F.; Lin, Y.; Berger, T.; Max, T.W.; Alcorn, J.F.; Randall, T.D.; Reinhart, T.A.; et al. Lipocalin 2 regulates inflammation during pulmonary mycobacterial infections. *PLoS ONE* **2012**, *7*, e50052. [CrossRef] [PubMed]

29. Francis, M.; Groves, A.M.; Sun, R.; Cervelli, J.A.; Choi, H.; Laskin, J.D.; Laskin, D.L. Editor's Highlight: CCR2 Regulates Inflammatory Cell Accumulation in the Lung and Tissue Injury following Ozone Exposure. *Toxicol. Sci.* **2017**, *155*, 474–484. [CrossRef] [PubMed]

30. Menoret, A.; Kumar, S.; Vella, A.T. Cytochrome b5 and cytokeratin 17 are biomarkers in bronchoalveolar fluid signifying onset of acute lung injury. *PLoS ONE* **2012**, *7*, e40184. [CrossRef] [PubMed]

31. Laskin, D.L.; Malaviya, R.; Laskin, J.D. Role of Macrophages in Acute Lung Injury and Chronic Fibrosis Induced by Pulmonary Toxicants. *Toxicol. Sci.* **2018**. [CrossRef] [PubMed]

32. Guo, C.; Atochina-Vasserman, E.; Abramova, H.; George, B.; Manoj, V.; Scott, P.; Gow, A. Role of NOS2 in pulmonary injury and repair in response to bleomycin. *Free Radic. Biol. Med.* **2016**, *91*, 293–301. [CrossRef] [PubMed]

33. Zhou, Y.; He, C.H.; Yang, D.S.; Nguyen, T.; Cao, Y.; Kamle, S.; Lee, C.M.; Gochuico, B.R.; Gahl, W.A.; Shea, B.S.; et al. Galectin-3 Interacts with the CHI3L1 Axis and Contributes to Hermansky-Pudlak Syndrome Lung Disease. *J. Immunol.* **2018**, *200*, 2140–2153. [CrossRef] [PubMed]

34. Bonham, C.A.; Strek, M.E.; Patterson, K.C. From granuloma to fibrosis: Sarcoidosis associated pulmonary fibrosis. *Curr. Opin. Pulm. Med.* **2016**, *22*, 484–491. [CrossRef] [PubMed]

35. Patterson, K.C.; Strek, M.E. Pulmonary fibrosis in sarcoidosis. Clinical features and outcomes. *Ann. Am. Thorac. Soc.* **2013**, *10*, 362–370. [CrossRef] [PubMed]

36. Zissel, G.; Prasse, A.; Muller-Quernheim, J. Immunologic response of sarcoidosis. *Semin. Respir. Crit. Care Med.* **2010**, *31*, 390–403. [CrossRef]

37. Hillerdal, G.; Nou, E.; Osterman, K.; Schmekel, B. Sarcoidosis: Epidemiology and prognosis. A 15-year European study. *Am. Rev. Respir. Dis.* **1984**, *130*, 29–32. [PubMed]

38. Ungprasert, P.; Crowson, C.S.; Matteson, E.L. Smoking, obesity and risk of sarcoidosis: A population-based nested case-control study. *Respir. Med.* **2016**, *120*, 87–90. [CrossRef] [PubMed]

39. Blanchet, M.R.; Israel-Assayag, E.; Cormier, Y. Inhibitory effect of nicotine on experimental hypersensitivity pneumonitis in vivo and in vitro. *Am. J. Respir. Crit. Care Med.* **2004**, *169*, 903–909. [CrossRef] [PubMed]

40. Di Lorenzo, G.; Di Bona, D.; Belluzzo, F.; Macchia, L. Immunological and non-immunological mechanisms of allergic diseases in the elderly: Biological and clinical characteristics. *Immun. Ageing* **2017**, *14*, 23. [CrossRef] [PubMed]

41. Martin-Romero, C.; Santos-Alvarez, J.; Goberna, R.; Sanchez-Margalet, V. Human leptin enhances activation and proliferation of human circulating T lymphocytes. *Cell. Immunol.* **2000**, *199*, 15–24. [CrossRef] [PubMed]

42. Mattoli, S.; Kleimberg, J.; Stacey, M.A.; Bellini, A.; Sun, G.; Marini, M. The role of CD8+ Th2 lymphocytes in the development of smoking-related lung damage. *Biochem. Biophys. Res. Commun.* **1997**, *239*, 146–149. [CrossRef] [PubMed]

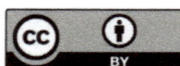

International Journal of
*Environmental Research
and Public Health*

MDPI

Article

Pulmonary Fibrosis among World Trade Center Responders: Results from the WTC Health Registry Cohort

Jiehui Li *, James E. Cone, Robert M. Brackbill, Ingrid Giesinger, Janette Yung and Mark R. Farfel

New York City Department of Health and Mental Hygiene, World Trade Center Health Registry, New York City, NY 10013, USA; jcone@health.nyc.gov (J.E.C.); rbrackbi@health.nyc.gov (R.M.B.); igiesinger@health.nyc.gov (I.G.); jyung@health.nyc.gov (J.Y.); mfarfel@health.nyc.gov (M.R.F.)
* Correspondence: jli3@health.nyc.gov; Tel.: +1-646-632-6669

Received: 12 February 2019; Accepted: 4 March 2019; Published: 7 March 2019

Abstract: Dust created by the collapse of the World Trade Center (WTC) towers on 9/11 included metals and toxicants that have been linked to an increased risk of pulmonary fibrosis (PF) in the literature. Little has been reported on PF among WTC responders. This report used self-reported physician diagnosis of PF with an unknown sub-type to explore the association between levels of WTC dust exposure and PF. We included 19,300 WTC responders, enrolled in the WTC Health Registry in 2003–2004, who were followed for 11 years from 2004 to 2015. Exposure was defined primarily by intensity and duration of exposure to WTC dust/debris and work on the debris pile. Stratified Cox regression was used to assess the association. We observed 73 self-reported physician-diagnosed PF cases, with a PF incidence rate of 36.7/100,000 person-years. The adjusted hazard ratio (AHR) of PF was higher in those with a medium (AHR = 2.5, 95% CI = 1.1–5.8) and very high level of exposure (AHR = 4.5, 95% CI = 2.0–10.4), compared to those with low exposure. A test for exposure—response trend was statistically significant (P_{trend} = 0.004). Future research on WTC dust exposure and PF would benefit from using data from multiple WTC Health Program responder cohorts for increased statistical power and clinically confirmed cases.

Keywords: World Trade Center disaster; pulmonary fibrosis; dust

---

1. Introduction

The collapse of the World Trade Center (WTC) towers resulting from the terrorist attack on 11 September 2001 (9/11) produced a dense cloud of dust and debris that spread widely and contained toxic substances including heavy metals (e.g., titanium), silica, asbestos fibers, and wood dust [1,2]. WTC responders were potentially highly exposed as a result of performing rescue and recovery work on the WTC site including searching for remains, firefighting and debris removal work that continued through June 2002 [3]. Of those involved in the rescue/recovery activities, nearly half were directly exposed to the dust cloud (blackout conditions) on 9/11 [3]. In total, 93% of WTC responders had commenced work on the site by the end of September, 2001 [3].

Short and longer-term health effects of 9/11 associated with intense dust/fume exposure include a number of respiratory diseases or symptoms, such as asthma, chronic obstructive pulmonary disease (COPD) and upper or lower respiratory symptoms [4–9]. A small number of cases of pulmonary fibrosis (PF) among WTC responders were reported in the first eight years following 9/11 [4,10,11]. PF is an interstitial lung disease, characterized by scarring (fibrosis) formed over time in the structural lung tissue between alveoli (or air sacs) [12]. Lung biopsies in four out of seven previously healthy WTC responders in a case series study revealed histologic patterns that were consistent with interstitial disease, following imaging that identified suspected interstitial disease after 9/11 exposure [10].

In another case series from the WTC Environmental Health Center (WTC EHC), five of six patients, who underwent surgical biopsy based on CT findings suggestive of diffuse interstitial disease of fibrosis, had pathologic findings of mild to moderate patchy interstitial fibrosis [11]. Moreover, these two case series that included mineralogical analyses of the available tissues found the presence of metals, silica, aluminum silicates, carbon nanotubes, chrysotile asbestos and calcium phosphate or sulfate [10,11]. Four cases of bilateral pulmonary fibrosis were also reported among New York City firefighters [4]. All of these initial observations from individual patients provided important clues to the occurrence of this rare disease among 9/11-exposed individuals.

WTC dust may be responsible for the reported PF cases as the substances known to be associated with PF in occupational studies include heavy metals (e.g., titanium), silica, and wood dust [13–19], which were also found in WTC dust [1,2]. However, little is known about the occurrence of PF in this population over time and whether the level of WTC dust exposure would be associated with PF in an observational study in which WTC responders with PF could be compared to those who do not have PF.

Using self-reported survey data on PF from the World Trade Center Health Registry [20], we investigated the incidence of PF and assessed the association between WTC dust exposure and PF in a large longitudinal cohort of WTC responders during an 11-year median follow-up period. We hypothesized that the intensity of WTC dust exposure is associated with increased risk of PF.

2. Materials and Methods

2.1. Study Population

The World Trade Center Health Registry (Registry) was established in 2003–2004 as an exposure cohort study designed to monitor the long-term health effects of the September 11 attacks among rescue/recovery workers and persons who lived, worked, or attended school in lower Manhattan. The Registry's methods have been published elsewhere [5,20]. Briefly, in 2003–2004 (enrollment, Wave 1 survey) over 71,000 people were enrolled and completed a telephone (95%) or in-person (5%) interview. Participants were identified either through lists provided by employers, government agencies, and other entities or by responding to an outreach campaign (30% list identified, 70% self-identified). At enrollment, data on demographics, exposure incurred during and after 9/11, and health information were collected. Since Wave 1 (W1), three follow-up surveys have been conducted, in 2006–2007 (Wave 2, W2), 2011–2012 (Wave 3, W3), and 2015–2016 (Wave 4, W4).

Physician diagnosis of PF was first inquired about in W3 and repeated in W4; therefore, only those who participated in W3 or W4 and completed a question related to PF diagnosis were included in this study. To test our hypothesis, we focused our study sample on WTC responders, who presumably experienced more intense dust exposure than those not involved with rescue/recovery. We defined WTC responders in this present study as those who worked at least one shift at the WTC site providing rescue, recovery, clean-up, construction, or support services from 11 September 2001 to 30 June 2002, and who provided information related to work and exposure at the WTC site anytime during the 9 months of rescue/recovery operations. Those younger than 18 years on 11 September 2001 or of unknown age were excluded. The final sample of responders included firefighters, police, emergency medical services/medical/disaster personnel, construction/engineering workers, affiliated or unaffiliated volunteers, other government workers, and sanitation workers.

The Centers for Disease Control and Prevention (CDC) and the New York City Department of Health and Mental Hygiene institutional review boards approved the World Trade Center Health Registry protocol.

2.2. PF Definition

Self-reported physician-diagnosed PF between 2004 and 2015 was the endpoint of interest. In W3 and W4, we inquired about whether the enrollee had ever been told by a physician that they had PF and the associated year of diagnosis. If WTC responders participated in both W3 and W4, the first report of the year of diagnosis was used, and PF was defined as consistent PF information being provided on both surveys. If responders participated in W3 or W4 but not both, the year of diagnosis reported at the respective survey was used. As we only had the year of diagnosis available, the midpoint of the reported year (June 30) was used as the diagnosis date. To reduce the subjectivity of self-reported physician-diagnosed PF, we added self-reported shortness of breath in the 30 days prior to reporting PF to the case definition. Shortness of breath is one of the most common symptoms presented by PF patients, due to scarring and thickening in the lung tissue. We excluded self-reported PF cases diagnosed prior to Registry enrollment or 2004 and those participants who had no symptoms of shortness of breath in the 30 days prior to reporting PF, had missing years of diagnosis, or inconsistent information on PF diagnosis. Individuals with sarcoidosis were excluded because not all cases of sarcoidosis are pulmonary and we were unable to differentiate these cases within our study. These included sarcoidosis identified either from the Registry's in-depth study through a medical record review [21], or from the New York State Department of Health's SPARCS (Statewide Planning and Research Cooperative System) inpatient data (2000–2015) using ICD-9 diagnosis code 135 or ICD-10 D86. Only 20% of persons with sarcoidosis develop fibrotic lung disease [22], although there has been a demonstrated association between WTC exposure and sarcoidosis among responders [21,23,24].

2.3. WTC Dust Exposure and Covariates

Physical exposure to dust at the WTC site was based on self-reported WTC exposures that were collected at enrollment [25]. The WTC dust exposure composite score, developed using a modified Delphi method, took information on date of arrival, duration of work at the site, dates or time period working on the pile and being near the WTC site, or exposure to dust/debris resulting from the collapse of buildings on 9/11 into account. The sum of WTC dust exposure scores for each WTC responder was analyzed both as a continuous variable (actual sum scores) for trend and as an ordinal scale variable for analysis of PF risk at each exposure quartile. The latter, based on quartiles of the summed points, was categorized as: Low (Q1 $\leq$ 25%), medium (Q2), high (Q3), and very high (Q4 > 75%).

Covariates identified in the literature as potential risk factors were included in the multivariable analysis, including age, gender, race and ethnicity, income, and smoking status (current, former or never), which were reported at enrollment. We also examined the prevalence of comorbidities in our WTC responders by PF status, as some physical and mental health conditions frequently co-exist or are highly prevalent in persons with idiopathic PF which is the most common type of PF [26]. Medical conditions were based on self-reports in W3 or W4 of having been told by a medical professional that the participant had the condition. Conditions included chronic obstructive pulmonary disease (COPD), diabetes, gastroesophageal reflux disease (GERD), obstructive sleep apnea (OSA), asthma, depression, anxiety, or post-traumatic stress disorder (PTSD).

2.4. Statistical Analysis

Incident rate of PF by characteristics and WTC exposure were summarized using crude incidence rates and expressed as PF per 100,000 person-years of follow-up. The association of WTC dust exposure with time to PF diagnosis was assessed using Cox proportional hazards regression modeling. To test for proportionality, we assessed time dependent covariates by creating interactions of all predictors and a function of survival time and included these in the model. We found that "smoking" did not satisfy the proportional hazard assumption, and therefore, carried out a stratified Cox proportional hazards regression for the analysis. In the stratified Cox model, "smoking" was controlled by stratification [27]. Results of multivariable analysis were expressed as adjusted hazard ratios (AHR) with 95% confidence intervals (CI). Person-years of follow-up began on the date of enrollment and ended at the time of PF diagnosis or were censored on the last follow-up (W3 or W4 survey completion date, whichever was most recent). All statistical analyses were performed using SAS software (SAS Institute, Cary, NC, USA V9.4). Two-sided p values of less than 0.05 were considered significant.

3. Results

Of a total of 29,721 WTC responders, enrolled in the Registry in 2003–2004, 19,300 WTC responders met eligibility criteria for data analyses. Excluded were those younger than 18 years old on 9/11 or deceased prior to enrollment (N = 205), non-participants of W3 and W4 (N = 8181), those with missing reports of PF or year of diagnosis (N = 1172), those with inconsistent reports, missing information on shortness of breath or pre-2004 PF (N = 837), sarcoidosis (N = 1), or missing data on WTC exposure (N = 25).

The characteristics of the study sample at enrollment are presented in Table 1. The median age of responders at enrollment was 41 years (interquartile range, 34–48 years). Responders included in this study were predominantly male (77.8%), non-Latino white (75.6%), and had an annual household income ≥$50,000 (70.2%). With respect to smoking status at baseline, the percent of former smokers was 29.3% among non-Latino whites, 19.9% in non-Latino blacks, 24.6% in Latinos, and 16.4% in Asians; the percent of current smokers was 15.2% among non-Latino whites, 15.7% in non-Latino blacks, 17.7% in Latinos, and 15.3% in Asians.

Table 1. Characteristics and World Trade Center (WTC) dust exposure of study sample at enrollment.

Variable at Enrollment	No.	%
Total	19,300	100
Age, year		
<45	10,564	54.7
45–64	8205	42.5
≥65	531	2.8
Gender		
Male	15,020	77.8
Female	4280	22.2
Race/Ethnicity		
Non-Latino white	14,586	75.6
Non-Latino black	1380	7.2
Latino	2265	11.7
Asian	426	2.2
Other/unknown	643	3.3
Household income ($)		
<50,000	4261	22.1
≥50,000	13,549	70.2
Missing	1490	7.7
Smoking status		
Never	10,849	56.2
Former	5332	27.6
Current	2996	15.5
Missing	123	0.6
WTC dust/debris exposure level		
Quantile 1 (Low)	4772	24.7
Quantile 2 (Medium)	4670	24.2
Quantile 3 (High)	4800	24.9
Quantile 4 (Very high)	5058	26.2

A total of 73 incident cases of PF were reported among 19,300 responders over the study period between 2004 and 2015, which totaled 199,113.6 person-years. The overall incidence rate of PF was 36.7 per 100,000 person-years. The PF incidence rate was higher in the older age groups, males, Latino or Asian, those with low household income, current smokers and those with higher WTC exposure (Table 2).

Table 2. Incidence rate of self-reported physician-diagnosed pulmonary fibrosis (PF) according to socio-demographics and WTC dust exposure (N = 19,300).

Variable at Enrollment	No. of PF	Person-Years (PY)	Rate (No. of PF/100,000 PY)	95% Confidence Interval
Total	73	199,113.6	36.7	29.2, 46.1
Age, year				
<45 (22–44)	29	107,890.0	26.9	18.7, 38.7
45–64	40	85,721.3	46.7	34.2, 63.6
≥65	4	5502.3	72.7	27.3, 193.6
Gender				
Male	61	154,690.0	39.4	30.7, 50.7
Female	12	44,427.5	27.0	15.3, 47.6
Race/Ethnicity				
Non-Latino white	45	151,627.3	29.7	22.2, 40.0
Non-Latino black	2	13,788.0	14.5	3.6, 58.0
Latino	17	22,846.3	74.4	46.3, 119.7
Asian	5	4334.8	115.3	48.0, 277.0
Other/unknown	4	6517.1	61.4	23.0, 163.5
Household income ($)				
<50,000	22	43,168.1	51.0	33.6, 77.4
≥50,000	46	140,651.4	32.7	24.5, 43.7
Missing	5	15,294.1	32.7	13.6, 78.5
Smoking status				
Never	31	112,062.1	27.7	19.5, 39.3
Former	19	55,556.1	34.2	21.8, 53.6
Current	22	30,295.1	72.6	47.8, 110.3
Missing	1	1200.3	83.3	11.8, 591.0
WTC dust/debris exposure level				
Quantile 1 (Low)	8	49,491.8	16.2	8.1, 32.3
Quantile 2 (Medium)	19	48,128.3	39.5	25.2, 61.9
Quantile 3 (High)	18	49,446.7	36.4	22.9, 57.8
Quantile 4 (Very high)	28	52,046.8	53.8	37.2, 77.9

In multivariable analysis, taking socio-demographics into account, we observed an exposure—response relationship between WTC dust exposure and PF (Table 3) (p for linear trend = 0.004). Compared to those with a low level (Q1) of exposure, approximately 2.5 times as many WTC responders in the 2nd and 3rd quantiles were experiencing PF, and those in Q4 (the highest level of exposure) experienced the highest AHR during the follow-up period. AHR at each quantile was significantly elevated compared to that at the lowest level.

Table 3. Adjusted hazard ratios (AHR) for self-reported physician-diagnosed pulmonary fibrosis (PF) according to socio-demographics and WTC dust exposure (*N* = 19,300).

Variable	AHR *	95% CI
Age at enrollment, year	1.05	1.03–1.08
Gender		
Female	referent	
Male	1.27	0.66–2.43
Race/Ethnicity		
Non-Latino white	referent	
Non-Latino black	0.47	0.11–1.95
Latino	2.45	1.37–4.37
Asian	4.62	1.81–11.79
Other/unknown	1.80	0.60–5.38
Household income at enrollment ($)		
<50,000	1.78	1.03–3.06
≥50,000	referent	
Missing	0.95	0.36–2.58
WTC dust/debris exposure level		
Quantile 1 (Low)	referent	
Quantile 2 (Medium)	2.51	1.09–5.80
Quantile 3 (High)	2.34	0.99–5.51
Quantile 4 (Very high)	4.51	1.96–10.38
P_{trend} for WTC exposure **	0.0043	

* Adjusted for demographic variables. ** Test for dose-response relationship.

Distribution of comorbidity by self-reported physician-diagnosed PF is presented in Table 4. The prevalence of co-existing physical conditions (e.g., GERD, OSA, asthma, COPD or emphysema, and diabetes) and mental disorders (e.g., depression, PTSD and anxiety) among PF patients was significantly higher than it was in those without PF (*p* = 0.030 for diabetes, and *p* < 0.001 for all other conditions). Of these comorbid conditions, GERD (69.4%) and OSA (68.5%) had the highest prevalence among individuals with PF.

Table 4. Distribution of comorbidity by self-reported physician-diagnosed pulmonary fibrosis (PF) status *.

Conditions Reported in W3 or W4	PF		No. PF	
	No.	%	No.	%
Physical conditions				
Gastroesophageal reflux disease (GERD)	50	69.4	6069	31.7
Obstructive sleep apnea (OSA)	50	68.5	4820	25.2
Asthma	44	60.3	4378	22.9
Chronic obstructive pulmonary disease (COPD) or emphysema	33	45.8	1406	7.3
Diabetes	15	20.8	2429	12.7
Mental disorders				
Depression	39	54.9	4583	26.0
PTSD	34	48.6	3593	20.6
Anxiety	25	36.8	2829	16.3

* Not mutually exclusive. *p* < 0.001 for all comorbidity listed in the table between two groups, except for diabetes (*p* = 0.030).

4. Discussion

In this longitudinal WTC exposure cohort of 19,300 responders, a total incidence rate of PF was 36.7 per 100,000 person-years between 2004 and 2015. Although little is reported on prevalence of PF in general populations, we do know that idiopathic pulmonary fibrosis (IPF), the most common type of PF, has an estimated prevalence of 14–63 cases per 100,000 population, and incidence of 6.8–17.4 per 100,000 population in the United States, dependent on the case definition [28]. Supporting our hypothesis, we observed that WTC dust exposure increased the risk of PF in an exposure—response relationship among WTC responders. AHR at each quartile was significantly elevated compared to that at the lowest quartile.

4.1. WTC Dust and PF

WTC dust may be a plausible source of PF risk due to its unique characteristics and components that are known to be linked to PF. Particle size (>90% between 2.5 and 100 μm) of WTC dust can be inhaled and deposited in the airways and lungs when the airborne concentrations are high [1,29]. Second, the highly alkaline nature of the pulverized building materials can cause both physical and chemical irritation to the respiratory and gastroesophageal epithelia [1,30]. Third, readily airborne resuspension can increase surface re-contamination levels of WTC dust both indoors and outdoors [30]. Of the 287 chemicals and chemical groups identified from environmental sampling of the area around the WTC in New York City [31], asbestos and glass fibers, crystalline silica, various metals, volatile organic compounds, polychlorinated polycyclic compounds, and polycyclic aromatic hydrocarbons were included. Some of the chemical toxic components identified from WTC dust, such as heavy metals (e.g., titanium), silica, asbestos fibers, and wood dust, have been linked to PF [2,32]. Taken together with early reports of PF among WTC exposed patients [10,11], the unique characteristics of WTC dust and its toxic components might explain our observed significant exposure—response effect of WTC dust exposure on PF among WTC responders.

Recently, a review of inflammatory response to inhalation of causative chemicals in WTC was suggested as a possible mechanism of a link between WTC dust and PF [32]. A dysregulated inflammatory response can gradually evolve into a pathogenic fibrotic response when inflammation becomes persistent [33]. Our findings of the association between WTC dust exposure and PF remain to be confirmed by an in-depth study using clinically confirmed cases over an extended follow-up period.

4.2. Comorbidity in PF

WTC responders with PF had significantly higher pulmonary and non-pulmonary comorbidities compared with those without PF, aligning with the high prevalence of co-existing physical or mental health conditions in idiopathic PF (IPF) patients in the literature. Raghu et al., in his review, found that prevalence of COPD in IPF patients ranged from 6 to 67%, of obstructive sleep apnea from 6 to 91%, of GERD from 0 to 94%, and of diabetes from 10 to 33% [26]. Depression and anxiety are also reported to be associated with dyspnea and other measures of fibrosis severity [34]; 50% of PF patients have depression and 30% have anxiety [34]. Consistent with the literature, PF in this study frequently co-existed with the physical or mental health conditions mentioned above. The comorbidities reported in responders with PF have also been reported to be significantly associated with WTC exposure among affected populations either in WTC rescue/recovery workers or local community members [7,30,35,36]. Although 9/11-exposed populations are at high risk for comorbidities [6,9,37], the much higher prevalence of comorbidities among PF cases than in those without PF further supports the association between WTC dust and PF observed in this study and warrants further study. Additionally, the significantly high comorbidity rate among PF patients may have an important clinical impact [26,38].

4.3. Possible Limitations with Self-Reported PF

Our findings should be interpreted with caution. The nonspecific self-reported physician-diagnosed PF is a fundamental limitation of this study. Lack of clinical information for case confirmation, such as high-resolution computed tomography (HRCT) findings, lung function and serologic tests, raises a concern with regard to the accuracy of PF ascertainment. To help mitigate the limitation, we defined PF by adding a concurrent symptom of shortness of breath. However, we do not have data on the severity of shortness of breath in the Registry cases, as this symptom is generally progressive in PF patients. We were also unable to identify types of PF due to lack of clinical information; there are over 200 types of PF [12]. Future study using clinical diagnosis of PF is needed to corroborate our findings.

In this study we observed similar socio-demographic differences that have been reported in the prevalence of PF, which provides some confidence in the use of self-reported PF. Females, non-Latino blacks and non-smokers tend to have a lower prevalence of PF than those who are male, of a non-African origin, and smokers [28,39]. Consistent with the literature, we observed that the PF incidence rate was lower among non-Latino blacks, and much higher among Latino compared to non-Latino whites [40]. However, the higher risk for PF among Asians in this study, compared to non-Latino whites, was not expected and not consistent with findings from other studies [41]. PF among Latino and Asians was significantly associated with WTC dust exposure, independent of smoking status and other demographics at baseline. Even though smoking is a known risk factor for PF and varied by race/ethnicity in this study, smoking did not explain our observed association between WTC dust exposure and PF. Further study is warranted to explain some inconsistent findings in racial differences in PF.

4.4. Other Potential Biases

Potential attrition bias due to non-response to W3 and W4 may have influenced the observed results. A previous Registry study by Yu found that compared to W3 participants, non-participants were younger, more likely to be male, non-white, and to have low household income [42]. The difference in demographics between participants and non-participants is a concern. However, the non-response to W3 was not associated with WTC exposures (e.g., injury as a result of the 9/11 attacks, witnessing of traumatic events and being caught in the dust cloud on 9/11 morning), or chronic diseases reported at enrollment (e.g., asthma, emphysema, diabetes and heart disease) [42]. Thus, attrition bias in our study may be minimal. In addition, knowing that early treatment is crucial to improve PF prognosis [43], participation in W3 or W4 might have been partly affected by the survival and severity of the PF condition, which we were not able to assess due to lack of information on PF treatment.

Some of the WTC responders enrolled in the Registry may also have enrolled in the WTC Health Program for medical monitoring and treatment. The availability of the WTC Health Program that provides health monitoring through periodic visits to responders and includes a chest radiograph [42,44] may have provided increased screening for lung disease to WTC responders compared to screening provided to those not exposed or the general public, and thus may lead to potential detection bias. However, such bias would not be expected to differ between those with a lower exposure level and those with a higher level of exposure, as all WTC responders meet the WTC Health Program criteria for monitoring.

The development of PF is considered to be multifactorial [45]; environmental or occupational exposure prior to, or outside of, 9/11 rescue recovery efforts may have contributed to disease development and progression. Lack of control for potential confounders among responders such as other occupational exposure, family history, history of viral infections [46] or genetic factors might bias the observed results. However, data on these potential confounders were not available.

5. Conclusions

Despite the limitations, this study found evidence of the association between WTC dust and PF risk among WTC responders, adding evidence to the literature of occupational exposure and self-reported PF. Specifically, PF may be another 9/11-related health condition among the exposed population. PF is an uncommon but serious condition that often co-exists with other health conditions that the 9/11-exposed population is at risk of developing. Awareness and early detection of PF among at-risk 9/11-exposed populations may slow the progress of the condition by early intervention. While on-going surveillance of PF is needed, in-depth research using medically-verified cases and pooled cases from multiple WTC Health Program cohorts (to increase sample size) would help to better understand the relationship between WTC dust exposure and PF.

Author Contributions: All authors made substantial contributions to the conception or design of the work; and interpretation of data for the work. J.L. conducted data analysis and drafted the manuscript with input from J.E.C., R.M.B., I.G., J.Y. and M.R.F. All authors edited and finalized the manuscript, and approved the final manuscript.

Funding: This publication was supported by Cooperative Agreement Numbers 2U50/OH009739 and 5U50/OH009739 from the National Institute for Occupational Safety and Health (NIOSH) of the Centers for Disease Control and Prevention (CDC); U50/ATU272750 from the Agency for Toxic Substances and Disease Registry (ATSDR), CDC, which included support from the National Center for Environmental Health, CDC, and by the New York City Department of Health and Mental Hygiene (NYC DCHMH). Its contents are solely the responsibility of the authors and do not necessarily represent the official views of NIOSH, CDC or the Department of Health and Human Services.

Acknowledgments: We thank Melanie Jacobson, from NYCDOHMH and Germania Pinheiro, from ATSDR, CDC for advice on study design; Charon Gwynn, James Hadler, and Sharon Perlman, MPH for thorough review of the manuscript.

Conflicts of Interest: The authors declare no conflict of interest.

References

1. Lioy, P.J.; Weisel, C.P.; Millette, J.R.; Eisenreich, S.; Vallero, D.; Offenberg, J.; Buckley, B.; Turpin, B.; Zhong, M.; Cohen, M.D.; et al. Characterization of the dust/smoke aerosol that settled east of the World Trade Center (WTC) in lower Manhattan after the collapse of the WTC 11 September 2001. *Environ. Health Perspect.* **2002**, *110*, 703–714. [CrossRef] [PubMed]

2. Kostrubiak, M. *World Trade Center Dust: Composition and Spatial-Temporal Considerations for Health*; Springer: Cham, Switzerland, 2018.

3. Woskie, S.R.; Kim, H.; Freund, A.; Stevenson, L.; Park, B.Y.; Baron, S.; Herbert, R.; de Hernandez, M.S.; Teitelbaum, S.; de la Hoz, R.E.; et al. World Trade Center disaster: Assessment of responder occupations, work locations, and job tasks. *Am. J. Ind. Med.* **2011**, *54*, 681–695. [CrossRef] [PubMed]

4. Prezant, D.J.; Levin, S.; Kelly, K.J.; Aldrich, T.K. Upper and lower respiratory diseases after occupational and environmental disasters. *Mt. Sinai J. Med.* **2008**, *75*, 89–100. [CrossRef] [PubMed]

5. Brackbill, R.M.; Hadler, J.L.; DiGrande, L.; Ekenga, C.C.; Farfel, M.R.; Friedman, S.; Perlman, S.E.; Stellman, S.D.; Walker, D.J.; Wu, D.; et al. Asthma and posttraumatic stress symptoms 5 to 6 years following exposure to the World Trade Center terrorist attack. *JAMA* **2009**, *302*, 502–516. [CrossRef] [PubMed]

6. Wisnivesky, J.P.; Teitelbaum, S.L.; Todd, A.C.; Boffetta, P.; Crane, M.; Crowley, L.; de la Hoz, R.E.; Dellenbaugh, C. Harrison, D.; Herbert, R.; et al. Persistence of multiple illnesses in World Trade Center rescue and recovery workers: A cohort study. *Lancet* **2011**, *378*, 888–897. [CrossRef]

7. Perlman, S.E.; Friedman, S.; Galea, S.; Nair, H.P.; Eros-Sarnyai, M.; Stellman, S.D.; Hon, J.; Greene, C.M. Short-term and medium-term health effects of 9/11. *Lancet* **2011**, *378*, 925–934. [CrossRef]

8. Yip, J.; Webber, M.P.; Zeig-Owens, R.; Vossbrinck, M.; Singh, A.; Kelly, K.; Prezant, D.J. FDNY and 9/11: Clinical services and health outcomes in World Trade Center-exposed firefighters and EMS workers from 2001 to 2016. *Am. J. Ind. Med.* **2016**, *59*, 695–708. [CrossRef] [PubMed]

9. Friedman, S.M.; Farfel, M.R.; Maslow, C.; Jordan, H.T.; Li, J.; Alper, H.; Cone, J.E.; Stellman, S.D.; Brackbill, R.M. Risk factors for and consequences of persistent lower respiratory symptoms among World Trade Center Health Registrants 10 years after the disaster. *Occup. Environ. Med.* **2016**, *73*, 676–684. [CrossRef] [PubMed]

10. Wu, M.; Gordon, R.E.; Herbert, R.; Padilla, M.; Moline, J.; Mendelson, D.; Litle, V.; Travis, W.D.; Gil, J. Case report: Lung disease in World Trade Center responders exposed to dust and smoke: Carbon nanotubes found in the lungs of World Trade Center patients and dust samples. *Environ. Health Perspect.* **2010**, *118*, 499–504. [CrossRef] [PubMed]

11. Caplan-Shaw, C.E.; Yee, H.; Rogers, L.; Abraham, J.L.; Parsia, S.S.; Naidich, D.P.; Borczuk, A.; Moreira, A.; Shiau, M.C.; Ko, J.P.; et al. Lung pathologic findings in a local residential and working community exposed to World Trade Center dust, gas, and fumes. *J. Occup. Environ. Med.* **2011**, *53*, 981–991. [CrossRef] [PubMed]

12. American Lung Association. Types, Causes and Risk Factors of Pulmonary Fibrosis. Available online: https://www.lung.org/lung-health-and-diseases/lung-disease-lookup/pulmonary-fibrosis/introduction/types-causes-and-risk-factors.html (accessed on 3 January 2019).

13. Baumgartner, K.B.; Samet, J.M.; Coultas, D.B.; Stidley, C.A.; Hunt, W.C.; Colby, T.V.; Waldron, J.A. Occupational and environmental risk factors for idiopathic pulmonary fibrosis: A multicenter case-control study. *Am. J. Epidemiol.* **2000**, *152*, 307–315. [CrossRef] [PubMed]

14. Hubbard, R. Occupational dust exposure and the aetiology of cryptogenic fibrosing alveolitis. *Eur. Respir. J. Suppl.* **2001**, *32*, 119s–121s. [PubMed]

15. Hubbard, R.; Cooper, M.; Antoniak, M.; Venn, A.; Khan, S.; Johnston, I.; Lewis, S.; Britton, J. Risk of cryptogenic fibrosing alveolitis in metal workers. *Lancet* **2000**, *355*, 466–467. [CrossRef]

16. Gustafson, T.; Dahlman-Hoglund, A.; Nilsson, K.; Strom, K.; Tornling, G.; Toren, K. Occupational exposure and severe pulmonary fibrosis. *Respir. Med.* **2007**, *101*, 2207–2212. [CrossRef] [PubMed]

17. Pinheiro, G.A.; Antao, V.C.; Wood, J.M.; Wassell, J.T. Occupational risks for idiopathic pulmonary fibrosis mortality in the United States. *Int. J. Occup. Environ. Health* **2008**, *14*, 117–123. [CrossRef] [PubMed]

18. Sack, C.; Vedal, S.; Sheppard, L.; Raghu, G.; Barr, R.G.; Podolanczuk, A.; Doney, B.; Hoffman, E.A.; Gassett, A.; Hinckley-Stukovsky, K.; et al. Air pollution and subclinical interstitial lung disease: The Multi-Ethnic Study of Atherosclerosis (MESA) air-lung study. *Eur. Respir. J.* **2017**, *50*, 1700559. [CrossRef] [PubMed]

19. Sack, C.S.; Doney, B.C.; Podolanczuk, A.J.; Hooper, L.G.; Seixas, N.S.; Hoffman, E.A.; Kawut, S.M.; Vedal, S.; Raghu, G.; Barr, R.G.; et al. Occupational Exposures and Subclinical Interstitial Lung Disease. The MESA (Multi-Ethnic Study of Atherosclerosis) Air and Lung Studies. *Am. J. Respir. Crit. Care Med.* **2017**, *196*, 1031–1039. [CrossRef] [PubMed]

20. Farfel, M.; DiGrande, L.; Brackbill, R.; Prann, A.; Cone, J.; Friedman, S.; Walker, D.J.; Pezeshki, G.; Thomas, P.; Galea, S.; et al. An overview of 9/11 experiences and respiratory and mental health conditions among World Trade Center Health Registry enrollees. *J. Urban Health* **2008**, *85*, 880–909. [CrossRef] [PubMed]

21. Jordan, H.T.; Stellman, S.D.; Prezant, D.; Teirstein, A.; Osahan, S.S.; Cone, J.E. Sarcoidosis diagnosed after 11 September 2001, among adults exposed to the World Trade Center disaster. *J. Occup. Environ. Med.* **2011**, *53*, 966–974. [CrossRef] [PubMed]

22. Patterson, K.C.; Strek, M.E. Pulmonary fibrosis in sarcoidosis. Clinical features and outcomes. *Ann. Am. Thorac. Soc.* **2013**, *10*, 362–370. [CrossRef] [PubMed]

23. Webber, M.P.; Yip, J.; Zeig-Owens, R.; Moir, W.; Ungprasert, P.; Crowson, C.S.; Hall, C.B.; Jaber, N.; Weiden, M.D.; Matteson, E.L.; et al. Post-9/11 sarcoidosis in WTC-exposed firefighters and emergency medical service workers. *Respir. Med.* **2017**, *132*, 232–237. [CrossRef] [PubMed]

24. Hena, K.M.; Yip, J.; Jaber, N.; Goldfarb, D.; Fullam, K.; Cleven, K.; Moir, W.; Zeig-Owens, R.; Webber, M.P.; Spevack, D.M.; et al. Clinical Course of Sarcoidosis in World Trade Center-Exposed Firefighters. *Chest* **2018**, *153*, 114–123. [CrossRef] [PubMed]

25. Li, J.; Brackbill, R.M.; Liao, T.S.; Qiao, B.; Cone, J.E.; Farfel, M.R.; Hadler, J.L.; Kahn, A.R.; Konty, K.J.; Stayner, L.T.; et al. Ten-year cancer incidence in rescue/recovery workers and civilians exposed to the 11 September 2001 terrorist attacks on the World Trade Center. *Am. J. Ind. Med.* **2016**, *59*, 709–721. [CrossRef] [PubMed]

26. Raghu, G.; Amatto, V.C.; Behr, J.; Stowasser, S. Comorbidities in idiopathic pulmonary fibrosis patients: A systematic literature review. *Eur. Respir. J.* **2015**, *46*, 1113–1130. [CrossRef] [PubMed]

27. Kleinbaum, D.G. *Survival Analysis: A Self-Learning Text*, 3rd ed.; Springer: New York, NY, USA, 2012.

28. Nalysnyk, L.; Cid-Ruzafa, J.; Rotella, P.; Esser, D. Incidence and prevalence of idiopathic pulmonary fibrosis: Review of the literature. *Eur. Respir. Rev.* **2012**, *21*, 355–361. [CrossRef] [PubMed]

29. Lioy, P.J.; Georgopoulos, P. The anatomy of the exposures that occurred around the World Trade Center site: 9/11 and beyond. *Ann. N. Y. Acad. Sci.* **2006**, *1076*, 54–79. [CrossRef] [PubMed]

30. Lippmann, M.; Cohen, M.D.; Chen, L.C. Health effects of World Trade Center (WTC) Dust: An unprecedented disaster's inadequate risk management. *Crit. Rev. Toxicol.* **2015**, *45*, 492–530. [CrossRef] [PubMed]
31. Connick, K.D.; Enright, P.L.; Middendorf, P.J.; Piacentino, J.; Reissman, D.B.; Sawyer, T.; Souza, K. *First Periodic Review of Scientific and Medical Evidence Related to Cancer for the World Trade Center Health Program*; National Institute for Occupational Safety and Health: Columbia, DC, USA, 2011.
32. Szeinuk, J. *Interstitial Pulmonary Disease after Exposure at the World Trade Center Disaster Site*; Springer: Cham, Switzerland, 2018.
33. Wilson, M.S.; Wynn, T.A. Pulmonary fibrosis: Pathogenesis, etiology and regulation. *Mucosal Immunol.* **2009**, *2*, 103–121. [CrossRef] [PubMed]
34. Fulton, B.G.; Ryerson, C.J. Managing comorbidities in idiopathic pulmonary fibrosis. *Int. J. Gen. Med.* **2015**, *8*, 309–318. [PubMed]
35. Jordan, H.T.; Stellman, S.D.; Reibman, J.; Farfel, M.R.; Brackbill, R.M.; Friedman, S.M.; Li, J.; Cone, J.E. Factors associated with poor control of 9/11-related asthma 10–11 years after the 2001 World Trade Center terrorist attacks. *J. Asthma* **2015**, *52*, 630–637. [CrossRef] [PubMed]
36. Liu, X.; Yip, J.; Zeig-Owens, R.; Weakley, J.; Webber, M.P.; Schwartz, T.M.; Prezant, D.J.; Weiden, M.D.; Hall, C.B. The Effect of World Trade Center Exposure on the Timing of Diagnoses of Obstructive Airway Disease, Chronic Rhinosinusitis, and Gastroesophageal Reflux Disease. *Front. Public Health* **2017**, *5*, 2. [CrossRef] [PubMed]
37. Li, J.; Zweig, K.C.; Brackbill, R.M.; Farfel, M.R.; Cone, J.E. Comorbidity amplifies the effects of post-9/11 posttraumatic stress disorder trajectories on health-related quality of life. *Qual. Life Res.* **2018**, *27*, 651–660. [CrossRef] [PubMed]
38. Ley, B.; Collard, H.R.; King, T.E., Jr. Clinical course and prediction of survival in idiopathic pulmonary fibrosis. *Am. J. Respir. Crit. Care Med.* **2011**, *183*, 431–440. [CrossRef] [PubMed]
39. Oh, C.K.; Murray, L.A.; Molfino, N.A. Smoking and idiopathic pulmonary fibrosis. *Pulm. Med.* **2012**, *2012*, 1–13. [CrossRef] [PubMed]
40. Swigris, J.J.; Olson, A.L.; Huie, T.J.; Fernandez-Perez, E.R.; Solomon, J.; Sprunger, D.; Brown, K.K. Ethnic and racial differences in the presence of idiopathic pulmonary fibrosis at death. *Respir. Med.* **2012**, *106*, 588–593. [CrossRef] [PubMed]
41. Hutchinson, J.; Fogarty, A.; Hubbard, R.; McKeever, T. Global incidence and mortality of idiopathic pulmonary fibrosis: A systematic review. *Eur. Respir. J.* **2015**, *46*, 795–806. [CrossRef] [PubMed]
42. Yu, S.; Brackbill, R.M.; Stellman, S.D.; Ghuman, S.; Farfel, M.R. Evaluation of non-response bias in a cohort study of World Trade Center terrorist attack survivors. *BMC Res. Notes* **2015**, *8*, 42. [CrossRef] [PubMed]
43. Molina-Molina, M.; Aburto, M.; Acosta, O.; Ancochea, J.; Rodriguez-Portal, J.A.; Sauleda, J.; Lines, C.; Xaubet, A. Importance of early diagnosis and treatment in idiopathic pulmonary fibrosis. *Expert Rev. Respir. Med.* **2018**, *12*, 537–539. [CrossRef] [PubMed]
44. Herbert, R.; Moline, J.; Skloot, G.; Metzger, K.; Baron, S.; Luft, B.; Markowitz, S.; Udasin, I.; Harrison, D.; Stein, D.; et al. The World Trade Center disaster and the health of workers: Five-year assessment of a unique medical screening program. *Environ. Health Perspect.* **2006**, *114*, 1853–1858. [CrossRef] [PubMed]
45. Richeldi, L.; Collard, H.R.; Jones, M.G. Idiopathic pulmonary fibrosis. *Lancet* **2017**, *389*, 1941–1952. [CrossRef]
46. Moore, B.B.; Moore, T.A. Viruses in Idiopathic Pulmonary Fibrosis. Etiology and Exacerbation. *Ann. Am. Thorac. Soc.* **2015**, *12* (Suppl. 2), S186–S192. [PubMed]

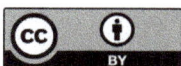

International Journal of
Environmental Research and Public Health

MDPI

Article

An Assessment of Long-Term Physical and Emotional Quality of Life of Persons Injured on 9/11/2001

Robert M. Brackbill [1,*], Howard E. Alper [1], Patricia Frazier [2], Lisa M. Gargano [1], Melanie H. Jacobson [1] and Adrienne Solomon [1]

[1] World Trade Center Registry, New York Department of Health and Mental Hygiene, New York, NY 10013, USA; halper@health.nyc.gov (H.E.A.); lgargano1@health.nyc.gcv (L.M.G.); mjacobson@health.nyc.gov (M.H.J.); asolomon1@health.nyc.gov (A.S.)
[2] Department of Psychology, University of Minnesota, Minneapolis, MN 55455, USA; Pfraz@umn.edu
*   Correspondence: rbrackbi@health.nyc.gov, Tel.: +1-646-632-6609; Fax: +1-646-632-6175

Received: 15 February 2019; Accepted: 21 March 2019; Published: 23 March 2019

Abstract: Fifteen years after the disaster, the World Trade Center Health Registry (Registry) conducted The Health and Quality of Life Survey (HQoL) assessing physical and mental health status among those who reported sustaining an injury on 11 September 2001 compared with non-injured persons. Summary scores derived from the Short Form-12 served as study outcomes. United States (US) population estimates on the Physical Component Score (PCS-12) and Mental Component Score (MCS-12) were compared with scores from the HQoL and were stratified by Post-traumatic Stress Disorder (PTSD) and injury status. Linear regression models were used to estimate the association between both injury severity and PTSD and PCS-12 and MCS-12 scores. Level of injury severity and PTSD history significantly predicted poorer physical health (mean PCS-12). There was no significant difference between injury severity level and mental health (mean MCS-12). Controlling for other factors, having PTSD symptoms after 9/11 predicted a nearly 10-point difference in mean MCS-12 compared with never having PTSD. Injury severity and PTSD showed additive effects on physical and mental health status. Injury on 9/11 and a PTSD history were each associated with long-term decrements in physical health status. Injury did not predict long-term decrements in one's mental health status. Although it is unknown whether physical wounds of the injury healed, our results suggest that traumatic injuries appear to have a lasting negative effect on perceived physical functioning.

Keywords: injury; physical health; mental health; World Trade Center disaster; Short Form-12 (SF-12); HQoL; 9/11

1. Introduction

The World Trade Center (WTC) disaster on 11 September 2001 exposed thousands of persons to both environmental pollutants and psychological trauma, which have had long-term physical and psychological ramifications. Having been injured on 9/11 has emerged as a common risk factor for both physical and mental health conditions [1–3]. For example, one study found that, among those injured on the day of the 9/11 disaster, the likelihood of having been diagnosed with a physical health condition, including respiratory disease problems (i.e., asthma, chronic bronchitis, emphysema) and/or circulatory disease (i.e., heart attack, angina, stroke) increased with the number of types of injuries they sustained (e.g., burn, head injury, and musculoskeletal) [4]. Injury on 9/11 also increased the likelihood of posttraumatic stress disorder (PTSD) 2-fold to 3-fold, which was measured by a post-traumatic stress checklist (PCL) screening instrument after adjusting for demographic factors and other WTC-related exposures [2,3]. In addition, physical injury has been reported as a risk factor for psychological sequelae among persons directly affected by other disasters, such as Hurricane Ike [5] and the 2004 Southeast Asia tsunami [6].

In general, among those who experience serious injuries, psychological distress related to anxiety, depression, or post-traumatic stress disorder (PTSD) can persist for years after the injury [6]. For instance, in a meta-analysis of the long-term impacts of injuries incurred in motor vehicle crashes, ranging from serious spinal cord injuries to less life-threatening musculoskeletal injuries, showed that the injuries had large impacts on psychological distress that, in some cases, increased in magnitude over time [7].

Serious injuries can also result in increased vulnerability to physical health conditions in the absence of psychological pathology [8]. This suggests that an injury, in addition to its immediate physical damage, can have long-term effects on physical health without an intervening psychological factor.

Given that mortality from injury has declined substantially because of treatment advances, the primary focus for non-fatal injuries currently is the impact of injuries on functionality and quality of life. For instance, Danish patients injured between 1995 and 2005 were more likely than a non-injured group of people to experience poor/very poor health [9]. In the Netherlands, from 1999 to 2000, limitations in mobility, self-care, and the ability to conduct daily activities were self-reported by severely injured adult patients followed up between 12 and 18 months post-injury [10]. Long-term declines in overall physical and mental health status following trauma were found in studies in Oslo, Australia, and the United States (US) using standard instruments (e.g., Short Form 36, Brief Pain Inventory, and Short Form 12) [11–13]). In the Danish study, Toft observed the effects on overall health up to 10 years after the injury [9] and for at least 2 years for both physical and mental health when compared with national norms [12,14]. In most cases, a greater relative decline in physical health compared with mental health was observed. However, researchers typically do not include in their assessment the relationship between PTSD and functional health status, especially physical health, nor do they employ a non-injury comparison group.

A prior qualitative inquiry of persons who sustained an injury on 9/11 found injured persons reported that their injuries were debilitating and limited daily activities, especially musculoskeletal injuries that required multiple surgeries with physical therapy [15]. In addition, quality of life and social integration problems emerged among participants in the study regardless of whether they had a history of PTSD [15].

This study examines the long-term effects of injury sustained on 9/11, including functional effects and a comparison group without injury. Based on the findings from the qualitative study, we hypothesized that the severity of the 9/11 injury would predict deficits in health status for both physical and mental health domains. We also hypothesized that PTSD history would be sufficient —but not a necessary factor—in observed long-term detriments in physical and mental health, as measured by the Short Form-12 (SF-12). In addition, it was hypothesized that the presence of other factors, such as social support and self-efficacy, would ameliorate the impact of injury and PTSD on physical and mental health status.

2. Materials and Methods

The World Trade Center Health Registry (Registry) is a prospective cohort that monitors the physical and mental health of 71,426 persons exposed to the attacks on 11 September 2001. The populations at risk included rescue/recovery workers who were involved in rescue, recovery, and disaster clean-up from 11 September 2001 to 30 June 2002. This includes residents who lived south of Canal Street in lower Manhattan on 9/11, persons who worked and were present south of Canal Street on 9/11, passersby and others who were occupants of destroyed or damaged buildings on 9/11, and students who were registered at, or staff employed by, schools located south of Canal Street. The Registry enrolled 17% of an estimated 409,492 persons in the populations-at-risk identified by the Registry [16], which varied from 34% of rescue/recovery workers to 11% of passersby. Since the enrollment survey in 2003–2004 (Wave 1), the Registry has conducted three health surveys: Wave 2 in

2006–2007, Wave 3 in 2011–2012, and Wave 4 in 2015–2016 (See references 2 and 17 for more detail on methods and participation) [2,17,18]. The Registry was approved by the New York City Institutional Review Board and Federal Centers for Disease Control and Prevention (15005).

2.1. Study Sample

From 10 March 2017 to 30 June 2017, the Registry conducted the Health and Quality of Life Survey (HQoL). Eligibility for this survey included completing all four Registry survey waves, being at least 18 years of age, and speaking English. Two groups were invited by email or mail to participate in the survey. The first group (n = 2699) included persons who reported on Wave 1 that they sustained one or more of the following injuries on 9/11: cut, abrasion, or puncture wound; sprain or strain; burn; broken bone or dislocation; and concussion or head injury. Those who reported "other injury" or "eye injury" only were not included. The second group (n = 2598) consisted of a non-injured comparison group of randomly selected persons who did not report any type of injury, including "other injury" or "eye injury." The overall participation rate was 76%, with a final sample of n = 2038 for the injury group and n = 1995 for the comparison group. For the purposes of the current study, we further restricted the sample to persons who were south of Chambers Street on 9/11/2001 (n = 2583 excluded) and who inconsistently reported that they were injured or not injured on 9/11 in both the Wave 1 survey and the HQoL (n = 1185 excluded). This resulted in n = 948 for the injured group and 1818 for the non-injured comparison of SF-12 outcomes [19].

2.2. SF-12 Outcomes

The HQoL survey included a series of questions referred to as the Short Form Health Survey-12, Version 1 (SF-12) [20]. The SF-12 was derived from the SF-36 to provide an efficient method for assessing overall physical and mental health functioning through a mean physical health Component summary score (PCS-12) and a mean mental health component summary score (MCS-12). The summary scores are based on combinations of SF-36 questions that were identified as representing overall physical and mental status and that were highly correlated with the SF-36 overall physical and mental health summary scores. The SF-12 consists of physical health domains of *general health* (one question), *pain interferes with functioning* (one question), *role physical* (two questions, less able to perform routine tasks), and *overall physical functioning* (two questions). Mental health domains include *vitality* (one question), *social functioning* (one question), *mental health* (two questions), and *role emotional* (two questions) (less able to engage emotionally). Both of the SF-12 summary scores are highly correlated with SF-36 (r = 0.95) and have acceptable test-retest reliabilities (PCS-12 r = 0.89 and MCS-12, r = 0.76) [21].

2.3. Level of Injury Severity

An estimate of the level of injury severity was defined using follow-up questions on the HQoL questionnaire, which asks about the most serious injury sustained on 11 September 2001. Four categories were derived for this analysis, which are no injury, low severity, medium severity, and high severity. Low severity represents persons with superficial injuries not requiring medical intervention or care based on no reported need for medical care, use of support (e.g., crutch), or physical therapy. Medium severity applies to persons with injuries that required supportive and rehabilitative care, such as staying in bed for at least a day, requiring a crutch, or participating in physical therapy, but did not require using a wheelchair, going to a hospital, or surgery. High severity indicates that the injury required a hospital emergency department visit, surgery, or a wheelchair during recovery from the injury. The 'no injury' group included persons who reported no type of injury sustained on 9/11 on both the Registry Wave 1 and HQoL.

2.4. History of PTSD

We included the presence or absence of probable PTSD based on PCL scores of 44 or greater on any prior Registry survey waves (2003–2004, 2006–2007, 2010–2011, or 2015–2016). Probable PTSD was assessed in all Registry survey waves using a 17-item 9/11-specific PCL [22]. The 17 items correspond to the Diagnostic and Statistical Manual of Mental Disorders (DSM-IV) PTSD symptoms [23]. Each stressor-specific item, such as "feeling very upset when something reminded you of the events of 9/11," was scored on a 5-point scale for experience of the symptom during the past 30 days (1 = not at all to 5 = extremely). The PCL score has been shown to have good temporal stability, internal consistency (>0.75), test-retest reliability (0.66), and high convergent validity [24], with overall diagnostic efficiency = 0.90, sensitivity = 0.94, and specificity = 0.86 [25].

2.5. Other Covariates

Sociodemographic characteristics of the study sample such as gender, age at time of HQoL survey, race/ethnicity group, education level, eligibility group (rescue/recovery worker, resident, area worker, passerby), and marital status were included in the analytical models. Other covariates that have a potential association with physical and mental health functioning including smoking history (W4), social support, and self-efficacy were also controlled for in the analysis.

Because low levels of social support are associated with an increased burden of chronic PTSD [26], we included a measure of social support as a covariate. The presence of social support and/or self-efficacy described below also has a likely role in faster recovery from injury [27]. The instrument we used for measuring social support was the Medical Outcomes Study (MOS) Modified Social Support Survey [28,29]. Respondents were asked a series of questions about their support system, such as: "Is someone available to take you to the doctor if you need to go?", "to have a good time with?", "to hug you?", "to prepare your meals if you are unable to do it yourself?", and "to understand your problems?" Items were rated on "0" (none of the time) to "4" (all of the time) by the respondent. Out of a possible sum of 20 for the five questions, persons with scores <17 (median score for the entire sample) were assigned to a low social support category.

Self-efficacy, which is correlated with emotional health and optimism, was measured using five questions from the 10-item General Self-Efficacy Scale (GSE) [30]. The items were: "It is easy for me to stick to my aims and accomplish my goals", "I am confident that I could deal efficiently with unexpected events", "Thanks to my resourcefulness, I know how to handle unforeseen situations", "I can remain calm when facing difficulties because I can rely on my coping abilities", and "No matter what comes my way, I am usually able to handle it" [31]. The respondent rated each question using the following scale: 1 = not true at all, 2 = hardly true, 3 = moderately true, and 4 = exactly true. Scores ranged from 4 to 20 with a score equal to or greater than the median self-efficacy summary score of 17, which was used as the criterion for possessing self-efficacy. A variable representing diagnosed chronic conditions including asthma, heart disease, gastroesophageal reflux syndrome (GERS), and other non-neoplastic lung conditions was examined in relation to the outcomes in bivariate analyses. The variable was not controlled for in analytical models because these could have been on the causal pathway between injury and physical or mental health functioning [32].

2.6. Statistical Analysis

The primary outcomes of this analysis were physical and mental health summary component scores (PCS-12 and MCS-12). First, age-standardized mean PCS-12 and MCS-12 scores by gender and injury and PTSD status were compared with national data obtained from a study of a normative, non-institutionalized US sample [33]. The HQoL scores of those without injury or PTSD were age standardized to the age distribution (by 10-year age groups) provided by Hanmer et al., 2006 [33]. Internal comparisons were then done using persons with no injury and no PTSD as a comparison to persons with injury and no PTSD, persons with no injury and ever PTSD, and persons with injury and ever PTSD. Paired t-tests of PCS-12 and MCS-12 means at $p < 0.05$ level of significance were used to identify differences in these comparisons.

In addition, mean MCS-12 and PCS-12 scores and standard deviations were calculated for descriptive results stratified by injury severity levels and PTSD status as well as other covariates included in this study. Analysis of variance was used to determine if the means for each variable were significantly different in the bivariate analysis.

Multivariable analysis consisted of linear regression models of PCS-12 and MCS-12 scores with an injury severity level and PTSD ever and never included as primary predictors, controlling for age at the time of HQoL survey, gender, race/ethnicity, education, smoking status, eligibility group, marital status, social support, and self-efficacy. Negative or positive betas represented the amount of change in the PCS-12 or MCS-12 score relative to the referent for the factor of interest.

Additional analysis was done to assess the interaction between injury severity and PTSD in their association with PCS-12 and MCS-12 means. A cross-product interaction term for injury severity and PTSD status was included in linear regression models for PCS-12 and MCS-12. In addition, a composite variable (variable representing the cross-product term in the regression model) was also created that combined the four levels of injury severity and PTSD (ever/never) with no injury and never PTSD as the reference for the following groups: no injury and ever PTSD, low severity injury and ever PTSD, medium severity injury and ever PTSD, high severity injury and ever PTSD in order to represent the combined effects of level of injury severity and PTSD.

3. Results

The mean Physical Component Score (PCS-12) for the entire HQoL sample was 43.3. The Mental Component Score (MCS-12) was 46.6. However, when the means were restricted to the 'no injury and never PTSD' group, they provided an approximate comparison to population-level measures of PCS-12 and MCS-12 (such as those provided by Hanmer, 2006 [33]), which were based on a US nationally representative sample (Table 1).

Table 1. Mean PCS-12 and MCS-12 for the US population and mean PCS-12 and MCS-12 for selected HQoL groups by gender.

Source	Male			Female		
	N	PCS-12	MCS-12	*N*	PCS-12	MCS-12
Non-institutionalized US adults *	7463	48.9	52.0	8819	47.0	50.4
HQoL: No injury and never PTSD **	768	45.5	50.7	589	44.1	49.4
HQoL: No injury and never PTSD ***	768	44.4	52.4	589	43.6	49.7
HQoL: Injury and never PTSD	200	39.8	52.5	95	41.4	48.8
HQoL: No injury and ever PTSD	156	40.8	39.7	198	40.9	39.0
HQoL: Injury and ever PTSD	343	34.8	38.5	263	35.4	36.9

* [33] ** Age standardized based on age distribution from Hanmer, 2006. *** Underlined are Non-age standardized for a comparison.

Specifically, men in the HQoL 'no injury and never PTSD' group had an age standardized mean PCS-12 of 45.5 compared with 48.9 from Hanmer. For this same group, the age standardized mean MCS-12 for men from the HQoL study was 50.7 compared to 52.0 in the Hanmer sample [33]. Women had mean scores that were less than three points different between HQoL and Hanmer for both PCS-12 and MCS-12. The mean PCS-12 for 'no injury and never PTSD' for women was 44.1 compared with 47.0 for Hanmer and 49.4 for mean MCS-12 compared with 50.4 based on Hanmer estimates [33].

Within our sample, injury of any severity level without PTSD diminished physical health by five points for men (PCS-12 mean: 39.8 vs. 44.6, t = 6.6, $p < 0.0001$ for injury and never PTSD vs. for no injury and never PTSD, respectively) and two points for women (PCS-12 mean: 41.9 vs. 43.6, t = 2.2, $p < 0.029$ for injury and never PTSD vs. for no injury and never PTSD, respectively) (Table 1). However, injury without PTSD did not produce a significant difference for either men or women for mean MCS-12 compared with no injury and never PTSD. Among men and women without injuries, those with PTSD had lower mental and physical health scores than those without PTSD (for men: PCS-12: 40.8 vs. 44.4, t = 4.8, $p < 0.0001$, MCS-12: 39.7 vs. 52.4, t = 4.4, $p < 0.0001$, for women: PCS-12: 40.9 vs. 43.6, t = 3.7, $p < 0.0001$, MCS-12: 39.0 vs. 49.7, t = 11.9, $p < 0.0001$). The injury and ever PTSD group PCS-12 and MCS-12 mean scores for men and women had lower values than the other groups.

Overall, 380 (13.7%) of study enrollees had high severity injuries on 9/11/2001 and 960 (36.8%) reported symptoms indicative of ever having PTSD (Table 2). Both PCS-12 and MCS-12 mean scores were lower for persons with more severe injuries (F = 105.6, $p < 0.0001$ for PCS-12: F = 53.9, $p < 0.0001$ for MCS-12) and a history of PTSD (F = 271.9, $p < 0.0001$ for PCS-12: F = 27.7, $p < 0.0001$ for MCS-12). Persons with high injury severity had the lowest PCS-12 mean score (37.0) compared with those with no injury (46.6) and those with ever PTSD had a lower MCS-12 mean score (38.4) compared with those with never PTSD (51.2).

Table 2. Mean SF-12 Physical Health Component Scores (PCS-12) and mean Mental Health Component Scores (MCS-12) by injury severity, PTSD history, and other covariates.

Characteristic	Total		Physical Functioning Total		Mental Functioning Total	
	N	%	Mean	SD	Mean	SD
Total Sample	2766	100	41.3	9.2	46.9	12.1
Injury Severity *						
None	1818	65.7	43.6	8.2	48.8	11.2
Low	120	4.3	40.9	10.2	45.6	13.1
Medium	448	16.2	37.0	9.1	42.5	12.7
High	380	13.7	37.0	8.7	42.1	12.8
PTSD **						
Ever	960	36.8	37.8	8.8	38.6	11.5
Never	1652	63.2	43.7	8.4	51.2	9.9
Gender						
Male	1547	55.9	41.6	9.2	47.9	12.0
Female	1219	44.1	41.7	8.7	45.5	12.1
Age at Injury Survey (Years)						
30–44	313	11.3	45.7	6.8	45.6	11.9
45–54	708	25.6	43.0	9.0	45.6	11.9
55–64	935	33.8	40.8	9.2	46.5	12.2
65–99	810	29.3	39.6	8.7	49.1	11.8
Race/Ethnicity						
White	2056	74.3	42.1	9.0	47.4	12.1
Black	261	9.4	40.9	8.9	45.6	12.5
Hispanic	264	9.5	39.5	8.9	43.6	11.6
Asian	109	3.9	41.0	8.7	48.1	12.4
Other	76	2.8	40.3	9.1	46.5	11.4
Education at Wave 1						
High School or Less	407	14.7	38.5	8.6	45.1	13.1
Some College	566	20.5	39.4	9.1	45.5	12.6
College and Post-Grad	1787	64.7	42.9	8.7	47.7	11.7
Eligibility Group						
Rescue/Recovery	626	22.6	38.7	9.6	47.4	12.3
Resident	317	11.5	42.6	8.1	46.5	12.2
Area Worker	1591	57.5	42.6	8.7	47.1	11.9
Passerby	232	8.4	41.6	9.1	44.6	12.5

Table 2. *Cont.*

Characteristic	Total		Physical Functioning Total		Mental Functioning Total	
	N	%	Mean	SD	Mean	SD
Marital Status at Wave 4						
Married/Cohabitating	1873	68.4	42.0	9.0	47.8	11.8
Divorced/Separated/Widowed/Never Married	867	31.6	40.9	8.9	44.7	12.6
Social Support at Wave 4						
Low	1191	44.1	40.4	9.2	42.2	12.5
High	1512	55.9	42.6	8.7	50.4	10.5
Self-Efficacy at Wave 4						
Yes	1189	43.5	43.3	8.7	52.4	9.8
No	1544	56.5	40.4	9.0	42.5	12.0
Smoking—Wave 4						
Current	159	5.8	40.1	9.0	43.4	11.5
Former	853	31.3	41.3	9.0	46.8	12.4
Never	1713	62.9	42.0	9.0	47.3	12.0
Any Chronic Disease—Wave 4 ***						
Yes	211	8.6	37.8	9.0	44.2	13.3
No	2241	91.4	42.0	8.9	47.1	12.0

* Severity was missing on 55 individuals due to missing data on medical intervention after injury. ** PTSD checklist score ≥44 on any prior WTCHR survey, *** Diagnosed chronic conditions included asthma, heart disease, GERS, and non-neoplastic lung conditions.

With regard to demographic characteristics, the mean PCS-12 and MCS-12 scores for females were slightly lower than for males (Table 2), which indicates slightly worse physical and mental health status for females when compared with men. In addition, PCS-12 mean scores decreased with age (i.e., physical health status worsened with increasing age), while MCS-12 mean scores increased with age (i.e., mental health status was relatively better with increasing age). Hispanic individuals had the lowest mean PCS-12 score (39.5) compared with other race/ethnicity groups. Persons with less than a high school education also exhibited the lowest mean score for PCS-12 (38.5) when compared with those with a college degree or higher. The same patterns were seen with the mean MCS-12 scores with the exception of age for which individuals younger than 45 years of age had the lowest mean MCS-12 score (45.6). Among Registry eligibility groups, rescue/recovery workers had a lower PCS-12 mean score (38.7) relative to other registry groups, but there was no significant difference between the eligibility groups for MCS-12 mean scores (F = 1.98, p = 0.115). In addition, persons with low social support and low self-efficacy had lower PCS-12 and MCS-12 mean scores when compared with those with high social support and self-efficacy.

The estimated betas (β) represent the results of linear regression as either increases or decreases of PCS-12 and MCS-12 mean scores relative to a reference category for each characteristic after controlling for other factors (Figures 1 and 2). PCS-12 mean scores were significantly lower for persons with medium or high severity injuries than for those with no injury (medium severity β = −4.4, 95% confidence interval (CI), −5.4 to −3.3, high severity β = −4.1 95% CI, −5.2 to −3.0). In contrast, there was no significant relationship between MCS-12 mean score and injury severity on 9/11 in multivariable models, which was similar to results from the bivariate analysis.

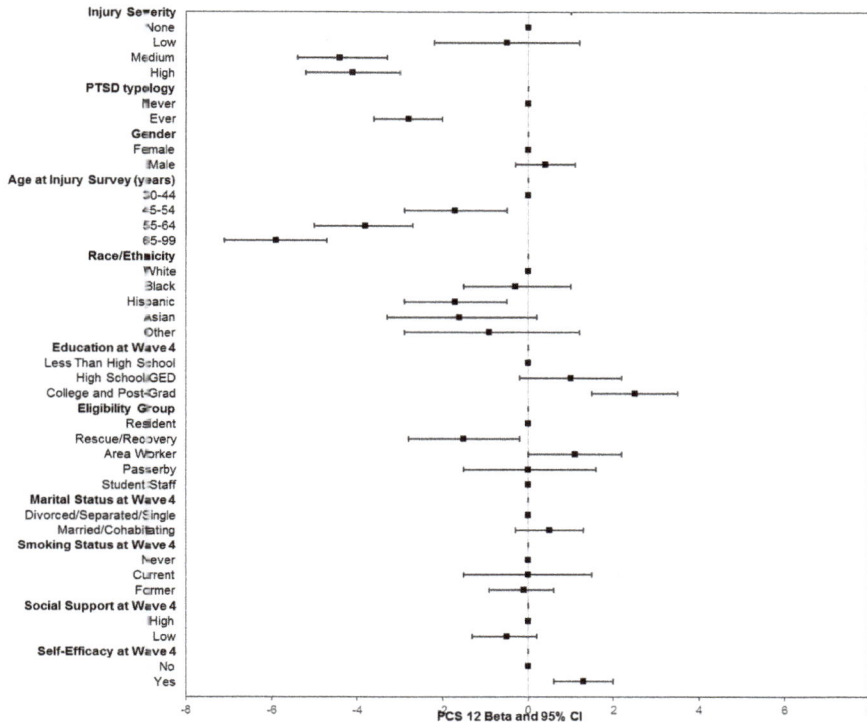

Figure 1. Linear regression of PCS-12 (physical health functioning) as a function of injury severity, PTSD history, demographic, and other factors. The betas are the predicted changes in mean scores relative to the reference category. Controlled for all variables included in figure. PTSD check list score ≥44 on any prior WTCHR survey.

Persons who had a history of probable PTSD had significantly lower summary scores for both PCS-12 and MCS-12 when compared with those with no history of PTSD. However, the beta coefficients for PTSD predicting mental health functioning were three times greater than those for predicting physical health functioning (β = −9.7, 95% confidence interval (CI) −10.6 to −8.7 for MCS-12 and PTSD, β = −2.8, 95%, CI −3.6 to −2.0 for PCS and PTSD).

Linear regression estimates of PCS-12 or MCS-12 differences for other factors in Figures 1 and 2 mirrored the results of bivariate comparisons for covariates represented in Table 2. For instance, persons with more than a high school education had significantly higher PCS-12 mean scores than those with less than a high school education, but there was no statistically significant relationship between education and mental health functioning. With regard to eligibility groups, rescue/recovery workers had significantly lower PCS-12 mean scores relative to residents, area workers, and passerby groups, but they had a significantly higher MCS-12 mean score (*p* < 0.001). Other notable findings for covariates included social support at Wave 4 that was predictive of mental functioning but not physical functioning, and self-efficacy significantly predicted both physical and mental health functioning. In addition, smoking history was not associated with PCS-12, but being a former smoker was a statistically significant predictor of lower MCS-12 mean scores (*p* < 0.001). Being diagnosed with a chronic disease prior to the assessment of physical and mental health functioning was not included in the model because it has been shown to be in the pathway for health, as measured by SF-12 [34]. In a sensitivity analysis, the inclusion of this measure in the model did not substantively alter the results.

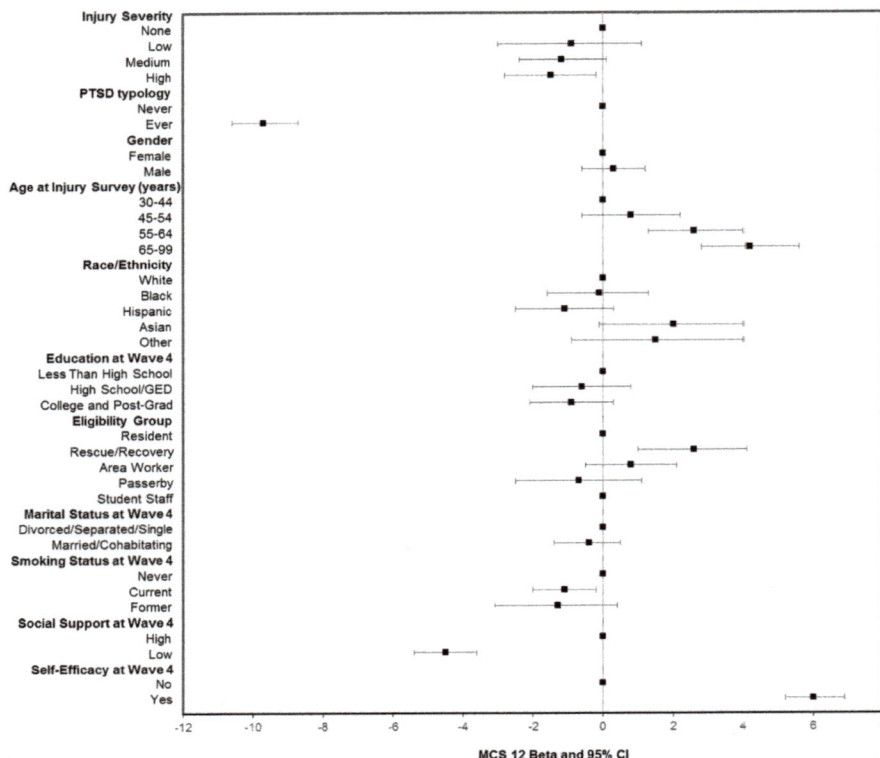

Figure 2. Linear regression of MCS-12 (mental health functioning) as a function of injury severity, PTSD history, demographic, and other factors. The betas are the predicted changes in mean scores relative to the reference category. Controlled for all variables included in the figure. PTSD checklist score ≥44 on any prior WTCHR survey.

The interaction between the injury severity level and probable PTSD on physical and mental health functioning was evaluated in a separate linear regression model in which the results are depicted in Figure 3 (PCS-12) and Figure 4 (MCS-12). Overall, although the interaction was not statistically significant, the combination of greater injury severity level and having a history of PTSD were associated with declines in the physical health status. However, injury severity had minimal influence on the association between PTSD history and mental health status. Specifically, people who had both a history of probable PTSD and medium or high severity injury had a substantially lower overall physical health status when compared with those with no injury and no PTSD (Figure 3). With regard to one's mental health status, PTSD had a dominant impact on mental health functioning in comparison with any severity level of injury. Those with a history of PTSD (ever PTSD) had mean scores of up to 12 points lower when compared with those without PTSD regardless of the injury status or level (Figure 4).

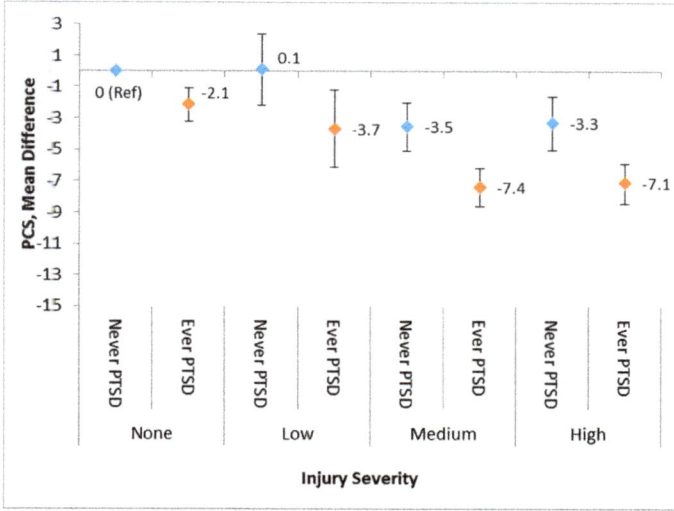

Figure 3. Adjusted regression beta coefficients for PCS-12 predicted by a combination of PTSD and the injury severity level.

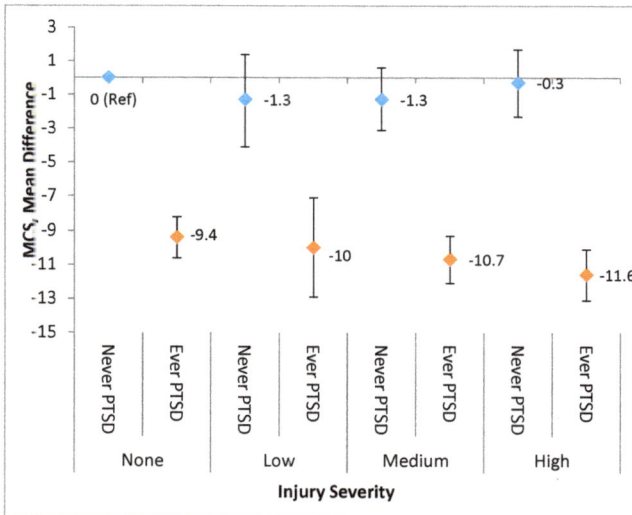

Figure 4. A combination of PTSD history and the injury severity level predicted adjusted regression beta coefficients for MCS-12.

4. Discussion

Based on prior research, we hypothesized that being injured on 11 September 2001 due to attacks on the World Trade Center would have long-term consequences on quality of life. In this study, we assessed both physical and mental health functioning using the well validated SF-12 health status instrument. The assessment demonstrated significant deficits for both the physical and mental health status among those who were injured on 9/11 and/or those with ensuing PTSD symptoms. For instance, there was a 7 to 10 point (women and men, respectively) deficit in SF-12 physical health summary score for those with an injury on 9/11 and no history of probable PTSD compared with population-based measures of the physical health status. Moreover, levels of injury severity, as defined by the degree of medical intervention following the 9/11 injury, had a dose-response association with a magnitude of the physical health function decrement but no association with mental health functioning. Thus, being injured on 9/11 is a major risk factor for long-term physical health effects among those directly exposed to the attacks, which represents a continued impact on a substantial population of affected persons.

Our finding that injury on 9/11 had an impact on physical functioning 15 years after sustaining an injury on 11 September 2001 indicates the extent to which an injury can diminish a person's long-term capacity to function. Few other studies have assessed the functional health status after this length of time following an injury even though some have found significant deficits after shorter periods. For example, one study reported an 80% increased likelihood of reporting poor health among injured individuals when compared with non-injured individuals five years after the injury occurrence [9]. There are a number of plausible mechanisms for a disaster-related injury to have long-term effects on physical health. First, the physical damage of the injury could persist as chronic pain and interfere with normal activity. Second, an injured person may be vulnerable for developing chronic disease, such as cardiovascular disease, due to inactivity secondary to the injury [1,35]. Third, people who are injured are more likely to engage in behavioral risks (e.g., smoking, alcohol consumption, or lack of exercise), which can result in diminished physical health through a number of possible pathways [36]. However, we did not find an association between smoking and physical health, as measured by PCS-12.

A history of probable PTSD was also the primary factor associated with the decline of both physical and mental health functioning. Specifically, PTSD had a significant effect on physical functioning with a three-point decrement in a physical health composite score between those with ever PTSD versus those with no history of PTSD after controlling for other factors, including injury severity. However, there was a three-fold greater likelihood of a history of probable PTSD predicting adjusting for injury severity and other covariates. This is in accord with several studies that have assessed the impact of mental health stress on overall mental health using SF-12 domain mean scores. For instance, a study on veterans of the 1991 Gulf War reported a negative correlation between the level of military stressors and mean MCS, as measured by the SF-12 and Military Service Experience questionnaire [37]. Another study reported that the mental health checklist scores that assessed the presence of psychological disorders including PTSD, depression, or general anxiety disorder, which were significantly negatively correlated with MCS-12 [38].

Other studies have similarly reported that injury impacts physical health more than mental health [11]. Two explanations are that the presence of comorbid conditions is associated with reduced capacity for self-care among injured persons [12], or that chronic conditions fully mediate the impact of 9/11 exposure on physical health status and partially mediate mental health status, as measured by SF-12 [34]. However, models run in our sensitivity analyses indicated that the regression coefficients for injury or PTSD were not altered for PCS-12 means, regardless of whether the number of diagnosed conditions were included in the models, which indicates that a history of the measured chronic conditions was not necessary for the injury and physical health relationship.

While injury severity was significantly related to a physical health decrement but not mental health decrement, a history of PTSD increased the likelihood of worse functioning for each level of injury severity for both physical and mental health. The obverse was evident when injury increased the PTSD-related decline in mental health.

The findings from a prior qualitative study on the same population represented in this study suggested that being injured diminished the quality of life both physically and mentally regardless of PTSD status [15]. By using a much larger sample with standardized measures of physical and mental health functioning, we did not discern an independent relationship between injury severity and mental health functioning, but rather that PTSD symptoms were a dominant factor for overall mental health functioning, as measured by the SF-12.

Many of the associations between demographic characteristics and other factors (e.g., social support) with physical and mental health summary scores were similar to those that have been reported for other populations. For instance, physical health functioning declined with age, but not mental health status, as exemplified by a mean PCS-12 score of 49 for 30-year-olds to 44-year-olds and a mean score of 42 for those 65 years and older. Similarly, another study based on a large US national survey reported a PCS-12 mean score that was −0.85 less than the population norm for 30–39 year olds and −5.1 for those aged 65 to 69. However, there was an increase by age for MCS-12 mean scores from −0.12 less than the population norm for those aged 30 to 39 to +2.4 years for those aged 60 to 69 years [39]. Gopinath [14] also reported a −1.5 decline in PCS-12 mean for each additional 10 years of age, but no change for the mean MCS-12 based on persons with minor musculoskeletal injuries. With regard to gender, other studies have noted that men have higher mean scores on PCS-12 than women, but similar mean MCS-12 scores [33,39] consistent with results from this study. Although we did not specifically evaluate the association between PTSD history for men and women separately with mental health status, the finding that there were no differences between men and women is surprising because women generally have higher PTSD rates than men [40,41]

With regard to other factors, Soberg [11] reported a three-fold higher level of physical and mental health summary scores within a year following injury for those with post-high school education compared with those with a high school-only education. However, in our study, we did not find a significant association between the educational level and MCS-12 or PCS-12. Other factors, such as social support or self-efficacy, were not typically included as factors in studies using PCS-12 or MCS-12. However, Kiely [42] reported that less social support among injured persons six months after injury was associated with a mental health deficit, as measured by the MCS-36, but not with physical health, as measured by the PCS-36. Our study had similar results.

The findings from this study indicate that both PCS-12 and MCS-12 are sensitive to long-term changes in health status and general health functioning many years after the disaster. The patterns of association between demographic and socio-behavioral factors concur with the magnitude of change in the PCS-12 and MCS-12 in various reports based on general population data and in studies specific to injured persons. The degree to which SF-12 is a strong indicator of health status is evident by the SF-12 having a dose-response relationship to a biologically based assessment of physical health referred to as a frailty index [43].

This study has several key strengths. First, we were able to assess physical and mental health status after a much longer period since the original event was compared with other studies. Second, we had a sufficient sample of persons injured on 11 September 2001 as well as a comparison group of non-injured persons to assess the combined influence of multiple characteristics longitudinally on physical and mental health status.

However, the study is also subject to some limitations. First, there is likely self-selection bias on a number of dimensions. For example, we only included persons who had participated in all of the registry follow-up surveys. A large proportion of persons in the cohort were also self-selected for original enrollment in the registry. An assessment of the impact of follow-up survey participation in the registry found that an increased propensity to participate in surveys was related to an absence of chronic conditions [17]. However, the overall physical and mental health of those who had no injury and never had PTSD in this study were not substantively different from the general US population. Second, we relied on self-report, which is especially problematic for key predictors in this study including having been injured on 9/11 and probable PTSD. Nonetheless, we defined being injured and injury severity in a way that minimized the bias of self-report by eliminating persons who provided inconsistent responses concerning their injury on 9/11 between what was reported at the registry enrollment survey and what was reported in the HQoL survey. Lastly, we do not have information on psychiatric conditions or vulnerabilities prior to the 9/11 trauma, which would have permitted controlling for this factor in the association of PTSD history with physical and mental health status.

5. Conclusions

In this study, we documented convincing evidence that many persons injured on 11 September 2001 were experiencing diminished physical health 15 years after the event. To put it into context, the mean PCS-12 score for persons injured without PTSD is comparable to reported mean PCS-12 scores for those with cerebral aneurysms (39.5) or congestive heart failure (42.8) [44,45]. Given that many persons who sustained an injury on 11 September 2001 also subsequently suffered from symptoms of PTSD, we found that, after adjusting for other factors, the combined effect of severe injury with PTSD yielded significant deficits in both physical and mental health functioning when compared with those who were not injured and did not experience PTSD. Even though, over the course of years since the injury, the physical wounds of the injury could have healed in some cases, our results suggest that traumatic injuries appear to have a lasting effect on perceived physical functioning. The discontinuity between adequate physical functioning and significantly lower quality of life is a phenomenon that has been observed among injured persons and could occur in this population [39] even though we do not have evidence that directly supports this relationship. Nonetheless, the results from this study can be generalized to the long-term health burden at both the individual and societal level from nonfatal injuries sustained in natural or man-made disasters.

Author Contributions: Conceptualization: R.M.B., H.E.A., P.F., L.M.G., and M.H.J. Formal analysis: H.E.A., R.M.B., and M.H.J. Methodology: R.M.B., H.E.A., M.H.J., and L.M.G. Project Administration: R.M.B. and L.M.G. Writing: R.M.B., M.H.J., P.F., and A.S. Reviewing and editing: R.M.B., M.H.J., L.M.G., H.E.A., P.F., and A.S.

Funding: This study was supported by the Cooperative Agreement U50/ATU272750 from the Agency for Toxic Substances and Disease Registry (ATSDR) and the Centers for Disease Control and Prevention (CDC), which included support from the National Center for Environmental Health and by Cooperative Agreement U50/OH009739 from the National Institute for Occupational Safety and Health (NIOSH) and the New York City Department of Health and Mental Hygiene. The findings and conclusions in this report are those of the authors and do not necessarily represent the views of the ATSDR or CDC/NIOSH.

Conflicts of Interest: The authors declare that they have no competing financial interests.

References

1. Alper, H.E.; Yu, S.; Stellman, S.D.; Brackbill, R.M. Injury, Intense Dust Exposure, and Chronic Disease among Survivors of the World Trade Center Terrorist Attacks of September 11, 2001. *Inj. Epidemiol.* **2017**, *4*, 17. [CrossRef] [PubMed]

2. Brackbill, R.M.; Hadler, J.L.; DiGrande, L.; Ekenga, C.C.; Farfel, M.R.; Friedman, S.; Perlman, S.E.; Stellman, S.D.; Walker, D.J.; Wu, D.; et al. Asthma and Posttraumatic Stress Symptoms 5 to 6 Years Following Exposure to the World Trade Center Terrorist Attack. *JAMA* **2009**, *302*, 502–516. [CrossRef] [PubMed]

3. DiGrande, L.; Neria, Y.; Brackbill, R.M.; Pulliam, P.; Galea, S. Long-term Posttraumatic Stress Symptoms Among 3,271 Civilian Survivors of the September 11, 2001, Terrorist Attacks on the World Trade Center. *Am. J. Epidemiol.* **2011**, *173*, 271–281. [CrossRef] [PubMed]

4. Brackbill, R.M.; Cone, J.E.; Farfel, M.R.; Stellman, S.D. Chronic Physical Health Consequences of Being Injured During the Terrorist Attacks on World Trade Center on September 11, 2001. *Am. J. Epidemiol.* **2014**, *179*, 1076–1085. [CrossRef] [PubMed]

5. Norris, F.H.; Sherrieb, K.; Galea, S. Prevalence and Consequences of Disaster-Related Illness and Injury from Hurricane Ike. *Rehabil. Psychol.* **2010**, *55*, 221–230. [CrossRef]

6. Dyster-Aas, J.; Arnberg, F.K.; Lindam, A.; Johannesson, K.B.; Lundin, T.; Michel, P.-O. Impact of Physical Injury on Mental Health After the 2004 Southeast Asia Tsunami. *Nord. J. Psychiatry* **2012**, *66*, 203–208. [CrossRef] [PubMed]

7. Craig, A.; Tran, Y.; Guest, R.; Gopinath, B.; Jagnoor, J.; Bryant, R.A.; Collie, A.; Tate, R.; Kenardy, J.; Middleton, J.W.; et al. Psychological Impact of Injuries Sustained in Motor Vehicle Crashes: Systematic Review and Meta-analysis. *BMJ Open* **2016**, *6*, e011993. [CrossRef] [PubMed]

8. Sumner, J.A.; Kubzansky, L.D.; Elkind, M.S.; Roberts, A.L.; Agnew-Blais, J.; Chen, Q.; Cerdá, M.; Rexrode, K.M.; Rich-Edwards, J.W.; Spiegelman, D.; et al. Trauma Exposure and Posttraumatic Stress

Disorder Symptoms Predict Onset of Cardiovascular Events in Women. *Circulation* **2015**, *132*, 251–259. [CrossRef] [PubMed]

9. Toft, A.M.H.; Moller, H.; Laursen, B. The Years after an Injury: Long-term Consequences of Injury on Self-rated Health. *J. Trauma* **2010**, *69*, 26–30. [CrossRef] [PubMed]

10. Holtslag, H.R.; van Beeck, E.F.; Lindeman, E.; Leenen, L.P. Determinants of Long-term Functional Consequences After Major Trauma. *J. Trauma* **2007**, *62*, 919–927. [CrossRef] [PubMed]

11. Soberg, H.L.; Finset, A.; Roise, O.; Bautz-Holter, E. The Trajectory of Physical and Mental Health from Injury to 5 Years after Multiple Trauma: A Prospective, Longitudinal Cohort Study. *Arch. Phys. Med. Rehabil.* **2012**, *93*, 765–774. [CrossRef]

12. Ioannou, L.J.; Cameron, P.A.; Gibson, S.J.; Gabbe, B.J.; Ponsford, J.; Jennings, P.A.; Arnold, C.A.; Gwini, S.M.; Georgiou-Karistianis, N.; Giummarra, M.J. Traumatic injury and perceived injustice: Fault attibrutions matter in a 'no-fault' compensation state. *PLoS ONE* **2017**, *12*, e0178894. [CrossRef] [PubMed]

13. Rios-Diaz, A.J.; Herrera-Escobar, J.P.; Lilley, E.J.; Appelson, J.R.; Gabbe, B.; Brasel, K.; deRoon-Cassini, T.; Schneider, E.B.; Kasotakis, G.; Kaafarani, H.; et al. Routine Inclusion of Long-term Functional and Patient-reported Outcomes into Trauma Registries: The FORTE Project. *J. Trauma Acute Care Surg.* **2017**, 97–104. [CrossRef]

14. Gopinath, B.; Jagnoor, J.; Harris, I.A.; Nicholas, M.; Casey, P.; Blyth, F.; Maher, C.G.; Cameron, I.D. Health-Related Quality of Life 24 Months After Sustaining a Minor Musculoskeletal Injury in a Road Traffic Crash: A Prospective Cohort Study. *Traffic Inj. Prev.* **2017**, *18*, 251–256. [CrossRef] [PubMed]

15. Gargano, L.M.; Gershon, R.R.; Brackbill, R.M. Quality of Life of Persons Injured on 9/11: Qualitative Analysis from the World Trade Center Health Registry. *PLoS Curr.* **2016**, *8*. [CrossRef] [PubMed]

16. Murphy, J.; Brackbill, R.M.; Thalji, L.; Dolan, M.; Pulliam, P.; Walker, D.J. Measuring and Maximizing Coverage in the World Trade Center Health Registry. *Stat. Med.* **2007**, *26*, 1688–1701. [CrossRef]

17. Yu, S.; Brackbill, R.M.; Stellman, S.D.; Ghuman, S.; Farfel, M.R. Evaluation of Non-response Bias in a Cohort Study of World Trade Center Terrorist Attack Survivors. *BMC Res. Notes* **2015**, *8*, 42. [CrossRef]

18. Jacobson, M.H.; Norman, C.; Nguyen, A.; Brackbill, R.M. Longitudinal Determinants of Depression Among World Trade Center Health Registry Enrollees, 14–14 years After the 9/11 attacks. *J. Affect. Disord.* **2018**, *229*, 483–490. [CrossRef]

19. Jacobson, M.H.; Brackbill, R.M.; Frazier, P.; Gargano, L.M. Conducting a study to assess the long-term impacts of injury after 9/11: Participation, recall, and description. *Inj. Epidemiol.* **2019**. [CrossRef]

20. Jenkinson, C.; Layte, R.; Jenkinson, D.; Lawrence, K.; Petersen, S.; Paice, C.; Stradling, J. A Shorter Form Health Survey: Can the SF-12 Replicate Results from the SF-36 in Longitudinal Studies? *J. Public Health Med.* **1997**, *19*, 179–186. [CrossRef] [PubMed]

21. Busija, L.; Pausenberger, E.; Haines, T.P.; Haymes, S.; Buchbinder, R.; Osborne, RH. Adult Measures of General Health and Health-Related Quality of Life: Medical Outcomes Study Short Form 36-Item (SF-36) and Short Form 12-Item (SF-12) health surveys, Nottingham Health Profile (NHP), Sickness Impact Profile (SIP), Medical Outcomes Study Short Form 6D (SF-6D), Health Utilities Index Mark 3 (HUI3), Quality of Well-Being Scale (QWB), and Assessment of Quality of Life (AQoL). *Arthritis Care Res. (Hoboken)* **2011**, *63*, S383–S412. [CrossRef] [PubMed]

22. McDonald, S.D.; Calhoun, P.S. The Diagnostic Accuracy of the PTSD Checklist: A Critical Review. *Clin. Psychol. Rev.* **2010**, *30*, 976–987. [CrossRef] [PubMed]

23. American Psychiatric Association. *Diagnostic and Statistical Manual of Mental Disorders*, 4th ed.; American Psychiatric Publishing, Inc.: Arlington, VA, USA, 1994.

24. Wilkins, K.C.; Lang, A.J.; Norman, S.B. Synthesis of the Psychometric Properties of the PTSD Checklist (PCL) Military, civilian, and specific versions. *Depress. Anxiety* **2011**, *28*, 596–606. [CrossRef] [PubMed]

25. Blanchard, E.B.; Jones-Alexander, J.; Buckley, T.C.; Forneris, A. Psychometric Properties of the PTSD Checklist (PCL). *Behav. Res. Ther.* **1996**, *34*, 669–673. [CrossRef]

26. Maslow, C.B.; Caramanica, K.; Welch, A.E.; Stellman, S.D.; Brackbill, R.M.; Farfel, M.R. Trajectories of Scores on a Screening Instrument for PTSD Among World Trade Center Rescue, Recovery, and Clean-up Workers. *J. Trauma Stress* **2015**, *28*, 198–205. [CrossRef]

27. Bouillon, B.; Kreder, H.J.; Eypasch, E.; Holbrook, T.L.; Kreder, H.J.; Mayou, R.; Nast-Kolb, D.; Pirente, N.; Schelling, G.; Tiling, T.; et al. Quality of Life in Patients with Multiple Injuries—Basic Issues, Assessment, and Recommendations. *Restor. Neurol. Neurosci.* **2002**, *20*, 125–134. [PubMed]

28. Sherbourne, C.D.; Stewart, A.L. The MOS Social Support Survey. *Soc. Sci. Med.* **1991**, *32*, 705–714. [CrossRef]

29. Ritvo, P.G.; Fisk, J.D.; Archibald, C.J.; Murray, T.J.; Field, C. Psychosocial and Neurological Predictors of Mental Health in Multiple Sclerosis Patients. *J. Clin. Epidemiol.* **1996**, *49*, 467–472. [CrossRef]

30. Schwarzer, R.; Jerusalem, J. Generalized Self-Efficacy scale. In *Measures in Health Psychology: A User's Portfolio; Causal and Control Beliefs*, Weinman, J., Johnston Wright, S., Eds.; NFER-NELSON: Windsor, UK, 1995; pp. 35–37.

31. Luszczynska, A.; Scholz, U.; Schwarzer, R. The General Self-efficacy Scale: Multicultural Validation Studies. *J. Psychol.* **2005**, *139*, 439–457. [CrossRef]

32. Yip, J.; Zeig-Owens, R.; Webber, M.P.; Kablanian, A.; Hall, C.B.; Vossbrinck, M.; Liu, X.; Weakley, J.; Schwartz, T.; Kelly, K.J.; et al. World Trade Center-related Physical and Mental Health Burden Among New York City Fire Department Emergency Medical Service Workers. *Occup. Environ. Med.* **2016**, *73*, 13–20. [CrossRef] [PubMed]

33. Hanmerxed, J.; Lawrence, W.F.; Anderson, J.P.; Kaplan, R.M.; Fryback, D.G. Report of Nationally Representative Values for the Noninstitutionalized US Adult Population for 7 Health-related Quality-of-Life Scores. *Med. Decis. Making* **2006**, *26*, 391–400. [CrossRef] [PubMed]

34. Yip, J.; Zeig-Owens, R.; Hall, C.B.; Webber, M.P.; Olivieri, B.; Schwartz, T.; Kelly, K.J.; Prezant, D.J. Health Conditions as Mediators of the Association Between World Trade Center Exposure and Health-related Quality of Life in Firefighters and EMS Workers. *J. Occup. Environ. Med.* **2016**, *58*, 200–206. [CrossRef] [PubMed]

35. Karacabey, K. Effect of Regular Exercise on Health and Disease. *Neuroendocrinol. Lett.* **2005**, *26*, 617–623. [PubMed]

36. McKenzie, D.P.; Ikin, J.F.; McFarlane, A.C.; Creamer, M.; Forbes, A.B.; Kelsall, H.L.; Glass, D.C.; Ittak, P.; Sim, M.R. Psychological Health of Australian Veterans of the 1991 Gulf War: An Assessment Using the SF-12, GHQ-12 and PCL-S. *Psychol. Med.* **2004**, *34*, 1419–1430. [CrossRef] [PubMed]

37. Tsai, J.; Ford, E.S.; Li, C.; Zhao, G.; Pearson, W.S.; Balluz, L.S. Multiple Healthy Behaviors and Optimal Self-related Health: Findings from the 2007 Behavioral Risk Factor Surveillance System. *Prev. Med.* **2010**, *51*, 268–274. [CrossRef] [PubMed]

38. Ball, K.; Macpherson, C.; Hurowitz, G.; Settles-Reaves, B.; DeVeaugh-Geiss, J.; Weir, S.; Schulberg, H.C.; Lawson, W.B.; Gaynes, B.N. M3 Checklist and SF-12 Correlation Study. *Best Pract. Ment. Health* **2015**, *11*, 83–89.

39. Fleishman, J.A.; Selim, A.J.; Kazis, L.E. Deriving SF-12v2 Physical and Mental Health Summary Scores: A Comparison of Different Scoring Algorithms. *Qual. Life Res.* **2010**, *19*, 231–241. [CrossRef] [PubMed]

40. Bowler, R.M.; Harris, M.; Li, J.; Goheva, V.; Stellman, S.D.; Wilson, K.; Alper, H.; Schwarzer, R.; Cone, J.E. Longitudinal mental health impact among police responders to the 9/11 terrorist attack. *Am. J. Ind. Med.* **2012**, *55*, 297–312. [CrossRef] [PubMed]

41. Gogos, A.; Ney, L.J.; Seymour, N.; Van Rheenen, T.E.; Felmingham, K.I. Sex differences in schizophrenia, bipolar disorder, and post-traumatic stress disorder: Are gonadal hormones the link? *Br. J. Pharmacol* **2019**. [CrossRef] [PubMed]

42. Kiely, J.M.; Brasel, K.J.; Weidner, K.L.; Guse, C.E.; Weigelt, J.A. Predicting Quality of Life Six Months after Traumatic Injury. *J. Trauma* **2006**, *61*, 791–798. [CrossRef] [PubMed]

43. Bello, G.A.; Lucchini, R.G.; Teitelbaum, S.L.; Shapiro, M.; Crane, M.A.; Todd, A.C. Development of a Physiological Frailty Index for the World Trade Center General Responder Cohort. *Curr. Gerontol. Geriatr. Res.* **2018**, *2018*, 3725926. [CrossRef] [PubMed]

44. King, J.T., Jr.; Horowitz, M.B.; Kassam, A.B.; Yonas, H.; Roberts, M.S. The Short Form-12 and the Measurement of Health Status in Patients with Cerebral Aneurysms: Performance, Validity, and Reliability. *J. Neurosurg.* **2005**, *102*, 489–494. [CrossRef] [PubMed]

45. Ware, J.E.; Kosinski, M.; Keller, S.D. A 12-item Short Form: Construction of scales and preliminary tests of reliability and validity. *Med. Care* **1996**, *34*, 220–233. [CrossRef] [PubMed]

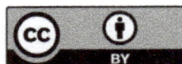

International Journal of
*Environmental Research
and Public Health*

MDPI

Article

Handgrip Strength of World Trade Center (WTC) Responders: The Role of Re-Experiencing Posttraumatic Stress Disorder (PTSD) Symptoms

Soumyadeep Mukherjee [1], Sean Clouston [2,*], Roman Kotov [3], Evelyn Bromet [3] and Benjamin Luft [4]

[1]   Community Health and Wellness, Health & Physical Education Department, Rhode Island College, Providence, RI 02908, USA; smukherjee@ric.edu
[2]   Program in Public Health, Department of Family, Population, and Preventive Medicine, Renaissance School of Medicine at Stony Brook University, Stony Brook, NY 11794, USA
[3]   Department of Psychiatry, Renaissance School of Medicine at Stony Brook University, Stony Brook, NY 11794, USA; roman.kotov@stonybrookmedicine.edu (R.K.); evelyn.bromet@stonybrookmedicine.edu (E.B.)
[4]   World Trade Center Health and Wellness Program Director, Department of Medicine, Renaissance School of Medicine at Stony Brook University, Stony Brook, NY 11794, USA; Benjamin.Luft@stonybrookmedicine.edu
*   Correspondence: sean.clouston@stonybrookmedicine.edu

Received: 18 February 2019; Accepted: 26 March 2019; Published: 29 March 2019

Abstract: *Background*: This study sought to examine whether handgrip strength (HGS), a measure of muscle strength and a biomarker of aging, was associated with post-traumatic stress disorder (PTSD) in a cohort of World Trade Center (WTC) responders at midlife. *Methods*: HGS was assessed utilizing a computer-assisted hand dynamometer administered to a consecutive sample of men and women ($n = 2016$) who participated in rescue and recovery efforts following the World Trade Center (WTC) attacks and subsequently attended monitoring appointments in Long Island, NY. PTSD symptom severity and depressive symptoms were assessed using the PTSD specific-trauma checklist (PCL-S) and the Patient Health Questionnaire (PHQ-9). General linear models were used to examine the association of WTC-related PTSD with HGS after adjusting for confounders. *Results*: The sample was at midlife (mean age = 53.3) when assessed, and 91.3% were men. Nearly 10% of the sample had probable PTSD (PCL $\geq$ 44) with concomitant depression (PHQ $\geq$ 10), while 5.1% had probable PTSD without depression. Average HGS was 57.4 lbs. (95% confidence interval (95% CI): 56.6–58.1) among men and 36.1 lbs. (95% CI = 33.8–38.5) among women. Mean HGS of those with probable PTSD with concomitant depression was lower (45.9 lbs., 95% CI = 43.6–48.2) than responders with only PTSD (49.1 lbs., 95% CI = 46.0–52.4) and those without PTSD or depression (57.5 lbs., 95% CI = 56.2–57.8). Subdomain analyses of PTSD symptoms revealed that re-experiencing symptoms at enrollment ($p = 0.003$) was associated with lower HGS after adjusting for depressive symptoms and other confounders. *Discussion*: Results suggested that higher WTC-related PTSD symptom severity was associated with lower HGS. Results support ongoing work suggesting that PTSD may be associated with more rapid physical aging. The potential for developing interventions that might simultaneously improve physical and mental health in the aftermath of trauma may be considered.

Keywords: 9/11 disaster; handgrip strength; WTC responders; PTSD; depression; aging

---

1. Introduction

Hand grip strength (HGS) is an indicator of upper body strength that quantifies the amount of static force with which a person's hand can squeeze a dynamometer [1]. Often used as a marker of overall muscular strength, HGS is negatively associated with physical frailty [2]. Diminishing HGS is associated with muscle wasting and is commonly observed in older age, suggesting that it may act as a biomarker for aging. Poorer HGS is also associated with increased disability and mortality [3].

In addition to physical health, HGS has shown association with mental health outcomes. For example, a number of studies examining adults in midlife and older have reported that depressive symptoms were associated with HGS [4,5], while another study among Australians aged 85 years and older also found that lower HGS was associated with worse functional, psychological, and social health [3]. Additionally, higher HGS was shown to be associated with better cognitive performance among older participants with major depression, and those with bipolar disorder, as well as among healthy controls [6] and, in a second study maximal HGS was found to be associated with cognitive performance in the general population, and among those with schizophrenia [7].

Despite associations with a variety of health outcomes, to date no work has examined associations between HGS and symptoms of posttraumatic stress disorder (PTSD) in individuals who have experienced a severe trauma. Our recent work has suggested that PTSD may increase risk of cognitive aging [8] and physical functional limitations [9], suggestive of the potential for more rapid aging. This study therefore sought to determine whether weaker HGS is also associated with PTSD. Since PTSD is often comorbid with depression, we further examined whether the association, if any, of HGS with PTSD was magnified by the presence of depression. Lastly, since PTSD is a heterogeneous disorder, we further examined whether HGS had differential associations with PTSD symptom domains.

2. Materials and Methods

2.1. Participants and Procedure

The Centers for Disease Control and Prevention, in the year 2002, established a monitoring and treatment program for those who responded to the World Trade Center (WTC) terrorist attacks of 11 September 2001 by participating in rescue and recovery efforts. Since then, more than 33,000 responders have enrolled in the WTC general responder population (GRP) [10]. The WTC Wellness Program at Stony Brook University (SBU) monitors more than 8000 of these responders primarily residing on Long Island, NY. This SBU cohort is similar in terms of exposure, sex, and age to those enrolled in the GRP [10], with the majority being males (92.0%), most of them working in law enforcement (71.5%) during 9/11, with an average age of 38.9 years at the time of the WTC attack. Most SBU responders (85.0%) have continued to return to either Nassau or Suffolk county clinics within 18 months of their prior visit.

In 2016, the SBU WTC Wellness program began assessing responders' HGS as a part of their functional assessment. The current study includes a consecutive sample of responders ($n = 2016$) who were monitored between April 2016 and September 2017. The study was approved by the Stony Brook University Ethics Review Board (IRB approval No. 604113); responders provided informed, written consent. In comparison with the SBU population of responders who were eligible for research but did not complete the functional assessment, those who completed the functional assessment were 0.85 years younger ($p < 0.001$) and were less likely to be women ($p = 0.004$), but had similar occupations on 11 September 2001 ($p = 0.115$), showed similar levels of current PTSD ($p = 0.521$), and similar baseline PTSD Checklist (PCL) scores ($p = 0.455$).

2.2. Assessment of HGS

HGS was assessed for both hands only if responders did not self-report any trouble with their hands, shoulders, or wrists and if they felt that they would be able to safely complete the assessment. Vernier dynamometers were administered by trained healthcare providers to measure and record HGS among responders sitting upright in chairs with arm rests such that their elbow formed close to a right angle while they squeezed the dynamometer between their thumb and other fingers with maximum strength for 10 s. Each responder completed two trials for each hand beginning with the left hand. Force was measured in pounds (lbs.) and recorded in a computer with Logger Pro software

(Vernier®Software & Technology, Beaverton, OR, USA). The data were exported as. csv files, cleaned and the maximum HGS was used for this study. The average of two trials were computed, followed by the average of two hands which was the outcome for this study.

2.3. Assessment of PTSD Symptoms

PTSD symptoms were assessed at each monitoring visit using the PTSD checklist, specific trauma version tailored to the WTC disaster (PCL-S trauma specific version) [11]. At each monitoring visit, respondents rated the extent to which they were bothered by 17 DSM-IV WTC-related PTSD symptoms during the past month on a scale from 1 (not at all) to 5 (extremely). The PCL has good internal consistency and convergent validity [12]. The total PCL score was used to categorize respondents into those who had or did not have probable WTC-related PTSD, using a cut-off of 44 [11]. Four PTSD symptom clusters were also analyzed: avoidance, hyperarousal, negative affect and re-experiencing symptoms.

2.4. Assessment of Depressive Symptoms

Symptoms of depression were measured by the Patient Health Questionnaire with nine items (PHQ-9). Probable depression was indicated by a PHQ-9 score of 10 or higher. WTC responders were categorized based on whether they had both probable PTSD and probable depression; probable PTSD without depression; or neither PTSD nor depression. Depression only group was not considered because of very few responders who had depression without PTSD symptoms.

2.5. Covariates

A number of variables that could be potentially associated with health and functional status were considered including age in years at the time of HGS assessment and gender. According to educational attainment, responders were categorized into those who did not finish high school, those who graduated high school, those with some college education, those with an undergraduate degree, and those who have been to graduate school. Race/ethnicity was categorized as non-Hispanic White, non-Hispanic Black, Hispanic, Asian, and others. Responders were categorized as single, married, and separated or divorced or widowed depending on their marital status. Current employment status was given as working full time, working part time, being disabled or on medical leave, retired, and laid off or unemployed. Annual household income (US$) was categorized as 50,000 or less, more than 50,000 to 70,000, more than 70,000 to 100,000 and higher than 100,000. According to their self-reported general health, responders had excellent, very good, good, fair, or poor general health. Responders' self-reported hand-dominance was taken into account to classify them as right-handed, left-handed, or ambidextrous.

Taking into account the severity of responders' exposure to the WTC disaster, four exposure groups—very high, high, intermediate, and low—were created based on the work of Wisnivesky et al. [13]. The very high exposure group comprised of those who worked more than 90 days at the WTC site, were exposed to the dust cloud due to the collapse of WTC buildings, and worked at least some time on the pile of debris. Rescue workers who were exposed to the dust cloud but either worked on-site less than 90 days or did not work on the debris pile, were categorized to have had high exposure. Workers with intermediate exposure were exposed to the dust cloud and either worked between 40 days and 90 days or did not work on the debris pile. Workers in the lowest exposure group worked less than 40 days on-site, were not exposed to dust from the collapse, and did not work on the debris pile.

2.6. Statistical Analysis

Descriptive sample statistics, including means and standard deviations of maximum HGS were computed. Average of two runs from each hand was calculated followed by the average from both hands. Means and/or proportions were computed for all independent variables and covariates.

Linear regression was performed to examine bivariate associations of mean HGS with WTC-related probable PTSD and all other independent variables. Mean HGS were compared between different levels of each variable and 95% confidence intervals (CI) were computed for the means. Estimates of regression coefficients and their respective p-values were reported. A two-tailed $\alpha = 0.05$ was utilized to determine statistical significance. Multivariable general linear models were used to examine the association of WTC-related PTSD with HGS after adjusting for covariates.

In separate analyses, scores for individual PTSD domains were used to examine whether re-experiencing symptoms, avoiding situations reminiscent of the WTC event, negative changes in beliefs and feelings, or hyperarousal symptoms were associated with HGS, after adjusting for depression (PHQ-9) scores and other covariates.

3. Results

The mean age of the sample was 53.3 (SD: 7.9) years with a range from 35.1 to 85.0 at the time of their HGS assessment, and 91.3% were men (Table 1).

Table 1. Distribution of handgrip strength (HGS) with independent variables among World Trade Center (WTC) responders (*n* = 2023).

Characteristics	Mean (SD)/Number (%)	Mean HGS (lbs.) (95% CI)
Age in years	53.3 (7.9)	55.5 (54.8–56.3)
Gender		
Men	1847 (91.3)	57.4 (56.6–58.1)
Women	176 (8.7)	36.1 (33.8–38.5)
Race/ethnicity		
Non-Hispanic White 0	1613 (85.8)	56.2 (55.3–57.0)
Non-Hispanic Black 1	86 (4.6)	50.8 (47.2–54.4)
Hispanic 2	156 (8.3)	52.7 (50.0–55.4)
Asian 3	19 (1.0)	52.6 (44.9–60.3)
Other 4	7 (0.4)	47.9 (35.3–60.5)
Hand dominance		
Right	1721 (85.1)	55.4 (54.6–56.2)
Left	208 (10.3)	55.5 (53.1–57.8)
Ambidextrous	94 (4.7)	58.4 (54.9–61.8)
Marital status		
Single	107 (5.3)	49.9 (46.6–53.1)
Married	1678 (83.0)	56.1 (55.3–56.9)
Separated/Divorced/Widowed	238 (11.8)	53.8 (51.6–56.0)
Education		
Did not finish high school	55 (2.8)	51.6 (47.0–56.1)
Graduated high school	349 (17.8)	53.5 (51.7–55.3)
Some college	935 (47.7)	55.6 (54.5–56.7)
Undergraduate degree	467 (23.8)	57.6 (56.1–59.2)
Graduate school	155 (7.9)	55.0 (52.3–57.7)
Current employment status		
Working full time	1153 (57.6)	58.8 (57.8–59.7)
Working part time	147 (7.3)	56.9 (54.2–59.6)
Disabled/on medical leave	106 (5.3)	50.6 (47.5–53.8)
Retired	572 (28.6)	50.1 (48.7–51.4)
Laid off/unemployed	25 (1.3)	51.3 (44.8–57.8)

Table 1. *Cont.*

Characteristics	Mean (SD)/Number (%)	Mean HGS (lbs.) (95% CI)
Annual income (USD)		
0 to 50,000	181 (11.7)	54.9 (52.5–57.4)
>50,000 to 70,000	428 (27.7)	55.2 (53.6–56.8)
>70,000 to 100,000	678 (43.9)	56.1 (54.8–57.4)
>100,000	258 (16.7)	56.4 (54.4–58.5)
Level of WTC exposure		
Low	331 (18.0)	53.9 (52.1–55.8)
Intermediate	1092 (59.4)	56.1 (55.1–57.1)
High	339 (18.5)	56.2 (54.4–58.0)
Very high	75 (4.1)	53.6 (49.8–57.5)
WTC-related PTSD		
Probable PTSD (PCL-S $\geq$ 44) with depression (PHQ-9 $\geq$ 10)	200 (9.9)	45.9 (43.6–48.2)
Probable PTSD without depression	104 (5.1)	49.2 (46.0–52.4)
No PTSD or depression	1719 (85.0)	57.0 (56.2–57.8)
Self-reported general health		
Excellent	87 (4.4)	61.4 (57.9–64.9)
Very good	461 (23.1)	59.6 (58.1–61.1)
Good	990 (49.7)	56.7 (55.7–57.7)
Fair	381 (19.1)	49.3 (47.6–50.9)
Poor	75 (3.8)	41.7 (38.0–45.5)

Total numbers vary between variables because only responders with valid response for each variable are included.

The majority (36%) were non-Hispanic White (NHW). The average maximal HGS was 55.5 lbs. (SD 17.1) with a minimum of 7.5 lbs. and a maximum of 109.0 lbs. There was no significant difference in HGS and hand dominance. There was a decrease in maximum HGS with increasing age: every year older age was associated with a decrease in maximum HGS by 0.5 lbs. ($p < 0.0001$) (Table 3). Women had mean maximum HGS being more than 21 lbs. lower than men. Among racial/ethnic groups, non-Hispanic Blacks had significantly lower HGS than NHWs. Those who were on disability or on medical leave and those who were retired at the time of the study had significantly lower HGS than those who were working full-time on 9/11/2001. Having fair or poor self-reported general health was associated with lower HGS than those with excellent health. Mean HGS of responders with probable PTSD with concurrent depression was 11 lbs. lower ($p < 0.0001$), whereas mean HGS of responders with probable PTSD without depression was 8 lbs. lower ($p < 0.0001$) than those without either PTSD or depression.

Table 2. Relationship of handgrip strength (HGS) with independent variables among WTC responders.

Characteristics	Bivariate Regression Coefficient (*p* Value)	Multivariable Regression Coefficient (*p* Value)
Age in years	−0.53 (<0.0001)	−0.52 (<0.0001)
Gender		
Men	Ref.	Ref.
Women	−21.23 (<0.0001)	−21.8 (<0.0001)
Race/ethnicity		
Non-Hispanic White	Ref.	Ref.
Non-Hispanic Black	−5.38 (0.04)	0.48 (0.81)
Hispanic	−3.44 (0.11)	−2.23 (0.15)
Asian	−3.58 (0.89)	−2.28 (0.53)
Other	−8.26 (0.70)	−15.74 (0.27)

Table 3. *Cont.*

Characteristics	Bivariate Regression Coefficient (*p* Value)	Multivariable Regression Coefficient (*p* Value)
Hand dominance		
Right	Ref.	Ref.
Left	0.09 (0.36)	−0.71 (0.54)
Ambidextrous	3.00 (0.22)	3.82 (0.05)
Marital status		
Single	Ref.	Ref.
Married	6.25 (0.0007)	0.91 (0.65)
Separated/Divorced/Widowed	3.94 (0.12)	1.46 (0.52)
Education		
Did not finish high school	Ref.	Ref.
Graduated high school	1.96 (0.93)	4.90 (0.06)
Some college	4.06 (0.42)	4.42 (0.08)
Undergraduate degree	6.07 (0.09)	4.59 (0.08)
Graduate school	3.47 (0.69)	3.01 (0.30)
Current employment status		
Working full time	Ref.	Ref.
Working part time	−1.84 (0.71)	−1.05 (0.51)
Disabled/on medical leave	−8.13 (<0.0001)	−5.04 (0.02)
Retired	−8.72 (<0.0001)	−2.17 (0.03)
Laid off/unemployed	−7.47 (0.17)	−6.41 (0.14)
Annual income (USD)		
0 to 50,000	Ref.	Ref.
>50,000 to 70,000	0.25 (0.99)	2.55 (0.08)
>70,000 to 100,000	1.18 (0.84)	2.90 (0.04)
>100,000	1.54 (0.78)	4.17 (0.01)
Level of WTC exposure		
Low	Ref.	Ref.
Intermediate	2.17 (0.18)	1.60 (0.15)
High	2.28 (0.31)	2.44 (0.07)
Very high	0.30 (0.99)	−3.93 (0.08)
WTC-related PTSD		
Probable PTSD (PCL-S ≥ 44) with depression (PHQ-9 ≥ 10)	−11.11 (<0.0001)	−5.33 (0.0005)
Probable PTSD without depression	−7.8 (<0.0001)	−3.04 (0.14)
No PTSD or depression	Ref.	Ref.
Self-reported general health		
Excellent	Ref.	Ref.
Very good	−1.76 (0.89)	−0.86 (0.69)
Good	−4.72 (0.08)	−1.72 (0.41)
Fair	−12.11 (<0.0001)	−7.27 (0.001)
Poor	−19.65 (<0.0001)	−15.52 (<0.0001)

Only responders with non-missing responses for each variable are included. Ref.: Reference category.

In multivariate analysis, being in fair or poor health was associated with lower HGS than those with excellent health (Table 3). Responders with both WTC-related probable PTSD and depression, but not those with PTSD without depression, had significantly (*p* = 0.0005) lower mean HGS than those without PTSD or depression. Higher age and female gender remained significantly associated with lower HGS, while race/ethnicity was no longer statistically significant. Mean HGS of those who were disabled or on medical leave and those retired was significantly lower than those working full-time. While income levels had no significant relationship in bivariate analyses, multivariable analysis revealed that HGS of responders with income between US$ 70,000 and 100,000, and those with annual income higher than US$ 100,000 were higher by 3lbs. ($p = 0.04$) and 4 lbs. ($p = 0.01$) respectively, in comparison with those earning US$ 50,000 or less. Levels of WTC exposure did not show significant relationship with mean HGS in either bivariate or multivariate analyses.

Subdomain Analyses

On further examination of the PTSD domains (results not shown in table), higher severity of re-experiencing symptoms was significantly associated with lower HGS while all other domains showed no such relationship after controlling for other domains and all other covariates. Increase in re-experiencing score by one point was associated with a decrease in HGS by 0.45 lbs. ($p = 0.0032$); since those with the worst symptom severity have symptom scores 15 or 20 points above those with no symptoms, this translates into substantial and large differences in HGS.

4. Discussion

Lower HGS, after adjusting for sex, is increasingly seen as a biomarker of aging [5,14–17]. Our study similarly revealed that max HGS was associated with older age, supporting this view. Additionally, our study revealed that those with probable WTC-PTSD, with and without concomitant depression had significantly lower maximal HGS than those without either PTSD or depression. Examining individual PCL domain scores revealed that the re-experiencing symptom cluster was specifically associated with HGS, a finding that remained significant even after adjusting for covariates and other PTSD symptoms.

A remarkable finding was that the mean HGS of WTC responders in this study, many of whom were in the law enforcement and are usually shown to have "healthy worker" effects, is not as high as might typically be expected. Based on normative data published by Mathiowetz et al., the mean HGS of adults in the 50–54 year-old age range—the mean age of our sample—was 102–114 lbs. for men and 57–66 lbs. for women [18]. Among respondents to the *Health and Retirement Survey* in 2006–2012, the mean HGS of 55–59-year-old men was 38–43 kg or 84–95 lbs., while it was 22–28 kg or 49–62 lbs. for women [17]. By comparison, the mean HGS was 57.4 lbs. for men and 36.1 lbs. for women in our sample. Unlike our sample, which comprised of responders with varying degrees of exposure to the WTC trauma, both of the aforementioned studies involved civilian populations. Moreover, adjustable-handle Jamar®dynamometer and Smedley®spring-type dynamometer were used as opposed to the Vernier dynamometer used in our study. Future research needs to examine whether lower HGS in our cohort can be attributed to their exposure to the traumatic WTC experiences, and/or due to differences in the instruments used. Our findings should be interpreted with caution, however, as lower HGS among WTC responders may also be attributed to PTSD-related weakness, easy fatigability, and neurasthenia, as evidenced from symptoms experienced by war veterans [19].

Our finding of lower maximal HGS among WTC responders with WTC-related PTSD and depression are along the lines of those reported by Clouston et al. when current PTSD was associated with a two-fold higher risk of functional limitations as indicated by Short Physical Performance Battery (SPPB) scores of 9 or lower [9]. Specifically, current PTSD showed strong adjusted associations with slower walking speeds (<0.8 m/s), slower chair-rise speed (<0.39 rises/s), and balance problems. Previous research by Keller-Ross and colleagues (2014) found that veterans with PTSD have greater fatigability as well as greater fluctuations in force exerted by their handgrip muscles [20]. It is possible that PTSD affects physical functioning and HGS through similar pathways. Furthermore, depending on their mental health and motivation, not all responders may have exerted adequate effort when asked to take the HGS test. However, this concern may have been partially addressed as our analyses took depressive symptoms, in addition to symptoms of PTSD, into consideration. It is notable that of all the PTSD domains, re-experiencing symptoms emerged as most significantly associated with lower HGS. This is comparable to prior work where re-experiencing symptoms were found to be consistently associated with cognitive impairment among WTC responders [8]. Re-experiencing symptoms that include sudden intrusive memories of the traumatic event, nightmares, flashbacks, and other feelings of distress, have been noted to be early markers of mental pathology [21,22]. Findings from our current study suggest that these symptoms can affect individuals both physically and mentally.

Future research may focus on the association between HGS and PTSD symptoms among populations with other traumatic experiences. There is some evidence that resistance training can lead to better cognitive functioning among the elderly through a posited reversal of age-related deterioration of the brain white matter [23,24]. It will be important to complete the clinical picture by examining other trauma-related symptoms, including depression. It might be useful to explore whether HGS improvement may help address some PTSD symptoms, in addition to the existing modes of management. It is also possible that changes in HGS precede changes in PTSD symptoms or higher HGS at baseline protects against psychological symptoms, as similar hypotheses have been postulated for cognitive decline as well. The integrity of white matter has been linked to optimum physical and mental functioning; therefore, the same underlying mechanisms could predispose responders to lower HGS as well as PTSD and depression symptoms.

Limitations

This is the first study to examine HGS in a large sample of WTC responders, and the first to report associations between PTSD and HGS. A key limitation of this study is its cross-sectional nature, limiting our ability to investigate possible reverse causation. Since we found associations between PTSD symptoms measured at program enrollment visits, which occurred on average 8–10 years before HGS was assessed, the potential for reverse causation is greatly reduced. However, the relationship could be bidirectional, and a potential common pathology that predisposes to both PTSD symptoms and muscular weakness might be the most valuable take-away from our study. It is, therefore, critical that future work examine associations between PTSD symptoms and changes to HGS over time. The generalizability of this study to the general population, given that responders in this study are residents of Long Island, NY, with a majority being highly educated White males. The WTC responders were exposed to a very unique event—the 9/11 attacks and its aftermath—which may not result in similar physical exposures and, therefore, concomitant PTSD complexity, severity, or chronicity that is similar to symptoms experienced after other traumatic exposures. This study does not, as well, consider the impact of childhood exposures to stressful events though such events have been found to worsen mental health [25]. Nevertheless, many of the findings among veterans and healthy adults from different countries provide similar overall conclusions.

5. Conclusions

This, to our knowledge, is the first study examining the association of HGS with PTSD with or without coexisting depressive symptoms in a large cohort exposed to a severe traumatic event. Our finding that PTSD symptoms in general, and re-experiencing in particular, are associated with lower HGS fifteen years after a significant traumatic event could have clinical implications in the potential for HGS to be a "biomarker" of aging in the context of severe and chronic PTSD. Furthermore, and similar to prior findings, this points out to the potential for interventions targeting physical strength also having a beneficial effect on responders' mental health, or vice versa.

Author Contributions: The research question was formulated by S.M. and S.C. The study was conceptualized and implemented by S.C. and B.L. Methodology was developed by S.C., E.B., R.K., and B.L. Resources were managed by S.C. and B.L. Data management and data analysis was done by S.M. and S.C. The article was drafted initially by S.M. and the initial draft was revised by S.C., E.B., R.K., and B.L. provided feedback and helped to improve the manuscript. S.M. was responsible for initial submission, making revisions according to comments by the journal editor and reviewers, and for resubmission. S.C., E.B., and B.L. provided inputs for addressing the reviewers' comments and helped in the revision process.

Funding: Funding for this study was provided by the National Institutes of Health (R01 AG049953; PI: Clouston), and by the Centers for Disease Control and Prevention's National Institute of Occupational Safety and Health to administer the monitoring survey and diagnose and treat World Trade Center (WTC)-related diseases (CDC200-2011-39361).

Conflicts of Interest: The authors declare no conflict of interest. The funders had no role in the design of the study; in the collection, analyses, or interpretation of data; in the writing of the manuscript, or in the decision to publish the results.

References

1. Massy-Westropp, N.M.; Gill, T.K.; Taylor, A.W.; Bohannon, R.W.; Hill, C.L. Hand grip strength: Age and gender stratified normative data in a population-based study. *BMC Res. Notes* **2011**, *4*, 127. [CrossRef]
2. Ling, C.H.; Taekema, D.; de Craen, A.J.; Gussekloo, J.; Westendorp, R.G.; Maier, A.B. Handgrip strength and mortality in the oldest old population: The Leiden 85-plus study. *Can. Med. Assoc. J.* **2010**, *182*, 429–435. [CrossRef] [PubMed]
3. Taekema, D.G.; Gussekloo, J.; Maier, A.B.; Westendorp, R.G.; de Craen, A.J. Handgrip strength as a predictor of functional, psychological and social health. A prospective population-based study among the oldest old. *Age Ageing* **2010**, *39*, 331–337. [CrossRef] [PubMed]
4. Fukumori, N.; Yamamoto, Y.; Takegami, M.; Yamazaki, S.; Onishi, Y.; Sekiguchi, M.; Otani, K.; Konno, S.; Kikuchi, S.; Fukuhara, S. Association between hand-grip strength and depressive symptoms: Locomotive syndrome and health outcomes in aizu cohort study (LOHAS). *Age Ageing* **2015**, *44*, 592–598. [CrossRef]
5. Lino, V.T.S.; Rodrigues, N.C.P.; O'Dwyer, G.; de Noronha Andrade, M.K.; Mattos, I.E.; Portela, M.C. Handgrip strength and factors associated in poor elderly assisted at a primary care unit in Rio de Janeiro, Brazil. *PLoS ONE* **2016**, *11*, e0166373. [CrossRef]
6. Firth, J.; Firth, J.A.; Stubbs, B.; Vancampfort, D.; Schuch, F.B.; Hallgren, M.; Veronese, N.; Yung, A.R.; Sarris, J. Association between Muscular Strength and cognition in people with major depression or bipolar disorder and healthy controls. *JAMA Psychiatry* **2018**, *75*, 740–746. [CrossRef]
7. Firth, J.; Stubbs, B.; Vancampfort, D.; Firth, J.A.; Large, M.; Rosenbaum, S.; Hallgren, M.; Ward, P.B.; Sarris, J.; Yung, A.R. Grip strength is associated with cognitive performance in schizophrenia and the general population: A UK biobank study of 476,559 participants. *Schizophr. Bull.* **2018**, *44*, 728–736. [CrossRef] [PubMed]
8. Clouston, S.A.; Kotov, R.; Pietrzak, R.H.; Luft, B.J.; Gonzalez, A.; Richards, M.; Ruggero, C.J.; Spiro, A., III; Bromet, E.J. Cognitive impairment among world trade center responders: Long-term implications of re-experiencing the 9/11 terrorist attacks. *Alzheimers Dement.* **2016**, *4*, 67–75. [CrossRef] [PubMed]
9. Clouston, S.A.; Guralnik, J.M.; Kotov, R.; Bromet, E.J.; Luft, B.J. Functional limitations among responders to the world trade center attacks 14 years after the disaster: Implications of chronic posttraumatic stress disorder. *J. Trauma. Stress* **2017**, *30*, 443–452. [CrossRef] [PubMed]
10. Dasaro, C.R.; Holden, W.L.; Berman, K.D.; Crane, M.A.; Kaplan, J.R.; Lucchini, R.G.; Luft, B.J.; Moline, J.M.; Teitelbaum, S.L.; Tirunagari, U.S.; et al. Cohort profile: World trade center health program general responder cohort. *Int. J. Epidemiol.* **2015**, *46*, e9. [CrossRef] [PubMed]
11. Blanchard, E.B.; Jones-Alexander, J.; Buckley, T.C.; Forneris, C.A. Psychometric properties of the PTSD Checklist (PCL). *Behav. Res. Ther.* **1996**, *34*, 669–673. [CrossRef]
12. Wilkins, K.C.; Lang, A.J.; Norman, S.B. Synthesis of the psychometric properties of the PTSD checklist (PCL) military, civilian, and specific versions. *Depress. Anxiety* **2011**, *28*, 596–605. [CrossRef]
13. Wisnivesky, J.P.; Teitelbaum, S.L.; Todd, A.C.; Boffetta, P.; Crane, M.; Crowley, L.; de la Hoz, R.E.; Dellenbaugh, C.; Harrison, D.; Herbert, R.; et al. Persistence of multiple illnesses in world trade center rescue and recovery workers: A cohort study. *Lancet* **2011**, *378*, 888–897. [CrossRef]
14. Koopman, J.J.; van Bodegom, D.; van Heemst, D.; Westendorp, R.G. Handgrip strength, ageing and mortality in rural Africa. *Age Ageing* **2015**, *44*, 465–470. [CrossRef] [PubMed]
15. Ong, H.L.; Abdin, E.; Chua, B.Y.; Zhang, Y.; Seow, E.; Vaingankar, J.A.; Chong, S.A.; Subramaniam, M. Hand-grip strength among older adults in Singapore: A comparison with international norms and associative factors. *BMC Geriatr.* **2017**, *17*, 176. [CrossRef] [PubMed]
16. Hamasaki, H.; Kawashima, Y.; Katsuyama, H.; Sako, A.; Goto, A.; Yanai, H. Association of handgrip strength with hospitalization, cardiovascular events, and mortality in Japanese patients with type 2 diabetes. *Sci. Rep.* **2017**, *7*, 7041. [CrossRef] [PubMed]
17. Sanderson, W.C.; Scherbov, S. Measuring the speed of aging across population subgroups. *PLoS ONE* **2014**, *9*, e96289. [CrossRef] [PubMed]

18. Mathiowetz, V.; Kashman, N.; Volland, G.; Weber, K.; Dowe, M.; Rogers, S. Grip and pinch strength: Normative data for adults. *Arch. Phys. Med. Rehabil.* **1985**, *66*, 69–74. [PubMed]

19. Hyams, K.C.; Wignall, F.S.; Roswell, R. War syndromes and their evaluation: From the US civil war to the Persian gulf war. *Ann. Intern. Med.* **1996**, *125*, 398–405. [CrossRef] [PubMed]

20. Keller-Ross, M.L.; Schlinder-Delap, B.; Doyel, R.; Larson, G.; Hunter, S.K. Muscle fatigability and control of force in men with posttraumatic stress disorder. *Med. Sci. Sports Exerc.* **2014**, *46*, 1302–1313. [CrossRef]

21. Chaudieu, I.; Norton, J.; Ritchie, K.; Birmes, P.; Vaiva, G.; Ancelin, M.L. Late-life health consequences of exposure to trauma in a general elderly population: The mediating role of reexperiencing posttraumatic symptoms. *J. Clin. Psychiatry* **2011**, *72*, 929–935. [CrossRef] [PubMed]

22. Lawrence-Wood, E.; Van Hooff, M.; Baur, J.; McFarlane, A.C. Re-experiencing phenomena following a disaster: The long-term predictive role of intrusion symptoms in the development of post-trauma depression and anxiety. *J. Affect. Disord.* **2016**, *190*, 278–281. [CrossRef] [PubMed]

23. Cassilhas, R.C.; Viana, V.A.; Grassmann, V.; Santos, R.T.; Santos, R.F.; Tufik, S.; Mello, M.T. The impact of resistance exercise on the cognitive function of the elderly. *Med. Sci. Sports Exerc.* **2007**, *39*, 401–1407. [CrossRef] [PubMed]

24. Suo, C.; Singh, M.F.; Gates, N.; Wen, W.; Sachdev, P.; Brodaty, H.; Saigal, N.; Wilson, G.C.; Meikeljohn, J.; Singh, N.; et al. Therapeutically relevant structural and functional mechanisms triggered by physical and cognitive exercise. *Mol. Psychiatry* **2016**, *21*, 1633–1642. [CrossRef]

25. Mukherjee, S.; Clouston, S.; Bromet, E.; Leibowitz, G.S.; Scott, S.B.; Bernard, K.; Kotov, R.; Luft, B.J. Past experiences of getting bulled and assaulted and posttraumatic stress disorder (PTSD) after a severe traumatic event in adulthood: A study of World Trade Center (WTC) responders. *J. Aggress. Maltreat. Trauma* **2019**, 1–19. [CrossRef]

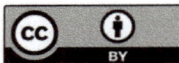

International Journal of
*Environmental Research
and Public Health*

MDPI

Article

Impact of Health on Early Retirement and Post-Retirement Income Loss among Survivors of the 11 September 2001 World Trade Center Disaster

Shengchao Yu *, Kacie Seil and Junaid Maqsood

World Trade Center Health Registry, Division of Epidemiology, New York City Department of Health and Mental Hygiene, New York, NY 10013, USA; kseil@health.nyc.gov (K.S.); jmaqsood1@health.nyc.gov (J.M.)
* Correspondence: syu@health.nyc.gov; Tel.: +1-646-632-6668

Received: 28 February 2019; Accepted: 29 March 2019; Published: 2 April 2019

Abstract: The health consequences of the 9/11 World Trade Center (WTC) terrorist attacks are well documented, but few studies have assessed the disaster's impact on employment among individuals exposed to the disaster. We examined the association between 9/11-related health conditions and early retirement among residents and workers who resided and/or worked near the WTC site on 9/11, and the association between such conditions and post-retirement income loss. The study included 6377 residents and/or area workers who completed the WTC Health Registry longitudinal health surveys in 2003–2004 and 2006–2007, and the 2017–2018 Health and Employment Survey. Logistic regression models were used to examine the associations. We found that 9/11-related health conditions were significantly associated with the likelihood of early retirement. Residents and/or area workers with more physical health conditions, especially when comorbid with posttraumatic stress disorder (PTSD), were more likely to retire before age 60 than those with no conditions. For retirees, having PTSD or PTSD comorbid with any number of physical conditions increased the odds of reporting substantial post-retirement income loss. Disaster-related outcomes can negatively impact aging individuals in the form of early retirement and income loss. Long-term effects of major disasters must continue to be studied.

Keywords: 9/11 impact; retirement; chronic disease; PTSD; disaster; income loss

1. Introduction

Many studies have documented the short-term health impacts of the World Trade Center (WTC) 11 September 2001 attacks, while longer-term observations of various chronic physical and mental health conditions continue to be reported among individuals exposed to the disaster [1–3]. However, relatively few studies have assessed the economic impact of the 9/11 attacks. It was noted that New York City (NYC) earnings at an aggregate level had $2.8 billion losses in the first three months post-9/11 [4]. For NYC industries, losses ranged from $3.6 to $6.4 billion in the nine months following the disaster [5]. Despite the well-established association between disaster exposure and impaired health among the 9/11-exposed population, few studies have examined the economic impact of 9/11-related poor health. One such study found that during the seven years after 9/11, nearly half of accidental disability retirements for NYC firefighters were for 9/11-related injuries or illnesses [6]. Another study conducted by the WTC Health Registry found a significant association between 9/11-related poor health and early retirement or job loss [7].

Unlike our first published work that focused on the 9/11 economic impact for non-uniformed rescue and recovery workers [7], this analysis concentrated on retirement and post-retirement well-being for residents and area workers who resided and/or worked near the WTC site on 9/11. Previous research showed that different groups of survivors, such as rescue and recovery workers, local residents, area workers, passersby, and students and school staff, may have had different health outcomes, both physical and mental, due to their varying levels of disaster exposure [1,8,9]. Consequently, health-related retirement may also differ for different groups of survivors. Furthermore, retirement options available to rescue and recovery workers, especially uniformed workers, as compared to residents and area workers, can be a key factor in making retirement decisions and must be linked to the subsequent economic outcome [10–13].

Retirement trends were shifting during the mid-1990s into the 2000s irrespective of the effects of the 9/11 disaster, as fewer people were retiring at younger ages compared to the 1970s and 1980s [14]. Trends of employer pension plans becoming rarer, a healthier population overall, fewer labor-intensive jobs, less employer-sponsored health benefits for retirees under age 65, and an older full retirement age for Social Security have resulted in people retiring at older ages than earlier generations [15]. In tandem, retirement patterns have become more complex with many individuals transitioning from full-time to part-time work or working again after retirement [15]. Early retirement, therefore, is an important factor to consider for economic assessments, as it can strongly affect one's well-being (such as post-retirement income) for the remainder of one's life.

Poor health has been linked to early retirement in numerous studies for different population groups or countries. Self-perceived poor health was a risk factor for early exit from the labor force through early retirement, unemployment, or both [16–20]. Other studies found an association between a variety of health conditions, such as respiratory, cardiovascular, musculoskeletal diseases, cancer, and other chronic conditions, and premature labor force exit [16,17,19,21–23]. However, health problems are not the only factor that impacts decisions about early retirement; one's financial situation is another key factor in this decision-making process [24,25]. Experiencing a layoff or having a spouse who retires early increases one's likelihood of retiring early whereas being able to take a new job that requires fewer hours or offers higher pay is protective against retiring early [26]. Multiple studies have concluded, however, that health, even a subjective assessment of health, is the most important predictor of early retirement [24–26].

Previous studies of 9/11 health impact showed elevated prevalence of many chronic physical conditions, posttraumatic stress disorder (PTSD), and physical-mental comorbidity among disaster survivors [1,9,27–32]. We examined 9/11-related health conditions and PTSD comorbidity in the current analysis of health's impact on early retirement. We also went one step further and assessed whether or not those physically and/or mentally affected by the disaster continued to experience decline in their well-being after retirement in terms of substantial income loss.

In 2017–2018, the WTC Health Registry conducted an in-depth study on health and employment for a sub-sample of its enrollees. Detailed information on employment, retirement, health insurance, and other economic indicators collected from this survey, coupled with detailed health data collected from the Registry's longitudinal surveys administered in waves since 2003, provided an opportunity to further investigate the impact of 9/11-related health on retirement and post-retirement well-being. As in our previous study [7], the number of 9/11-related chronic physical health conditions and PTSD were used to measure post-9/11 health status. We hypothesized that the more 9/11-related health conditions an individual had, the more likely he or she would be to retire before age 60. Furthermore, for those who had already retired, the number of post-9/11 conditions they suffered was associated with the degree of their post-retirement income loss.

2. Materials and Methods

2.1. Study Population

The WTC Health Registry maintains a longitudinal cohort that was established in 2002 following the 11 September 2001 terrorist attacks with the aim of monitoring the long-term health outcomes in individuals exposed to the events of 9/11 in NYC. In 2003–2004, the Registry enrolled 71,426 rescue or recovery workers, Lower Manhattan residents, area workers, passersby, and students or school staff by conducting its first health survey (Wave 1). Eligible enrollees have since been invited to participate in three additional health surveys in 2006–2007 (Wave 2), 2011–2012 (Wave 3), and 2015–2016 (Wave 4) as well as a number of in-depth studies. Previous Registry publications provide a more detailed description of this cohort [1,8].

From September 2017 to March 2018, the Registry conducted the Health and Employment Survey (HES) with a sample pool of English-speaking enrollees under 75 years of age (as of 2017) who completed at least Waves 1 and 2. Enrollees who reported retirement or unemployment due to disability/health at any of the three follow-up surveys (Waves 2–4) were invited to participate in the HES study along with a roughly equivalent number of not-yet retired age-matched enrollees. In total, 23,036 enrollees were invited to complete the HES, and the response rate reached 65%. The US Centers for Disease Control and Prevention (3793) and the NYC Department of Health and Mental Hygiene (02058) institutional review boards approved the Registry protocol and the HES protocol (17047), including the use of the data.

This study used data collected from the HES and was limited to those who lived or worked near the WTC site on 11 September 2001. During analyses, the HES data were merged with the Registry's four waves of health survey data to obtain 9/11-related health information for the study sample. We excluded 341 enrollees who had retired before the 9/11 disaster, as our focus was on the link between 9/11-related health and retirement. The final study sample was 6377 enrollees, which included 3486 retired and 2891 not-yet-retired enrollees. Of the 3486 retirees, 1234 retired before age 60, 2143 retired at or after age 60, and 109 did not report time of retirement. Additionally, 2395 enrollees reported post-retirement income loss.

2.2. Study Outcomes: Early Retirement and Post-Retirement Income Loss

In the HES, enrollees were asked if they were currently retired and, if retired, for the month and year of retirement. This information was used to calculate retirement age. In the analytical model, a dichotomous outcome variable was created for early retirement which was defined as having retired before reaching the age of 60.

Those self-reporting retirement in the HES were also asked if their total post-retirement personal income after taxes changed as compared to pre-retirement and in which direction; if they responded that their income had decreased, a follow-up question asked for the percentage of decrease (<25%, 25% to 50%, >50%). A dichotomous outcome variable for post-retirement income loss was created for those who reported substantial income loss which was defined as having over 50% of income decrease.

2.3. Chronic Physical Health Conditions and PTSD Measure

Starting in Wave 1, Registry enrollees were asked in each of the follow-up wave surveys whether they had ever been told by a doctor or other health professional that they had any of more than a dozen listed health conditions and the year of first diagnosis if diagnosed. For this study, asthma, heart disease (coronary heart disease, angina, heart attack, or other heart disease), stroke, lung disease (emphysema, chronic bronchitis, reactive airways dysfunction syndrome, sarcoidosis, pulmonary fibrosis, or other lung disease), diabetes, gastroesophageal reflux disease, and autoimmune disease (multiple sclerosis or amyotrophic lateral sclerosis, rheumatoid arthritis, or other autoimmune disease) were selected, as all have been reported to be elevated among 9/11 exposed individuals [27,33–39]. If an enrollee reported a diagnosis for any of the seven selected types of conditions in or after 2001, we categorized them as having a 9/11-related chronic physical health condition. Probable PTSD was assessed at every wave of the Registry survey via a 9/11-specific PTSD Checklist-Civilian Version (PCL-17) scale. A cut-off score of 44 or greater at any wave was used to define probable PTSD as in prior published Registry studies [1]. Co-occurrence of any of the seven selected types of physical conditions and probable PTSD was then defined as 9/11-related physical–mental comorbidity in this study.

The total number of chronic physical conditions, comorbid with PTSD or not, was used as the health indicator in the analytical models.

2.4. Sociodemographic Characteristics and Other Covariate Measures

Sociodemographic characteristics of the study sample were measured by sex, age at 11 September 2001, race/ethnicity, household income, education, and marital status. A quantitative 9/11 exposure measure was also included in the analysis as it is closely associated with PTSD [1]. The exposure measure combines disaster information, such as dust cloud exposure, injury, witnessing horror, bereavement, and home evacuation experience, collected from both Waves 1 and 2 into a 12-item score that was collapsed into four categories: 0–1 as no/low exposure, 2–3 as medium, 4–5 as high, and six or greater as very high exposure.

2.5. Statistical Analyses

Two logistic regression models were used to calculate the adjusted odds ratio (AOR) and 95% confidence intervals (95% CI) to measure the association between 9/11-related health conditions and our study outcomes. The equation for these models is

$$\text{logit}(p) = \ln\left(\frac{p}{1-p}\right) = \beta_0 + \beta_1 X_1 + \beta_2 X_2 + \cdots + \beta_k X_k \tag{1}$$

where p is the probability of our outcome occurring, β_0 is the intercept, $\beta_1, \ldots, \beta_k$ are the regression coefficients, and $X_1, \ldots, X_k$ are the predictors or covariates included in the model (described above). The adjusted odds ratio was estimated by taking the exponential of the regression coefficients in the model.

The first model included 4125 non-retired enrollees and early retirees, and aimed to demonstrate the relationship between poor health (measured by the number of 9/11-related health conditions with and without PTSD) and the likelihood of retiring before age 60, while adjusting for sociodemographic factors and disaster exposure.

The second model included 2395 enrollees who reported income loss after retirement and investigated the association between 9/11-related health conditions and substantial post-retirement income loss while adjusting for disaster exposure and all sociodemographic characteristics included in the first model except for age at 11 September 2001. Even though post-retirement income decreases are common and subject to lower tax rates and less work-related expenses [40], this analysis aimed to reveal that substantial income decrease (percentage of decrease larger than 50%) was associated with health.

The analyses for this study were conducted in SAS version 9.4 (SAS Institute Inc., Cary, NC, USA).

3. Results

Among 4125 residents and area workers who lived or worked near the WTC site on 9/11, 1234 (29.9%) reported having retired before age 60 (Table 1). Sociodemographic characteristics that were significantly associated with early retirement included age, race/ethnicity, total household income, marital status, and education. Not surprisingly, younger enrollees were less likely to report that they had retired under age 60, as they may have not yet retired at all. Compared to non-Hispanic white residents and area workers, non-Hispanic black and Hispanic residents and area workers both had higher odds of reporting early retirement (AOR = 1.7, 95% CI: 1.3–2.1; AOR = 1.3, 95% CI: 1.0–1.7). Enrollees who were in the three higher household income groups ($50,000–<$75,000, $75,000–<$150,000, and ≥$150,000) each had higher likelihoods of experiencing early retirement. Those in the highest income group (≥$150,000) were more than twice as likely as those in the lowest income group (<$25,000) to have early retirement (AOR = 2.2, 95% CI: 1.5–3.2). On the contrary, the likelihood of reporting early retirement dropped by about 40% (AOR = 0.6, 95% CI: 0.4–0.7) and 70% (AOR = 0.3, 95% CI: 0.3–0.4), respectively, for those with a college or post-graduate degree compared to those with high school and below education. Enrollees who were widowed had a higher likelihood of experiencing early retirement compared to those who were married or living with a partner (AOR =

1.5, 95% CI: 1.0–2.3). Sex and 9/11-related disaster exposure did not show significant association with early retirement for residents and area workers.

Table 1. Early retirement, chronic physical health conditions and post-traumatic stress disorder (PTSD) comorbidity, and other characteristics among non-retired and early retired enrollees.

Sample Characteristics	Retirement Status				Likelihood of Early Retirement	
	Not Retired (N, %)		Retired Early (N, %)		AOR [a]	95% CI [b]
	2891	70.1	1234	29.9		
Sex						
Female	1481	68.1	693	31.9	Ref	
Male	1410	72.3	541	27.7	1.0	0.8, 1.1
Age on 9/11						
0–24	31	93.9	2	6.1	0.1	0.0, 0.6
25–44	1089	79.1	287	20.9	0.5	0.4, 0.6
45–64	1771	65.2	945	34.8	Ref	
Race/ethnicity						
Non-Hispanic white	2085	72.1	805	27.9	Ref	
Non-Hispanic black	304	59.3	209	40.7	1.7	1.3, 2.1
Hispanic	253	64.4	140	35.6	1.3	1.0, 1.7
Non-Hispanic Asian	155	77.9	44	22.1	0.9	0.6, 1.3
Other race or multi-racial	94	72.3	36	27.7	0.9	0.6, 1.4
Total household income in 2002, $						
<25,000	167	72.3	64	27.7	Ref	
25,000 to <50,000	473	70.0	203	30.0	1.1	0.8, 1.6
50,000 to <75,000	477	68.3	221	31.7	1.6	1.1, 2.3
75,000 to <150,000	924	71.2	373	28.8	1.6	1.1, 2.3
≥150,000	564	71.4	226	28.6	2.2	1.5, 3.2
Education						
High school diploma or lower	335	54.1	284	45.9	Ref	
Some college or college graduate	1583	70.0	677	30.0	0.6	0.4, 0.7
Post-graduate	964	78.2	268	21.8	0.3	0.3, 0.4
Marital status						
Married or Living with partner	1852	69.8	803	30.2	Ref	
Divorced or separated	415	69.5	182	30.5	0.9	0.7, 1.1
Widowed	57	53.8	49	46.2	1.5	1.0, 2.3
Never married	552	74.1	193	25.9	0.9	0.7, 1.2
Disaster exposure						
Low/none	630	70.6	262	29.4	Ref	
Medium	1264	70.9	520	29.1	0.9	0.8, 1.1
High	784	70.8	323	29.2	0.8	0.7, 1.1
Very high	213	62.3	129	37.7	1.1	0.8, 1.5
Number of chronic conditions [c] without PTSD						
0	1289	76.8	390	23.2	Ref	
1	527	68.7	240	31.3	1.5	1.2, 1.8
2	193	67.2	94	32.8	1.4	1.1, 1.9
≥3	61	59.8	41	40.2	1.9	1.2, 3.0
Number of chronic conditions [c] with PTSD						
0	324	73.6	116	26.4	1.2	0.9, 1.6
1	238	65.2	127	34.8	1.7	1.3, 2.2
2	153	57.1	115	42.9	2.5	1.9, 3.4
≥3	106	48.8	111	51.2	3.4	2.4, 4.7

[a] AOR: Adjusted odds ratio and was adjusted for all factors listed in this table. [b] 95% CI: 95% confidence interval. [c] Chronic physical health conditions include asthma, heart diseases, stroke, lung diseases, diabetes, gastroesophageal reflux disease (GERD), and autoimmune diseases.

Having chronic 9/11-related physical health conditions without PTSD was found to be significantly associated with early retirement in a dose-response manner with the odds of reporting early retirement increasing as the number of conditions increased (AOR = 1.5, 95% CI: 1.2–1.8; AOR = 1.4, 95% CI: 1.1–1.9; AOR = 1.9, 95% CI: 1.2–3.0 for those with one, two, and three or more conditions without PTSD, respectively) (Table 1). When chronic physical conditions were comorbid with PTSD, the likelihood of experiencing early retirement increased further and also in a dose-response manner. For example, for residents or area workers who had three or more 9/11-related physical conditions and PTSD, their odds of reporting early retirement were more than three times higher than those who did not have any of the selected conditions or PTSD (AOR = 3.4, 95% CI: 2.4–4.7). Interestingly, having PTSD alone did not significantly increase one's odds of early retirement as compared to those who did not have any physical conditions (AOR = 1.2, 95% CI: 0.9–1.6). To test the robustness of the association of 9/11-related health and early retirement, we performed a sensitivity analysis using an Ordinary Least Squares model by replacing the dichotomous early retirement outcome variable with a continuous variable measuring actual age at retirement. Our results showed findings consistent with the early retirement model results: The coefficients for enrollees who suffered one, two, or three or more physical conditions comorbid with PTSD (coefficients = −1.82, −2.89, and −2.92, respectively, and all with $p < 0.0001$) were all significant with the retirement age decreasing by an average of two to three years compared to those who did not have any 9/11-related chronic conditions (results not shown).

Approximately 73% of retirees in the study sample reported that their post-retirement income had decreased as compared to their pre-retirement income, while 19% reported no significant income changes, and 8% reported increased post-retirement income. Although post-retirement income loss seemed to be a norm for retirees regardless of their retirement age, among those who reported decreased income, a significantly higher proportion (45.9% vs. 33.7% in Table 2) of early retirees reported an income decrease of more than 50% ($p < 0.0001$). Because of the significant association of 9/11-related poor health and early retirement demonstrated in Table 1, we further tested if 9/11-related poor health was directly linked to retirees' post-retirement financial status.

Table 2. Percentage of post-retirement income loss among retirees reporting decreased income.

Retirement Age (Years)	Post-Retirement Income Loss, %		Total, N
	≤50% (N = 1437)	>50% (N = 889)	2326
<60	54.1	45.9	859
≥60	66.3	33.7	1467

Table 3 presents results on the association between 9/11-related health and the likelihood of having more than 50% of income decrease after retirement among enrollees who reported decreased income. Only three sociodemographic characteristics were associated with substantial post-retirement income loss: race/ethnicity, total household income, and education. More specifically, non-Hispanic black residents and area workers were 30% less likely to report income loss greater than 50% as compared to non-Hispanic white residents and area workers (AOR = 0.7, 95% CI: 0.6–1.0). Other racial/ethnic groups did not show significantly higher or lower odds of experiencing substantial income loss compared to non-Hispanic whites. Compared to the lowest income group (<$25,000), the three middle income groups ($25,000–<$50,000, $50,000–<$75,000, and $75,000–<$150,000) were less likely to have substantial income loss (AOR = 0.5, 95% CI: 0.3–0.8; AOR = 0.6, 95% CI: 0.3–0.9; AOR = 0.6, 95% CI: 0.4–1.0, respectively); however, the highest income group (≥$150,000) did not show significantly higher or lower odds of experiencing substantial income loss. Enrollees with some college experience or a college degree had a significantly higher likelihood of substantial income loss compared to enrollees with lower education attainment (AOR = 1.2, 95% CI: 1.0–1.6). Each level of 9/11-related disaster exposure was highly associated with post-retirement income loss in a dose-response manner. The highest level of exposure increased the odds of having substantial income loss by 2.5 times compared to those with little or no exposure (AOR = 2.5, 95% CI: 1.7–3.6).

Table 3. Post-retirement income loss, chronic physical health conditions and post-traumatic stress disorder (PTSD) comorbidity, and other characteristics among retirees reporting decreased income.

Sample Characteristics	Post-Retirement Income Loss more than 50%				Likelihood of Substantial Income Loss	
	No (N, %)		Yes (N, %)		AOR [a]	95% CI [b]
	1469	61.3	926	38.7		
Sex						
Female	787	63.3	456	36.7	Ref	
Male	682	59.2	470	40.8	1.0	0.8, 1.2
Race/ethnicity						
Non-Hispanic white	990	59.1	685	40.9	Ref	
Non-Hispanic black	234	69.6	102	30.4	0.7	0.6, 1.0
Hispanic	145	66.5	73	33.5	0.8	0.5, 1.1
Non-Hispanic Asian	57	58.8	40	41.2	1.1	0.7, 1.7
Other race or multi-racial	43	62.3	26	37.7	1.0	0.5, 1.7
Total household income in 2002, $						
<25,000	46	47.9	50	52.1	Ref	
25,000 to <50,000	255	68.5	117	31.5	0.5	0.3, 0.8
50,000 to <75,000	280	67.3	136	32.7	0.6	0.3, 0.9
75,000 to <150,000	499	64.4	276	35.6	0.6	0.4, 1.0
≥150,000	226	48.3	242	51.7	1.3	0.8, 2.1
Education						
High school diploma or lower	299	65.9	155	34.1	Ref	
Some college or college graduate	780	60.0	521	40.0	1.2	1.0, 1.6
Post-graduate	380	60.8	245	39.2	1.0	0.8, 1.4
Marital status						
Married or living with partner	961	60.7	623	39.3	Ref	
Divorced or separated	236	59.9	158	40.1	1.2	0.9, 1.6
Widowed	66	71.0	27	29.0	0.7	0.4, 1.1
Never married	195	63.1	114	36.9	1.0	0.8, 1.4
Disaster exposure						
Low/none	362	71.7	143	28.3	Ref	
Medium	653	63.6	373	36.4	1.4	1.0, 1.7
High	360	55.8	285	44.2	1.7	1.2, 2.2
Very high	94	42.9	125	57.1	2.5	1.7, 3.6
Number of chronic conditions [c] without PTSD						
0	546	65.7	285	34.3	Ref	
1	316	64.6	173	35.4	1.1	0.9, 1.5
2	129	68.6	59	31.4	0.9	0.6, 1.3
≥3	59	62.8	35	37.2	1.4	0.9, 2.2
Number of chronic conditions [c] with PTSD						
0	118	53.2	104	46.8	1.7	1.2, 2.5
1	114	53.0	101	47.0	1.8	1.2, 2.5
2	104	55.9	82	44.1	1.6	1.1, 2.3
≥3	83	48.8	87	51.2	1.9	1.3, 2.7

[a] AOR: Adjusted odds ratio and was adjusted for all factors listed in this table. [b] 95% CI: 95% confidence interval. [c] Chronic physical health conditions include asthma, heart diseases, stroke, lung diseases, diabetes, gastroesophageal reflux disease (GERD), and autoimmune diseases.

Substantial post-retirement income loss was also significantly associated with the number of 9/11-related health conditions but only for those who suffered from PTSD alone or PTSD comorbid with physical conditions. In other words, enrollees without PTSD who only had chronic physical health conditions did not have higher odds of losing more than 50% of their income post-retirement compared to those who had no health conditions. Once enrollees had PTSD, their likelihood of having substantial income loss increased significantly as compared to those without any health conditions (e.g., AOR = 1.7, 95% CI: 1.2–2.5). PTSD comorbid with one or more physical health conditions had a similar effect on enrollees' odds of experiencing substantial income loss as PTSD alone.

4. Discussion

The impact of the 9/11 disaster on early retirement and post-retirement well-being among survivors has rarely been studied until now. This study examined the association of 9/11-related health and early retirement for residents and area workers who resided and/or worked near the WTC site on 9/11. Furthermore, we assessed the longer-term impact of 9/11-related health on post-retirement income loss among survivors.

Sixteen years after the 9/11 disaster, among the 3486 retired residents and area workers in our study sample, about 35% had retired before reaching 60 years of age. Early retirement was found to be significantly associated with chronic 9/11-related physical health conditions in a dose-response manner, and a sensitivity analysis estimating the magnitudes of the effects in terms of years of work lost found consistent results. More specifically, the likelihood of reporting early retirement versus not-yet retired grew as the number of physical health conditions increased. The odds of reporting early retirement increased further when these conditions were comorbid with PTSD but not when PTSD was reported in the absence of any 9/11-related physical conditions. These findings suggest that residents or area workers who suffered from 9/11-related PTSD but not other chronic physical conditions were not more likely to retire early due to this mental health condition alone; several explanations may clarify this. One reason is that PTSD may not severely impact daily working life, especially if the PTSD is mild. Only 6% of the early retirees in this study sample reported having Accidental Disability Retirement (ADR), a benefit available to members of certain plans if they become permanently physically or mentally incapacitated and are unable to perform the duties of their job due to an accident that took place on the job [41]. The percentage of early retirees with ADR and PTSD but no other chronic condition is even lower (4%), which suggests the proportion of enrollees with severe PTSD alone is low. Another potential reason is that stigma associated with a mental health condition such as PTSD may prevent one from recognizing the condition, let alone coping with it by retiring early.

Despite the fact that PTSD alone did not show a significant association with reporting early retirement, this study found that residents and area workers with PTSD alone or PTSD comorbid with any number of physical conditions were significantly more likely to experience substantial income loss post-retirement. PTSD comorbid with one or more physical health conditions had a similar effect, in terms of significance and magnitude, on the odds of experiencing substantial income loss as PTSD alone. Having any number of physical conditions (including three or more conditions) in the absence of PTSD was not significantly associated with substantial post-retirement income loss, which suggests PTSD is the key and driving factor in this association. The economic impact of 9/11-related PTSD, although not directly reflected in the form of early retirement, tended to be stronger in the long-term as individuals suffering PTSD were less likely to assume income-generating activities that could ultimately lead to significant income loss. Like having PTSD alone, disaster exposure did not show a significant association with early retirement but was highly related to post-retirement income loss. The absence of exposure's effect in the model for early retirement is likely a result of having the 9/11-related health measure in the same model absorbing its effect. We re-ran our model for Table 1 without the health measure and found that disaster exposure at a very high level was significantly associated with 50% higher likelihood of early retirement (AOR = 1.5, 95% CI: 1.1–2.0, results not shown) compared to those who had low or no exposure during the disaster. This finding implies that the health measure we chose for this study represented the impact of this disaster well. A closer look at the data suggested that enrollees in the highest category of the 9/11 exposure scale were most likely to have suffered PTSD or PTSD comorbid with physical health conditions (results not shown) which made their comparable associations with the two outcomes unsurprising.

Similar to the findings in our earlier study [7], those with higher household income or lower education were more likely to report early retirement than staying in the labor force as compared to the low income group or higher education achievers. This seemingly contradictory impact of high income and low education reflects the complexity of the retirement decision-making process.

For residents and area workers with 9/11-related poor health, having a higher income may have allowed them to voluntarily retire early or made them more likely to afford early retirement without considerable additional financial concern compared to having a lower income. On the other hand, the early retirement decision for the lower education group was less likely to be a "choice", as their low education (usually accompanied with low income) and poor health may not have allowed them to maintain their work, especially when the work was more physical or manual in nature. The association of lower socioeconomic status and higher risk of involuntary labor force exit was also found in previous studies [42,43].

This study provided evidence of a strong association between 9/11-related poor health and early retirement among survivors who lived and worked near the WTC site. Furthermore, with additional information collected from the HES, we demonstrated, for the first time, the significant impact of 9/11-related PTSD and 9/11-related physical–mental comorbidity on substantial post-retirement income loss. Our findings suggest that after labor force exit, poor health, especially PTSD, continued to adversely affect survivors' overall well-being in the form of considerable income reduction. The compromised post-retirement well-being as a result of poor health did not come as a surprise because many of the affected people could have involuntarily experienced early retirement before securing their full retirement benefits; or, they might be less likely to participate in any income-generating activities, particularly if they experienced mental health or physical–mental comorbidity issues after retirement. This lasting effect of poor health, along with the fact that certain race/ethnicity (Hispanic and non-Hispanic black) and low education groups are more likely to retire early, should direct future 9/11-related resources by placing a greater focus on limiting sharp income loss and providing adequate and affordable health care services to retirees from various vulnerable groups to maintain a certain level of quality of life.

One notable advantage of this study is that we directly assessed the relationship between 9/11-related health and post-retirement income loss using statistical modeling. This investigation provides the first look at one aspect of survivors' well-being beyond retirement and will lead to additional exploration of the economic impact of 9/11, such as the relationship between substantial income loss and worsening health and its associated high medical cost, poor health reducing survivors' ability to re-enter the workforce to compensate for post-retirement income loss, and how survivors' retirement plans directly affect their post-retirement well-being. In addition, future research should also assess other aspects of post-retirement well-being such as retirees' current health status or health-related quality of life (as in an ongoing study by our group) and insurance coverage. These results will not only give us a broader picture of retirees' overall well-being but also help estimate the realistic gap on health care access in terms of making policy recommendations.

5. Conclusions

This study found that 9/11-related health conditions were significantly associated with the likelihood of early retirement among residents and area workers who survived the 9/11 attacks. The likelihood of reporting early retirement increased as the number of health conditions increased. Having PTSD alone was not associated with early retirement; however, PTSD was the driving factor out of all 9/11-related health conditions studied that was linked to substantial income loss post-retirement. For future studies of 9/11 economic impact, our findings emphasize the key role that PTSD may play in the longer-term.

Author Contributions: Conceptualization, S.Y. and K.S.; Methodology, S.Y. and K.S.; Formal Analysis, S.Y., K.S., and J.M.; Writing—Original Draft Preparation, S.Y.; Writing—Review and Editing, S.Y., K.S., and J.M.; Supervision, S.Y.; Project Administration, S.Y.

Funding: This work was supported by Cooperative Agreement Numbers 2U50/OH009739 and 5U50/OH009739 from the National Institute for Occupational Safety and Health (NIOSH) of the Centers for Disease Control and Prevention (CDC); U50/ATU272750 from the Agency for Toxic Substances and Disease Registry (ATSDR), CDC, which included support from the National Center for Environmental Health, CDC; and by the New York City Department of Health and Mental Hygiene (NYC DOHMH). Its contents are solely the responsibility of the authors and do not necessarily represent the official views of NIOSH, CDC, or the Department of Health and Human Services.

Conflicts of Interest: The authors declare no conflict of interest. The funders had no role in the design of the study; in the collection, analysis, or interpretation of data; in the writing of the manuscript, or in the decision to publish the results.

References

1. Brackbill, R.M.; Hadler, J.L.; DiGrande, L.; Ekenga, C.C.; Farfel, M.R.; Friedman, S.; Perlman, S.E.; Stellman, S.D.; Walker, D.J.; Wu, D.; et al. Asthma and posttraumatic stress symptoms 5 to 6 years following exposure to the world trade center terrorist attack. *JAMA* **2009**, *302*, 502–516. [CrossRef]

2. Jordan, H.T.; Stellman, S.D.; Morabia, A.; Miller-Archie, S.A.; Alper, H.; Laskaris, Z.; Brackbill, R.M.; Cone, J.E. Cardiovascular disease hospitalizations in relation to exposure to the 11 September 2001 world trade center disaster and posttraumatic stress disorder. *J. Am. Heart Assoc.* **2013**, *2*, e000431. [CrossRef]

3. Boffetta, P.; Zeig-Owens, R.; Wallenstein, S.; Li, J.; Brackbill, R.; Cone, J.; Farfel, M.; Holden, W.; Lucchini, R.; Webber, M.P.; et al. Cancer in world trade center responders: Findings from multiple cohorts and options for future study. *Am. J. Ind. Med.* **2016**, *59*, 96–105. [CrossRef] [PubMed]

4. Dolfman, M.L.; Wasser, S.F. 9/11 and the new york city economy: A borough-by-borough analysis. *Mon. Labor Rev.* **2004**, *127*, 3–33.

5. Bram, J.; Orr, J.; Rapaport, C. Measuring the effects of the September 11 attack on new york city. *Econ. Policy Rev.* **2002**, *8*, 5–20.

6. Niles, J.K.; Webber, M.P.; Gustave, J.; Zeig-Owens, R.; Lee, R.; Glass, L.; Weiden, M.D.; Kelly, K.J.; Prezant, D.J. The impact of the world trade center attack on fdny firefighter retirement, disabilities, and pension benefits. *Am. J. Ind. Med.* **2011**, *54*, 672–680. [CrossRef] [PubMed]

7. Yu, S.; Brackbill, R.M.; Locke, S.; Stellman, S.D.; Gargano, L.M. Impact of 9/11-related chronic conditions and ptsd comorbidity on early retirement and job loss among world trade center disaster rescue and recovery workers. *Am. J. Ind. Med.* **2016**, *59*, 731–741. [CrossRef]

8. Farfel, M.; DiGrande, L.; Brackbill, R.; Prann, A.; Cone, J.; Friedman, S.; Walker, D.J.; Pezeshki, G.; Thomas, P.; Galea, S.; et al. An overview of 9/11 experiences and respiratory and mental health conditions among world trade center health registry enrollees. *Urban Health* **2008**, *85*, 880–909. [CrossRef]

9. Perlman, S.E.; Friedman, S.; Galea, S.; Nair, H.P.; Erős-Sarnyai, M.; Stellman, S.D.; Hon, J.; Greene, C.M. Short-term and medium-term health effects of 9/11. *Lancet* **2011**, *378*, 925–934. [CrossRef]

10. Abbate, P.J.J. 2005–2006 Annual Report of the Committee on Governmental Employees. Available online: http://nyassembly.gov/comm/GovEmp/20061215/ (accessed on 31 January 2019).

11. Holloran, K.; Castet, R.-S. Summary Plan Description. The New York City Police Pension Fund, April 2014. Available online: https://www1.nyc.gov/html/nycppf/html/home/home.shtml (accessed on 31 January 2019).

12. Nigro, D.A. Comprehensive Annual Financial Report: A Pension Trust Fund of the City of New York for Fiscal Years Ended June 30, 2015 and June 30, 2014. Available online: http://comptroller.nyc.gov/wp-content/uploads/2016/02/FIRE-FY-2015.pdf (accessed on 7 July 2016).

13. NYCER. 22-Year Plan Fact Sheet. New York City Employees' Retirement System, 2016. Available online: https://www.cobanyc.org/sites/default/files/fact-sheet-720.pdf (accessed on 7 July 2016).

14. D'Addio, A.C.; Whitehouse, E. Trends in retirement and in working at older ages. In *Pensions at A Glance 2011: Retirement-Income Systems in OECD and G20 Countries*; OECD Publishing: Paris, France, 2011; pp. 39–47.

15. Johnson, R.W.; Butrica, B.A.; Mommaerts, C. *Work and Retirement Patterns for the G.I. Generation, Silent Generation, and Early Boomers: Thirty Years of Change*; CRR WP 2010-8; Center for Retirement Research at Boston College: Chestnut Hill, MA, USA, 2010.

16. Alavinia, S.M.; Burdorf, A. Unemployment and retirement and ill-health: A cross-sectional analysis across european countries. *Int. Arch. Occup. Environ. Health* **2008**, *82*, 39–45. [CrossRef] [PubMed]

17. Pit, S.W.; Shrestha, R.; Schofield, D.; Passey, M. Health problems and retirement due to ill-health among australian retirees aged 45–64 years. *Health Policy* **2010**, *94*, 175–181. [CrossRef]

18. van den Berg, T.; Schuring, M.; Avendano, M.; Mackenbach, J.; Burdorf. A. The impact of ill health on exit from paid employment in europe among older workers. *Occup. Environ. Med.* **2010**, *67*, 845–852. [CrossRef] [PubMed]

19. Rice, N.E.; Lang, I.A.; Henley, W.; Melzer, D. Common health predictors of early retirement: Findings from the english longitudinal study of ageing. *Age Ageing* **2011**, *40*, 54–61. [CrossRef]

20. van Rijn, R.M.; Robroek, S.J.; Brouwer, S.; Burdorf, A. Influence of poor health on exit from paid employment: A systematic review. *Occup. Environ. Med.* **2014**, *71*, 295–301. [CrossRef]

21. Haahr, J.P.L.; Frost, P.; Andersen, J.H. Predictors of health related job loss: A two-year follow-up study in a general working population. *J. Occup. Rehabil.* **2007**, *17*, 581–592. [CrossRef]

22. Lindbohm, M.L.; Kuosma, E.; Taskila, T.; Hietanen, P.; Carlsen, K.; Gudbergsson, S.; Gunnarsdottir, H. Early retirement and non-employment after breast cancer. *Psychooncology* **2014**, *23*, 634–641. [CrossRef]

23. Singer, S.; Meyer, A.; Wienholz, S.; Briest, S.; Brown, A.; Dietz, A.; Binder, H.; Jonas, S.; Papsdorf, K.; Stolzenburg, J.U.; et al. Early retirement in cancer patients with or without comorbid mental health conditions: A prospective cohort study. *Cancer* **2014**, *120*, 2199–2206. [CrossRef] [PubMed]

24. Dwyer, D.S.; Mitchell, O.S. Health problems as determinants of retirement: Are self-rated measures endogenous? *J. Health Econ.* **1999**, *18*, 173–193. [CrossRef]

25. McGarry, K. Health and retirement: Do changes in health affect retirement expectations? *J. Hum. Resour.* **2004**, *39*, 624–648. [CrossRef]

26. Munnell, A.H.; Sanzenbacher, G.T.; Rutledge, M.S. *What Causes Workers to Retire Before They Plan?* CRR WP 2015-22; Center for Retirement Research at Boston College: Chestnut Hill, MA, USA, 2015.

27. Stellman, J.M.; Smith, R.P.; Katz, C.L.; Sharma, V.; Charney, D.S.; Herbert, R.; Moline, J.; Luft, B.J.; Markowitz, S.; Udasin, I.; et al. Enduring mental health morbidity and social function impairment in world trade center rescue, recovery, and cleanup workers: The psychological dimension of an environmental health disaster. *Environ. Health Perspect.* **2008**, *116*, 1248–1253. [CrossRef]

28. Chiu, S.; Niles, J.K.; Webber, M.P.; Zeig-Owens, R.; Gustave, J.; Lee, R.; Rizzotto, L.; Kelly, K.J.; Cohen, H.W.; Prezant, D.J. Evaluating risk factors and possible mediation effects in posttraumatic depression and posttraumatic stress disorder comorbidity. *Public Health Rep.* **2011**, *126*, 201–209. [CrossRef] [PubMed]

29. Nair, H.P.; Ekenga, C.C.; Cone, J.E.; Brackbill, R.M.; Farfel, M.R.; Stellman, S.D. Co-occurring lower respiratory symptoms and posttraumatic stress disorder 5 to 6 years after the world trade center terrorist attack. *Am. J. Public Health* **2012**, *102*, 1964–1973. [CrossRef] [PubMed]

30. Friedman, S.M.; Farfel, M.R.; Maslow, C.B.; Cone, J.E.; Brackbill, R.M.; Stellman, S.D. Comorbid persistent lower respiratory symptoms and posttraumatic stress disorder 5–6 years post-9/11 in responders enrolled in the world trade center health registry. *Am. J. Ind. Med.* **2013**, *56*, 1251–1261. [CrossRef] [PubMed]

31. Caramanica, K.; Brackbill, R.M.; Liao, T.; Stellman, S.D. Comorbidity of 9/11-related ptsd and depression in the world trade center health registry 10–11 years postdisaster. *J. Trauma. Stress* **2014**, *27*, 680–688. [CrossRef]

32. Bromet, E.J.; Hobbs, M.J.; Clouston, S.A.; Gonzalez, A.; Kotov, R.; Luft, B.J. Dsm-iv post-traumatic stress disorder among world trade center responders 11–13 years after the disaster of 11 September 2001 (9/11). *Psychol. Med.* **2016**, *46*, 771–783. [CrossRef] [PubMed]

33. Li, J.; Brackbill, R.M.; Stellman, S.D.; Farfel, M.R.; Miller-Archie, S.A.; Friedman, S.; Walker, D.J.; Thorpe, L.E.; Cone, J. Gastroesophageal reflux symptoms and comorbid asthma and posttraumatic stress disorder following the 9/11 terrorist attacks on world trade center in new york city. *Am. J. Gastroenterol.* **2011**, *106*, 1933–1941. [CrossRef] [PubMed]

34. Jordan, H.T.; Miller-Archie, S.A.; Cone, J.E.; Morabia, A.; Stellman, S.D. Heart disease among adults exposed to the 11 September 2001 world trade center disaster: Results from the world trade center health registry. *Prev. Med.* **2011**, *53*, 370–376. [CrossRef]

35. Jordan, H.T.; Stellman, S.D.; Prezant, D.; Teirstein, A.; Osahan, S.S.; Cone, J.E. Sarcoidosis diagnosed after 11 September 2001, among adults exposed to the world trade center disaster. *J. Occup. Environ. Med.* **2011**, *53*, 966–974. [CrossRef]

36. Miller-Archie, S.A.; Jordan, H.T.; Ruff, R.R.; Chamany, S.; Cone, J.E.; Brackbill, R.M.; Kong, J.; Ortega, F.; Stellman, S.D. Posttraumatic stress disorder and new-onset diabetes among adult survivors of the world trade center disaster. *Prev. Med.* **2014**, *66*, 34–38. [CrossRef]

37. Webber, M.P.; Moir, W.; Zeig-Owens, R.; Glaser, M.S.; Jaber, N.; Hall, C.; Berman, J.; Qayyum, B.; Loupasakis, K.; Kelly, K.; et al. Nested case-control study of selected systemic autoimmune diseases in world trade center rescue/recovery workers. *Arthritis Rheumatol.* **2015**, *67*, 1369–1376. [CrossRef]

38. Jordan, H.T.; Stellman, S.D.; Reibman, J.; Farfel, M.R.; Brackbill, R.M.; Friedman, S.M.; Li, J.; Cone, J.E. Factors associated with poor control of 9/11-related asthma 10–11 years after the 2001 world trade center terrorist attacks. *J. Asthma* **2015**, *52*, 630–637. [CrossRef] [PubMed]

39. Yu, S.; Alper, H.E.; Nguyen, A.M.; Brackbill, R.M. Risk of stroke among survivors of the 11 September 2001, world trade center disaster. *J. Occup. Environ. Med.* **2018**, *60*, e371–e376. [CrossRef] [PubMed]

40. Aon Consulting. Replacement Ratio Study: A Measurement Tool for Retirement Planning. Aon Consulting, 2008. Available online: https://www.aon.com/about-aon/intellectual-capital/attachments/human-capital-consulting/RRStudy070308.pdf (accessed on 18 March 2019).

41. NYSLRS. Your Retirement Plan: Police and Fire Plan for Tier 1, 2, 5 and 6 Members, and Tier 3 Members Covered by Article 11 (Section 375-b and 375-c). New York State and Local Police and Fire Retirement System, 2012; pp. 26–28. Available online: https://www.osc.state.ny.us/retire/word_and_pdf_documents/publications/1500s/1512-noncont-pfrs.pdf (accessed on 31 January 2019).

42. McDonough, P.; Amick, B.C. The social context of health selection: A longitudinal study of health and employment. *Soc. Sci. Med.* **2001**, *53*, 135–145. [CrossRef]

43. Robroek, S.J.; Rongen, A.; Arts, C.H.; Otten, F.W.; Burdorf, A.; Schuring, M. Educational inequalities in exit from paid employment among dutch workers: The influence of health, lifestyle and work. *PLoS ONE* **2015**, *10*, e0134867. [CrossRef] [PubMed]

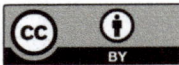

International Journal of
*Environmental Research
and Public Health*

MDPI

Article

Longitudinal Change of PTSD Symptoms in Community Members after the World Trade Center Destruction

Rebecca Rosen [1,2,*], Zhaoyin Zhu [2,3], Yongzhao Shao [2,4], Mengling Liu [2,3,4], Jia Bao [2,3], Nomi Levy-Carrick [1,2] and Joan Reibman [2,4,5]

[1] Department of Psychiatry, NYU School of Medicine, 550 First Ave, New York, NY 10016, USA; nlevy-carrick@bwh.harvard.edu
[2] Health and Hospitals World Trade Center Environmental Health Center, Bellevue Hospital Center, H7E, 462 First Ave, New York, NY 10016, USA; zhaoyin.zhu@nyu.edu (Z.Z.); yongzhao.shao@nyulangone.org (Y.S.); Mengling.Liu@nyulangone.org (M.L.); jia.bao@nyulangone.org (J.B.); joan.reibman@nyumc.org (J.R.)
[3] Department of Population Health, NYU School of Medicine, 180 Madison Ave., New York, NY 10016, USA
[4] Department of Environmental Medicine, NYU School of Medicine, 550 First Ave, New York, NY 10016, USA
[5] Department of Medicine, NYU School of Medicine, 550 First Ave, New York, NY 10016, USA
*   Correspondence: rebeccarosen18@gmail.com or RebeccaLRosen@nyumc.org; Tel.: +011-917-514-7587

Received: 1 March 2019; Accepted: 3 April 2019; Published: 4 April 2019

Abstract: The World Trade Center (WTC) Environmental Health Center (EHC) is a treatment program for community members with exposure to the 9/11 terrorist attack and its physical and emotional aftermath. Compared to the general responders program, the WTC EHC is diverse with equal gender distribution, representation of many races and ethnicities, and a wide range of social economic status. Patients in the WTC EHC were initially enrolled for physical symptoms, most of which were respiratory, however a large portion of the enrollees scored positive for probable posttraumatic stress disorder (PTSD). In this paper we identify patient characteristics associated with probable PTSD. We also determine the characteristics associated with the longitudinal change of PTSD symptoms, including persistence and remittance, using the widely used Posttraumatic Check List-17 (PCL) cut-off value of 44, as well as changes in PCL total score and symptom cluster scores in patients of Low and High PTSD symptom severity. Few patients with elevated scores achieved a score below 44. However, longitudinal improvement in PCL score at follow-up was identified for patients with High PTSD scores (PCL > 57.5). Changes in PCL symptom clusters differed between those with High and Low PCL scores. These data suggest improvement over time in PCL score that differs depending on the severity of the score and variable responses in the PCL symptom clusters.

Keywords: PTSD symptom change; PCL score; longitudinal analysis; PTSD cluster; WTC survivors; 9/11 disaster

1. Introduction

The terrorist attack on the World Trade Center (WTC) on 11 September 2001 resulted in a vast environmental disaster with the collapse of the WTC towers. Local community members and first responders had potential for both acute massive dust inhalation from the dust clouds created as the WTC buildings collapsed (WTC dust cloud), as well as chronic inhalation and topical exposure from re-suspended dust and fumes from the fires that burned for months [1–4]. Exposed community members include local residents, local workers, school children, and those passing by as tourists or commuters. Well-described adverse medical health effects in this population include persistent lower respiratory symptoms (LRS) [5–11]. Many of these community members witnessed destruction, death and dismemberment and often experienced fear of their own death as they escaped collapsing buildings or engulfment by blinding dust clouds. Some individuals were exposed to extended rescue and recovery efforts, or displacement from homes and workplaces due to clean up efforts of damaged or contaminated buildings. Well-described mental health symptoms in the community include those associated with posttraumatic stress disorder (PTSD), depression, and anxiety [6,12,13].

The World Trade Center Environmental Health Center (WTC EHC) was established to treat and monitor the health conditions of community members that resulted from exposure to the event and its aftermath [14]. The initial funding of the program limited inclusion in the treatment program to those with physical symptoms [4,11]. As a result, patients with exposure-based mental health symptoms but no physical symptoms were not eligible for enrollment in the treatment program during its initial years. Despite this, from the program's beginning, the Initial and Monitoring visit evaluations included assessment of both physical and mental health symptoms.

We have previously described mental health symptoms in the WTC EHC population [13]. We now report the longitudinal change of PTSD symptoms in our original cohort who self referred for physical complaints. Our goal was to identify factors associated with persistent or remitted PTSD symptoms over two time points including demographic characteristics, WTC exposures and baseline severity of a PTSD screening instrument score. We also examined differences among changes in symptom clusters consistent with PTSD heterogeneity.

2. Methods

2.1. Subjects

Patients who enrolled in the WTC EHC at Bellevue Hospital between August 2005 and February 2009 were included in the analysis. At that time, a physical complaint was the only criterion for enrollment [4,11]. The Institutional Review Board of New York University School of Medicine approved the research database (NCT00404898) and only data from patients who signed informed consent were used for analysis. Patients were included in the analysis if they had data including WTC exposure, physical and mental health questionnaires from an Initial visit between August 2005 and February 2009, and a subsequent Monitoring visit. All Monitoring visits were between October 2009 and May 2016.

2.2. WTC Exposures and Medical Assessment

Upon enrollment in the WTC EHC, patients completed a multi-dimensional, interviewer-administered questionnaire that included demographic information and characterizations of WTC-related exposure [11]. Individuals were classified as positive for dust cloud exposure if they reported having been in a WTC dust cloud created by the collapsing buildings on 11 September 2001. Potential for WTC acute and chronic exposures were characterized by classification into four additional categories: local resident (resident), local worker, cleanup worker and other.

Patients who reported more than 5 pack-year history of tobacco use were defined as ever smokers. Body mass index (BMI) of patients was calculated using information gathered during the Initial medical visit. The presence and severity of lower respiratory symptoms (LRS) of wheeze, cough, chest tightness and dyspnea, as well as the upper respiratory symptom of rhinitis or sinusitis were measured by standardized health questionnaires [11]. Patients with symptoms more than twice per week during the month preceding enrollment were considered positive for any LRS or sinus symptoms. Spirometry was performed in accordance with American Thoracic Society/European Respiratory Society standards [15] on a Viasys Vmax spirometer (Yorba Linda, CA). Patients were categorized as abnormal if they had a reduced forced vital capacity (FVC), reduced forced expiratory volume in one second (FEV_1), or a reduced ratio of FEV_1/FVC [16].

2.3. Mental Health Symptom and Treatment Assessments

The Posttraumatic Check List-17 (PCL) [17] was used to measure PTSD symptom presence and severity. A score ≥ 44 was considered positive for probable PTSD (PTSD+), and a score < 44 was considered negative for probable PTSD (PTSD−) [9]. We evaluated the longitudinal change in PCL score using a comparison of PCL scores at Initial and Monitoring visits. We defined those who scored positive for probable PTSD at both Initial and Monitoring visits as Persistent PTSD and those who scored positive at their Initial visit and negative at their Monitoring visit as Remitted PTSD. PTSD symptom severity was further defined by the level of the initial PCL score as follows: < 44, No PTSD; 44–57.5, Low PTSD; > 57.5, High PTSD. The "Low" and "High" categories were defined using 57.5 as the cut point as this number is the median score among those with a score $\geq$ 44. Questions from the PCL-17 were also matched to the DSM-V diagnostic criteria for characterization into four clusters as previously described [13], reflecting symptoms of re-experiencing, avoidance, negative cognitions/mood, and arousal. An average score for each patient was calculated for each cluster, ranging between 1–5.

We used the Hopkins Symptom Checklist for depression and anxiety (HSCL-25) [18]. These scales provided scores of depression (HSCL-D) and anxiety (HSCL-A) severity with a score $\geq$ 1.75 considered to suggest probable depression or probable anxiety. The CAGE Questionnaire was used to screen for problem alcohol use, with a score $\geq$ 2 used to categorize persons with probable alcohol abuse [19].

We collected self-reported mental health treatment information during the Monitoring examination. Treatment for a mental health condition was defined to include any type of reported treatment. Treatment was included if it was reported as individual psychotherapy for $\geq$ one month, group psychotherapy treatment for $\geq$ 2 months, or prescribed pharmacologic treatment.

2.4. Statistical Methods

Categorical variables were summarized using counts and percentages and the significance of between-group difference was assessed by Chi-square test. Continuous variables were summarized using median and interquartile range (IQR) and difference between independent groups was assessed by Wilcoxon rank-sum test (i.e., Mann-Whitney test), and between correlated groups using Wilcoxon signed rank test. Logistic regression was used to quantify the association between binary outcomes (e.g., probable PTSD) and covariates of interest. Linear regression was used to quantify the association between continuous outcome (e.g., PCL score) and covariates of interest. Multivariate models were constructed using selected covariates that were significant in univariate analyses. Observed mental health treatment was not randomized in this study cohort and therefore direct comparison of treated versus untreated groups would not be meaningful due to potential associated biases. To overcome this issue, we used the propensity score method to discuss potential existence of treatment effect on the longitudinal changes of PCL scores. A value of $P < 0.05$ was used to test for two-sided statistical significance. All statistical analyses were conducted using SAS, version 9.4 (SAS Institute, Cary, North Carolina, United States).

3. Results

3.1. Patient Characteristics

WTC exposure history, physical and mental health data gathered at Initial and Monitoring visits were available for 738 patients. The median time between visits was 3.43 years (Q1, Q3; 2.88, 4.32). Most patients (Table 1) were > age 45 (69%), with a similar number of males (49%) and females (51%). Many were Hispanic (44%), had an annual individual income of < $30,000 and had a $\leq$ 12th grade level of education (40%). Local workers comprised the largest exposure category (47%). Fifty per cent reported having been caught in the WTC dust cloud. Most patients (90%) had LRS, and 57% reported sinus symptoms. Lung function was within normal limits in most (64%).

Table 1. Patient characteristics at Initial visit and comparison of PTSD+ and PTSD− patients (*n* = 738).

Demographic Characteristics	Total	PTSD+ (*n* = 284)	PTSD− (*n* = 454)	*p*-Value
Gender, *n* (%)				0.24
Female	375 (51)	152 (53.5)	223 (49)	
Male	363 (49)	132 (46.5)	231 (51)	
Age, *n* (%)				0.24
<45	229 (31)	81 (29)	148 (33)	
≥45	509 (69)	203 (71)	306 (67)	
Race/ethnicity, *n* (%)				0.001
Hispanic	323 (44)	149 (52)	174 (38)	
Non-Hispanic white	205 (28)	66 (23)	139 (31)	
Non-Hispanic black	142 (19)	45 (16)	97 (21)	
Asian	49 (7)	14 (5)	35 (8)	
Other	19 (3)	10 (4)	9 (2)	
Education, *n* (%)				0.003
≤High school	292 (40)	132 (47)	160 (35)	
>High school	445 (60)	152 (54)	293 (65)	
Income, *n* (%)				<0.0001
≤$15,000/year	301 (42)	148 (54)	153 (35)	
$15,000–$30,000/year	145 (21)	49 (18)	96 (22)	
>$30,000/year	265 (37)	76 (28)	189 (43)	
BMI, *n* (%)				0.80
≤30	466 (64)	177 (63)	289 (64)	
>30	262 (36)	102 (37)	160 (36)	
Ever smoker, *n* (%)				0.21
yes	287 (39)	118 (42)	169 (37)	
no	451 (61)	163 (58)	284 (63)	
Exposures				
WTC dust cloud exposure, *n* (%)				0.14
yes	361 (49)	148 (53)	213 (48)	
no	377 (51)	130 (47)	234 (52)	
Exposure classification, *n* (%)				0.12
Local worker	340 (47)	127 (45)	213 (47)	
Resident	140 (19)	45 (16)	95 (21)	
Clean-up worker	171 (23)	77 (27)	94 (21)	
Other	80 (11)	33(12)	47 (10)	
Symptoms				
Lower respiratory symptoms				
Any Lower Respiratory Symptoms				0.001
yes	663 (90)	266 (95)	397 (87)	
no	75 (10)	15 (5)	57 (13)	
Spirometry				0.17
normal	472 (64)	173 (61)	299 (66)	
abnormal	266 (36)	111 (39)	155 (34)	
Upper respiratory symptoms				
Sinus congestion				0.79
yes	408 (56)	153 (56)	255 (57)	
no	330 (44)	122 (44)	195 (43)	
Positive mental health score				
PTSD, *n* (%)				
yes	284 (38)			
no	454 (62)			

Table 1. *Cont.*

Demographic Characteristics	Total	PTSD+ (n = 284)	PTSD− (n = 454)	p-Value
Depression, n (%)				<0.0001
yes	404 (55)	265 (93)	139 (31)	
no		19 (7)	315 (69)	
Anxiety, n (%)				<0.0001
yes	277 (38)	202 (71)	75 (17)	
no	461 (62)	82 (29)	379 (83)	
Cage, n (%)				0.02
yes	50 (7)	27 (10)	23 (5)	
no	688 (93)	250 (90)	428 (95)	

Univariate analysis. Categorical variables presented as frequencies and percentages and difference between 2 groups assessed by the Chi-Square test.

As noted above, the criterion for enrollment in this early program was the presence of physical, but not mental health symptoms. Despite this, many patients scored positive for probable PTSD (PTSD+; 38%, $n = 284$), depression (55%), and anxiety (38%) at their Initial visit. Symptoms suggestive of alcohol misuse were reported in 7% of the population. Categories were not mutually exclusive.

3.2. Characteristics Associated with PTSD Symptoms at Initial Visit

We compared demographic characteristics, medical symptoms, lung function and comorbid conditions in PTSD+ ($n = 284$) and PTSD− ($n = 454$) patients at their Initial visit (Table 1; see methods section for category description). Patients who self-reported as Hispanic ($p = 0.001$), had income $\leq$ $15,000/year or $\leq$ 12th grade education were more likely to score PTSD+ ($p < 0.001$, 0.003 respectively). The presence of any LRS symptom ($p = 0.001$) was associated with being PTSD+. Those PTSD+ were also more likely to report probable depression and anxiety (both $p < 0.0001$) and to report alcohol misuse ($p = 0.02$). In a multivariate logistical regression using any significant variable, the presence of physical symptoms of LRS (OR = 2.21; $p = 0.05$), as well as co-morbid mental health symptoms of probable depression (OR = 18.11; $p < 0.0001$), probable anxiety (OR = 4.64; $p < 0.001$), or alcohol misuse (OR = 2.45; $p = 0.05$), remained significant (data not shown).

3.3. Demographic and WTC Exposure Characteristics Associated with Persistent and Remitted PTSD

As shown (Table 2), 279 patients who scored PTSD+ at their initial visit could be classified as Persistent or Remitted as described in the methods section (5 patients with incomplete baseline characteristics were excluded from analysis). The majority of patients ($n = 214$) remained Persistent, while few patients ($n = 65$) fit criteria for Remitted. Race/ethnicity and baseline depression status were associated with being Persistent ($p = 0.01$ and 0.04 respectively) in univariate analysis. No covariates were significant in multivariate analysis (data not shown).

Table 2. Characteristics associated with Persistent and Remitted PTSD *.

Demographic Characteristics	Persistent PTSD (*n* = 214)	Remitted PTSD (*n* = 65)	*p*-Value
Gender, *n* (%)			0.20
Female	109 (51)	39 (60)	
Male	105 (49)	26 (40)	
Age, *n* (%)			0.91
<45	61 (28.5)	19 (29)	
≥45	153 (71.5)	46 (71)	
Race/ethnicity, *n* (%)			0.01
Hispanic	119 (56)	28 (43)	
Non-Hispanic white	52 (24)	12 (18)	
Non-Hispanic black	30 (14)	14 (22)	
Asian	6 (3)	8 (12)	
Other	7 (3)	3 (5)	
Education, *n* (%)			0.58
≤High school	97 (45)	32 (49)	
>High school	117 (55)	33 (51)	
Income, *n* (%)			0.16
≤$15,000/year	107 (52)	39 (63)	
$15,000 - $30,000/year	40 (19)	6 (10)	
>$30,000/year	59 (29)	17 (27)	
BMI, *n* (%)			0.25
≤30	138 (65)	36 (57)	
>30	74 (35)	27 (43)	
Ever smoker, *n* (%)			0.90
yes	89 (42)	28 (43)	
no	122 (58)	37 (57)	
Exposures			
WTC dust cloud exposure, *n* (%)			0.12
yes	117 (56)	28 (44)	
no	93 (44)	35 (56)	
Exposure classification, *n* (%)			0.37
Local worker	101 (48)	25 (38)	
Resident	32 (15)	11 (17)	
Clean-up worker	58 (27)	18 (28)	
Other	21(10)	11 (17)	
Symptoms			
Lower respiratory symptoms			
Any Lower Respiratory Symptoms			0.85
yes	200 (95)	62 (95)	
no	11 (5)	3 (5)	
Spirometry			0.30
normal	134 (63)	36 (55)	
abnormal	80 (37)	29 (45)	

Table 2. *Cont.*

Demographic Characteristics	Persistent PTSD (*n* = 214)	Remitted PTSD (*n* = 65)	*p*-Value
Upper respiratory symptoms			
Sinus congestion			0.052
yes	123 (59)	28 (45)	
no	85 (41)	34 (55)	
Positive mental health score			
Depression, *n* (%)			0.04
yes	203 (95)	57 (88)	
no	11 (5)	8 (12)	
Anxiety, *n* (%)			0.11
yes	157 (73)	41 (63)	
no	57 (27)	24 (37)	
Cage, *n* (%)			0.94
yes	21 (10)	6 (10)	
no	189 (90)	56 (90)	

* Univariate analysis, *n* = 279 (five subjects with incomplete baseline characteristics are excluded from analysis. Categorical variables presented as frequencies and percentages and difference between 2 groups assessed by the Chi-Square test.

3.4. Longitudinal Assessment of Severity of PTSD Symptoms

A dichotomous evaluation as Remitted or Persistent may be insensitive to a heterogeneous decrease of the PCL score. We therefore directly studied changes in the PCL score. Patients were grouped into severity categories based on their PCL score at Initial visit as No PTSD, Low PTSD, or High PTSD (Table 3; see methods section for description of grouping). High PTSD patients had a 9-point reduction in the median score between visits ($p < 0.0001$), consistent with a statistically significant improvement in PCL score. In contrast, the decrease in median PCL score in the Low PTSD patients did not reach significance. Despite these improvements, the median score at Monitoring remained $\geq$ 44 in both groups. There was a small but statistically significant increase of median PCL score among the No PTSD group, and the median score at Monitoring remained < 44.

Table 3. Longitudinal assessment of PTSD score in severity categories.

PCL Status	No PTSD (*n* = 454)	Low PTSD (*n* = 142)	High PTSD (*n* = 142)
Initial (PCL1)	27 (20, 35)	51 (47, 54)	66 (62, 70)
Monitoring (PCL2)	32 (23, 41)	49 (42, 58)	57 (49, 66)
Change (PCL1-PCL2)	−4 (−12, −2)	2 (−6, 9)	9 (2, 17)
p-value	<0.0001	0.11	<0.0001

Continuous variables presented as Median and IQR (Q1, Q3) and difference between 2 groups assessed by Wilcoxon signed rank test.

The possibility exists that treatment modified the PCL score over time. Our study was not designed to evaluate treatment, however we used the observed treatment status, as defined in the methods section, to develop propensity scores from logistic regression with relevant predictors including race/ethnicity, income, and initial mental health scores included in the model. High propensity scores of being treated were positively correlated with decreases in longitudinal PCL scores ($p < 0.0001$; data not shown).

3.5. PTSD Symptom Clusters Over Time

The heterogeneity within PTSD can also be described by the symptom clusters that comprise the overall score. We therefore examined change in score of each PTSD symptom cluster within our PTSD severity categories (Table 4). Patients with Low PTSD showed significant improvement only in the arousal cluster score ($p = 0.01$); we were unable to detect a significant change in the score of any of the other clusters. In contrast, those with High PTSD improved significantly on all clusters (re-experiencing, $p = 0.0003$; avoidance, $p = 0.001$; negative thoughts/emotions and arousal, $p < 0.0001$). A slight increase in all cluster scores was noted in those who scored below threshold on initial visit.

Table 4. PCL cluster scores at Initial and Monitoring visit in PTSD severity categories.

Symptom Severity Level	Visit	Re-Experiencing	Avoidance	NegativeThoughts/Mood	Arousal
No PTSD ($n = 454$)					
	Initial	1.4 (1.0, 2.0)	1.0 (1.0, 2.0)	1.2 (1.0, 1.8)	1.8 (1.1, 2.4)
	Monitoring	1.6 (1.2, 2.4)	2.0 (1.0, 3.0)	1.5 (1.0, 2.2)	2.0 (1.4, 2.8)
	p-value	<0.0001	<0.0001	<0.0001	<0.0001
Low PTSD ($n = 142$)					
	Initial	2.6 (2.2, 3.0)	3.0 (2.0, 4.0)	2.8 (2.4, 3.3)	3.6 (3.0, 3.8)
	Monitoring	2.8 (2.2, 3.4)	3.0 (2.5, 4.0)	2.7 (1.8, 3.2)	3.2 (2.6, 4.0)
	p-value	0.23	0.45	0.06	**0.01**
High PTSD ($n = 142$)					
	Initial	3.8 (3.4, 4.2)	4.0 (3.5, 5.0)	3.8 (3.2, 4.2)	4.2 (3.8, 4.6)
	Monitoring	3.2 (2.6, 4.0)	3.5 (3.0, 4.5)	3.1 (2.4, 3.8)	3.7 (3.0, 4.2)
	p-value	0.0003	0.001	<0.0001	<0.0001

Cluster scores are median of questions noted and IRQ (Q1, Q3) and difference between 2 groups assessed by Wilcoxon signed rank test.

4. Discussion

In this paper we characterize mental health scores in patients who had enrolled in a community program for physical symptoms after a traumatic event and describe characteristics associated with PTSD symptom scores in this population, as well as changes in scores over time. Our population was a diverse race/ethnic population with many of low income and education. Importantly, despite enrollment in the program for physical symptoms, many patients scored positive for probable PTSD. We did not observe many patients with remittance of PTSD symptoms defined as a score below 44, however we identified patients who had improvement in PCL scores, particularly in those who were more symptomatic as reflected in higher PCL scores on enrollment in the program. Moreover, we showed improvement in each PTSD symptom cluster score in patients with more severe PTSD symptoms, whereas those with milder PTSD symptoms had more limited improvement.

We identified many patients who scored positive for probable PTSD despite enrolling in a program for physical symptoms. High rates of PTSD have been well described in civilian populations who are not trained for trauma [9,20–22]. Our patients were recruited for physical symptoms and were not specifically seeking mental health treatment. High mental health scores were only incidentally reported, reinforcing the need to perform mental health screening in all disaster-exposed populations. Moreover, these high rates may in part be due to the diversity of the population, including many with low income and education, factors previously reported to be associated with the development of PTSD [21,23]. In addition, the presence of co-morbid physical symptoms, including lower respiratory symptoms, and mental health symptoms was also associated with probable PTSD, reinforcing the need to consider co-morbid presentations [6,24,25].

Few studies have examined the longitudinal change in mental health symptoms in WTC community members, [6,26–29] particularly in those who have sought care for physical, or even mental health symptoms as a result of their exposure. To begin to analyze the change in symptoms over time in our highly affected population we used a simple cut-off value that is often used to determine whether an individual should undergo further evaluation, and has been used in numerous epidemiologic studies in WTC-exposed populations [9]. Most (77%) of the patients in the study remained symptomatic when the group was dichotomized into Persistent or Remitted based on this score. This finding suggests that these symptoms were refractory as has been described in some WTC exposed populations [22,30] and underscores the importance of studying and improving patient management. Alternatively, this finding may suggest that this dichotomous evaluation is insensitive for the identification of more subtle changes in the level of PTSD symptoms. Indeed, we noted changes in PCL scores when evaluated as a continuous variable in subgroups of patients. In addition, the PCL may have low sensitivity in identifying functional improvement.

There was wide variation in the PCL score in our population, suggesting heterogeneity within the severity of symptoms. When we compared the change in PCL score as a continuous variable, patients who had a higher score at their Initial visit had a significant improvement in their score. This finding was not seen in those who began with a lower score. Importantly, neither group reduced their median score below our cut-off threshold. This finding suggests that there is improvement, although there may to be differences in responsivity.

Our study was not designed to evaluate treatment, however, we used the observed treatment status to develop propensity scores from logistic regression with relevant predictors and showed that high propensity scores of having received treatment were positively correlated with decreases in longitudinal PCL scores. These data suggest a relationship between treatment and improvement in PCL score and reinforce the need for clinical trials to study the role of individual treatment modalities and potential treatment effect.

We have previously suggested heterogeneity of PTSD within this community population [13]. However, few studies examine longitudinal changes in the individual components that comprise PTSD. Symptom cluster trajectories have been shown to have a variable course in, for example, traumatically injured populations [31]. We show an improvement in score in those with High PTSD at initial evaluation, suggesting that there may be differences in the components of these higher scores that can be modified. When we evaluated this question by examining changes within symptom clusters, patients with higher PCL scores at Initial visit showed improvement across all clusters. This finding suggests that patients with greater PTSD symptom severity at Initial visit have responsiveness across all components of PTSD. Patients with lower PCL scores reflecting less symptom severity only improved significantly on the arousal cluster, suggesting that this cluster of symptoms may more easily attenuated. Their failure to completely return to levels below threshold suggest the possibility of some level of intractability.

There are limitations to this study. We studied a civilian population at only two time points, limiting the ability to identify fluctuations in symptom presentation. The population under study was exposed to the same traumatic event, which is a strength of the study. However, this unique exposure may also limit the generalizability of these results. Participants were self-referred patients seeking treatment for physical symptoms related to exposure to the WTC disaster and were not selected from a wider group of WTC exposed community members, raising the potential for selection bias for these symptoms. The possibility exists, too, that the role of treatment was inadequately evaluated and patients with higher scores might have been more likely to have received treatment, with subsequent bias, in our evaluation. We used the PCL-17 to assess PTSD symptoms. Although this is a commonly used tool, it can be subject to recall bias, sensitivity, and specificity [32]. Certain variables were not completely assessed and included in the analysis, such as pre and post-trauma variables. These limitations reinforce the need for more studies.

5. Conclusions

Our goal was to understand longitudinal patterns of PTSD in a cohort of WTC exposed community members seeking help for physical ailments related to the exposure. Many patients scored positive for probable PTSD, which was associated with physical and mental health comorbidities. Few patients remitted, when analyzed as a threshold score, and no we could not identify variables associated with remittance or persistence after multivariate analysis. However, we detected improvement in scores in patients with persistence; the decrease was significant for those with more severe PTSD symptoms. Heterogeneity in response was also observed in changes in PTSD symptom clusters, where we showed improvement in each PTSD symptom cluster score for patients with more severe PTSD symptoms, whereas those with milder PTSD symptoms improved only on the arousal cluster.

An understanding of the patterns of longitudinal PTSD symptoms is important for trauma management in this and other populations. Identifying the variability in changes in PTSD symptom clusters can also help to target treatment. Moreover, studies suggest that PTSD symptoms do not remain stable over a lifetime, but may change and even reactivate with aging, suggesting the need for further study evaluation [33]. Understanding the patterns of longitudinal symptoms in this cohort will assist in identifying patients at high risk for chronicity and in guiding timely, effective interventions.

Author Contributions: Conceptualization, R.R., J.R., N.L.-C.; methodology, Y.S., M.L.; formal analysis, Z.Z., J.B., Y.S.; data curation, Z.Z., J.B.; writing—original draft preparation, R.R., J.R.; writing—review and editing, Y.S., Z.Z., M.L., N.L.-C.; funding acquisition, J.R.

Funding: This research was funded by American Red Cross Liberty Disaster Relief Fund, the City of New York National Institute of Occupational Safety and Health, Centers of Disease Control 200-2017-93327, 200-2017-93427, NIEHS Grant 5P30ES000260.

Acknowledgments: We graciously appreciate Edith Davis and Evelin Zumba, for their tireless administration of the program. We thank the mental health and medical staff of the WTC Environmental Health Center for their dedication to the treatment and support of our patients. We also thank members of the WTC Health Program Survivor Steering Committee for their invaluable advice and efforts on behalf of the community.

Conflicts of Interest: The authors declare no conflict of interest.

References

1. Lioy, P.J.; Georgopoulos, P. The anatomy of the exposures that occurred around the World Trade Center site: 9/11 and beyond. *Ann. N. Y. Acad. Sci.* **2006**, *1076*, 54–79. [CrossRef] [PubMed]

2. Lippmann, M.; Cohen, M.D.; Chen, L.C. Health effects of World Trade Center (WTC) Dust: An unprecedented disaster's inadequate risk management. *Crit. Rev. Toxicol.* **2015**, *45*, 492–530. [CrossRef] [PubMed]

3. Maslow, C.B.; Friedman, S.M.; Pillai, P.S.; Reibman, J.; Berger, K.I.; Goldring, R.; Stellman, S.D.; Farfel, M. Chronic and acute exposures to the world trade center disaster and lower respiratory symptoms: Area residents and workers. *Am. J. Public Health* **2012**, *102*, 1186–1194. [CrossRef] [PubMed]

4. Reibman, J.; Levy-Carrick, N.; Miles, T.; Flynn, K.; Hughes, C.; Crane, M.; Lucchini, R.G. Destruction of the World Trade Towers: Lessons Learned from an Environmental Health Disaster. *Ann. Am. Thorac. Soc.* **2016**, *13*, 577–583. [CrossRef]

5. Lin, S.; Jones, R.; Reibman, J.; Bowers, J.; Fitzgerald, E.F.; Hwang, S.A. Reported respiratory symptoms and adverse home conditions after 9/11 among residents living near the World Trade Center. *J. Asthma* **2007**, *44*, 325–332. [CrossRef]

6. Brackbill, R.M.; Hadler, J.L.; DiGrande, L.; Ekenga, C.C.; Farfel, M.R.; Friedman, S.; Perlman, S.E.; Stellman, S.D.; Walker, D.J.; Wu, D.; et al. Asthma and posttraumatic stress symptoms 5 to 6 years following exposure to the World Trade Center terrorist attack. *JAMA* **2009**, *302*, 502–516. [CrossRef] [PubMed]

7. Friedman, S.M.; Farfel, M.R.; Maslow, C.B.; Cone, J.E.; Brackbill, R.M.; Stellman, S.D. Comorbid persistent lower respiratory symptoms and posttraumatic stress disorder 5-6 years post-9/11 in responders enrolled in the World Trade Center Health Registry. *Am. J. Ind. Med.* **2013**, *56*, 1251–1261. [CrossRef]

8. Reibman, J.; Lin, S.; Hwang, S.-A.A.; Gulati, M.; Bowers, J.A.; Rogers, L.; Berger, K.I.; Hoerning, A.; Gomez, M.; Fitzgerald, E.F. The World Trade Center residents' respiratory health study: New-onset respiratory symptoms and pulmonary function. *Environ. Health Perspect.* **2005**, *113*, 406–411. [CrossRef] [PubMed]

9. Farfel, M.; DiGrande, L.; Brackbill, R.; Prann, A.; Cone, J.; Friedman, S.; Walker, D.J.; Pezeshki, G.; Thomas, P.; Galea, S.; et al. An overview of 9/11 experiences and respiratory and mental health conditions among World Trade Center Health Registry enrollees. *J. Urban Health Bull. N. Y. Acad. Med.* **2008**, *85*, 880–909. [CrossRef] [PubMed]

10. Lin, S.; Reibman, J.; Bowers, J.A.; Hwang, S.-A.; Hoerning, A.; Gomez, M.I.; Fitzgerald, E.F. Upper Respiratory Symptoms and Other Health Effects among Residents Living Near the World Trade Center Site after September 11, 2001. *Am. J. Epidemiol.* **2005**, *162*, 499–507. [CrossRef]

11. Reibman, J.; Liu, M.; Cheng, Q.; Liautaud, S.; Rogers, L.; Lau, S.; Berger, K.I.; Goldring, R.M.; Marmor, M.; Fernandez-Beros, M.E.; et al. Characteristics of a residential and working community with diverse exposure to World Trade Center dust, gas, and fumes. *J. Occup. Environ. Med.* **2009**, *51*, 534–541. [CrossRef]

12. DiGrande, L.; Perrin, M.A.; Thorpe, L.E.; Thalji, L.; Murphy, J.; Wu, D.; Farfel, M.; Brackbill, R.M. Posttraumatic stress symptoms, PTSD, and risk factors among lower Manhattan residents 2–3 years after the September 11, 2001 terrorist attacks. *J. Trauma. Stress* **2008**, *21*, 264–273. [CrossRef] [PubMed]

13. Rosen, R.L.; Levy-Carrick, N.; Reibman, J.; Xu, N.; Shao, Y.; Liu, M.; Ferri, L.; Kazeros, A.; Caplan-Shaw, C.E.; Pradhan, D.R.; et al. Elevated C-reactive protein and posttraumatic stress pathology among survivors of the 9/11 World Trade Center attacks. *J. Psychiatr. Res.* **2017**, *89*, 14–21. [CrossRef] [PubMed]

14. Kazeros, A.; Zhang, E.; Cheng, X.; Shao, Y.; Liu, M.; Qian, M.; Caplan-Shaw, C.; Berger, K.I.; Goldring, R.M.; Ghumman, M.; et al. Systemic Inflammation Associated With World Trade Center Dust Exposures and Airway Abnormalities in the Local Community. *J. Occup. Environ. Med.* **2015**, *57*, 610–616. [CrossRef] [PubMed]

15. Miller, M.R.; Hankinson, J.; Brusasco, V.; Burgos, F.; Casaburi, R.; Coates, A.; Crapo, R.; Enright, P.; van der Grinten, C.P.; Gustafsson, P.; et al. Standardisation of spirometry. *Eur. Respir. J.* **2005**, *26*, 319–338. [CrossRef]

16. Pellegrino, R.; Viegi, G.; Brusasco, V.; Crapo, R.O.; Burgos, F.; Casaburi, R.; Coates, A.; van der Grinten, C.P.; Gustafsson, P.; Hankinson, J.; et al. Interpretative strategies for lung function tests. *Eur. Respir. J.* **2005**, *26*, 948–968. [CrossRef]

17. Weathers, F.W.; Litz, B.T.; Herman, D.S.; Huska, J.A.; Keane, T.M. The PTSD Checklist (PCL): Reliability, validity, and diagnostic utility. In Proceedings of the Annual Convention of the international society for traumatic stress studies, San Antonio, TX, USA, 24–27 October 1993.

18. Derogatis, L.R.; Lipman, R.S.; Rickels, K.; Uhlenhuth, E.H.; Covi, L. The Hopkins Symptom Checklist (HSCL): A self-report symptom inventory. *Behav. Sci.* **1974**, *19*, 1–15. [CrossRef] [PubMed]

19. Ewing, J.A. Detecting alcoholism. The CAGE questionnaire. *JAMA* **1984**, *252*, 1905–1907. [CrossRef]

20. Perrin, M.A.; DiGrande, L.; Wheeler, K.; Thorpe, L.; Farfel, M.; Brackbill, R. Differences in PTSD prevalence and associated risk factors among World Trade Center disaster rescue and recovery workers. *Am. J. Psychiatry* **2007**, *164*, 1385–1394. [CrossRef] [PubMed]

21. Norris, F.H.; Friedman, M.J.; Watson, P.J.; Byrne, C.M.; Diaz, E.; Kaniasty, K. 60,000 disaster victims speak: Part I. An empirical review of the empirical literature, 1981-2001. *Psychiatry* **2002**, *65*, 207–239. [CrossRef] [PubMed]

22. Feder, A.; Mota, N.; Salim, R.; Rodriguez, J.; Singh, R.; Schaffer, J.; Schechter, C.B.; Cancelmo, L.M.; Bromet, E.J.; Katz, C.L.; et al. Risk, coping and PTSD symptom trajectories in World Trade Center responders. *J. Psychiatr. Res.* **2016**, *82*, 68–79. [CrossRef]

23. Kessler, R.C.; Sonnega, A.; Bromet, E.; Hughes, M.; Nelson, C.B. Posttraumatic stress disorder in the National Comorbidity Survey. *Arch. Gen. Psychiatry* **1995**, *52*, 1048–1060. [CrossRef] [PubMed]

24. Li, J.; Zweig, K.C.; Brackbill, R.M.; Farfel, M.R.; Cone, J.E. Comorbidity amplifies the effects of post-9/11 posttraumatic stress disorder trajectories on health-related quality of life. *Qual. Life Res.* **2018**, *27*, 651–660. [CrossRef] [PubMed]

25. Kotov, R.; Bromet, E.J.; Schechter, C.; Broihier, J.; Feder, A.; Friedman-Jimenez, G.; Gonzalez, A.; Guerrera, K.; Kaplan, J.; Moline, J.; et al. Posttraumatic stress disorder and the risk of respiratory problems in World Trade Center responders: Longitudinal test of a pathway. *Psychosom. Med.* **2015**, *77*, 438–448. [CrossRef] [PubMed]

26. Adams, R.E.; Boscarino, J.A. Predictors of PTSD and delayed PTSD after disaster: The impact of exposure and psychosocial resources. *J. Nerv. Ment. Dis.* **2006**, *194*, 485–493. [CrossRef] [PubMed]

27. Boscarino, J.A.; Adams, R.E. PTSD onset and course following the World Trade Center disaster: Findings and implications for future research. *Soc. Psychiatry Psychiatr. Epidemiol.* **2009**, *44*, 887–898. [CrossRef]

28. Neria, Y.; Olfson, M.; Gameroff, M.J.; DiGrande, L.; Wickramaratne, P.; Gross, R.; Pilowsky, D.J.; Neugebaur, R.; Manetti-Cusa, J.; Lewis-Fernandez, R.; et al. Long-term course of probable PTSD after the 9/11 attacks: A study in urban primary care. *J. Trauma. Stress* **2010**, *23*, 474–482. [CrossRef]

29. Galea, S.; Ahern, J.; Tracy, M.; Hubbard, A.; Cerda, M.; Goldmann, E.; Vlahov, D. Longitudinal determinants of posttraumatic stress in a population-based cohort study. *Epidemiology* **2008**, *19*, 47–54. [CrossRef]

30. Berninger, A.; Webber, M.P.; Cohen, H.W.; Gustave, J.; Lee, R.; Niles, J.K.; Chiu, S.; Zeig-Owens, R.; Soo, J.; Kelly, K.; et al. Trends of elevated PTSD risk in firefighters exposed to the World Trade Center disaster: 2001–2005. *Public Health Rep. (Washington D.C. 1974)* **2010**, *125*, 556–566. [CrossRef]

31. O'Donnell, M.L.; Elliott, P.; Lau, W.; Creamer, M. PTSD symptom trajectories: From early to chronic response. *Behav. Res.* **2007**, *45*, 601–606. [CrossRef]

32. Williams, J.L.; Monahan, C.J.; McDevitt-Murphy, M.E. Factor Structure of the PTSD Checklist in a Sample of OEF/OIF Veterans Presenting to Primary Care: Specific and Nonspecific Aspects of Dysphoria. *J. Psychopathol. Behav. Assess.* **2011**, *33*, 514–522. [CrossRef] [PubMed]

33. Hermes, E.D.; Rosenheck, R.A.; Desai, R.; Fontana, A.F. Recent trends in the treatment of posttraumatic stress disorder and other mental disorders in the VHA. *Psychiatr. Serv.* **2012**, *63*, 471–476. [CrossRef] [PubMed]

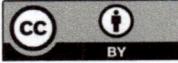

International Journal of
Environmental Research and Public Health

MDPI

Article

The Association between Health Conditions in World Trade Center Responders and Sleep-Related Quality of Life and Sleep Complaints

Indu Ayappa [1,*], Yingfeng Chen [2], Nisha Bagchi [1], Haley Sanders [1], Kathleen Black [3], Akosua Twumasi [1], David M. Rapoport [1], Shou-En Lu [2] and Jag Sunderram [4]

[1] Division of Pulmonary, Critical Care and Sleep Medicine Icahn School of Medicine at Mount Sinai, New York, NY 10029, USA; nb2229@nyu.edu (N.B.); haley.sanders@mssm.edu (H.S.); Akosua.Twumasi@mssm.edu (A.T.); david.rapoport@mssm.edu (D.M.R.)
[2] School of Public Health, Rutgers University, Piscataway, NJ 08854, USA; yingfengc123@gmail.com (Y.C.); sl1020@sph.rutgers.edu (S.-E.L.)
[3] Environmental and Occupational Health Sciences Institute, Rutgers Biomedical and Health Sciences, Piscataway, NJ 08854, USA; kgb3@eohsi.rutgers.edu
[4] Division of Pulmonary and Critical Care Medicine, Robert Wood Johnson Medical School, Rutgers University, New Brunswick, NJ 08901, USA; sunderja@rwjms.rutgers.edu
* Correspondence: indu.ayappa@mssm.edu; Tel.: +01-212-241-1967

Received: 27 February 2019; Accepted: 3 April 2019; Published: 6 April 2019

Abstract: *Background:* World Trade Center (WTC) dust-exposed subjects have multiple comorbidities that affect sleep. These include obstructive sleep apnea (OSA), chronic rhinosinusitis (CRS), gastroesophageal-reflux disorder (GERD) and post-traumatic stress disorder (PTSD). We examined the impact of these conditions to sleep-related outcomes. *Methods:* Demographics, co-morbidities and symptoms were obtained from 626 WTC (109F/517M), 33–87years, BMI = 29.96 ± 5.53 kg/m^2) subjects. OSA diagnosis was from a 2-night home sleep test (ARES^{TM}). Subjective sleep quality, sleep-related quality of life (QOL, Functional Outcomes of Sleep Questionnaire), excessive daytime sleepiness (Epworth Sleepiness Scale), sleep duration and sleep onset and maintenance complaints were assessed. *Results:* Poor sleep quality and complaints were reported by 19–70% of subjects and average sleep duration was 6.4 h. 74.8% of subjects had OSA. OSA diagnosis/severity was not associated with any sleep-related outcomes. Sleep duration was lower in subjects with all conditions ($p < 0.05$) except OSA. CRS was a significant risk factor for poor sleep-related QOL, sleepiness, sleep quality and insomnia; PTSD for poor sleep-related QOL and insomnia; GERD for poor sleep quality. These associations remained significant after adjustment for, age, BMI, gender, sleep duration and other comorbidities. *Conclusions:* Sleep complaints are common and related to several health conditions seen in WTC responders. Initial interventions in symptomatic patients with both OSA and comorbid conditions may need to be directed at sleep duration, insomnia or the comorbid condition itself, in combination with intervention for OSA.

Keywords: obstructive sleep apnea; comorbid insomnia; sleep-related quality of life; chronic sinusitis; sleepiness; WTC responders

1. Introduction

Following the World Trade Center (WTC) disaster, many responders who worked in rescue, recovery and debris removal were exposed to high concentrations (greater than 100,000 μm/m^3 total particles) of debris [1]. This exposure was associated with an increased risk of developing obstructive sleep apnea (OSA) [2], chronic rhinosinusitis (CRS) [3], post-traumatic stress disorder (PTSD), gastroesophageal reflux disease (GERD), anxiety and depression [4] all of which may be associated with sleep disruption. We recently reported a high prevalence of OSA in WTC responders related to chronic rhinosinusitis [5].

OSA is often associated with poor quality of life and sleepiness, likely from the associated sleep fragmentation and intermittent hypoxia. Although there is a weak relationship between presence of OSA and/or severity of OSA and sleep complaints and daytime outcomes, this correlation appears to be quite variable [6–10]. Sleep duration and insomnia may be additional factors affecting the relationship of OSA to sleepiness [6,9]. There is also increasing evidence that medical conditions that often coexist with OSA, such as CRS, anxiety, depression, PTSD and GERD, are associated with sleep complaints [11–17] and may confound the relationship between OSA and sleep-related quality of life outcomes. The independent contribution of each of these conditions to sleep-related complaints and the associated quality of life has not been closely examined.

Data on sleep-related quality of life, sleepiness and sleep duration were collected as part of a larger study (WTCSNORE) examining the role of nasal pathology in the pathophysiology of OSA in 643 WTC responders. We evaluated the relative contribution of sleep duration and comorbid illness to these outcomes in this population.

2. Materials and Methods

Study Population: The WTCSNORE study is a recently completed National Institute for Occupational Safety and Health (NIOSH) funded (#U01OH01415) study to examine the effect of nasal pathology on OSA in WTC responders. Between March 2013 and December 2016 we enrolled 643 subjects with no history of OSA and without reported loud and frequent snoring prior to 11 September 2001 from the WTC health programs at Rutgers Robert Wood Johnson Medical School, New York University School of Medicine and Icahn School Medicine at Mt. Sinai. The study protocol was approved by the Institutional Review Boards of Rutgers RBHS (Pro2012002164), NYU School of Medicine (I12-02578) and the Icahn School of Medicine at Mount Sinai (HS#16-00511) and all subjects signed informed consent. Subjects were considered ineligible if they had been diagnosed with gross skeletal alterations affecting the upper airway (e.g., micrognathia) or unstable chronic medical conditions known to affect OSA (chronic heart failure, stroke), were pregnant or had intent to become pregnant within the period of the protocol, were unable to sign informed consent form, were currently on treatment for OSA, were a habitual snorer prior to 9/11/2001, or had a diagnosis of OSA prior to 9/11/2001. In all subjects we obtained demographic data and the following metrics were assessed:

(1) Sleep-related Quality of life (QOL) was assessed using the Functional Outcomes of Sleep Questionnaire (FOSQ) [18]. The FOSQ is a validated 30-item questionnaire that is used to assess the impact of disorders of excessive sleepiness on activity of daily living. It consists of 5 subscales evaluating activity level, vigilance, intimacy, general productivity and social outcomes and has a possible combined score that ranges from 5 (poor) to 20 (excellent). A score < 17 is taken to indicate poor sleep-related quality of life.

(2) Excessive daytime sleepiness was evaluated with the Epworth Sleep Scale (ESS), a well-validated questionnaire that asks the subject to rate the likelihood of falling asleep in 8 commonly encountered situations [19]. Possible scores range from 0 (the least sleepy) to 24 (the most sleepy). A score of > 10 defines presence of excessive daytime sleepiness.

(3) A questionnaire regarding sleep and snoring was administered that included questions regarding bed and wake up times, duration of sleep (hours/night), frequency of difficulty falling and maintaining sleep per week, and overall quality of sleep. Quality of sleep was rated on a 4-point scale (1: excellent, 2: good, 3: fair, and 4: poor); poor sleep quality was defined as ≥ 3. Sleep onset insomnia was defined as present when the subject reported having trouble falling asleep at least 1–2 times a week, and sleep maintenance insomnia was recorded when a subject reported waking up early and not being able to go back to sleep at least 1–2 days per week.

(4) Home monitoring for OSA: Subjects wore an ARES^{TM} Unicorder (SleepMed, Inc., West Palm Beach, FL, USA) at home for 2 nights, with a pre-addressed mailer to return the device to the sleep lab. The ARES^{TM} Unicorder is a home sleep test device that has been validated against full in-lab polysomnography [20,21], shows high sensitivity for OSA (0.98) and is routinely used in clinical practice for home monitoring of OSA. It is worn on the forehead and does not require additional wires to external devices. It measures oxygen saturation and pulse rate from reflectance oximetry, airflow from a nasal cannula/pressure transducer, snoring via acoustic microphone and head movement actigraphy and head position from accelerometers. The ARES^{TM} respiratory data were analyzed as follows: Data from the monitor were autoscored and then manually edited by a single trained sleep technician and reviewed by a sleep expert. Apneas were scored when there was a reduction in airflow to less than 10% of baseline for >10 s. Hypopneas 4% were scored for >30% reduction in airflow associated with 4% or more decrease in oxygen saturation. Hypopneas with arousals (HypopneasArsl) were scored for visible reduction (>30% reduction) in airflow associated with surrogates of arousal (head movement, changes in snoring, or changes in pulse rate combined with disappearance of inspiratory flow limitation and a marked (>150%) increase in flow amplitude) at the end of the event, but <4% decrease in oxygen saturation [22]. AHI4% was calculated as Apneas+Hypopneas4% divided by total valid recording time in hours (h). The Respiratory Disturbance Index (RDI) was calculated as Apneas + Hypopneas 4% + HypopneasArsl divided by total valid recording time. Using these metrics, we define OSA as present when AHI4% $\geq$ 5/h or when RDI $\geq$ 15/h. When OSA is present by this definition, severity was graded by the AHI4%: mild (AHI4% < 15/h), moderate (AHI4% $\geq$ 15/h but < 30/h) or severe (AHI4% $\geq$ 30/h) [23].

(5) Chronic rhinosinusitsis (CRS): CRS was defined based on epidemiological criteria used in the European Position Paper on Rhinosinusitis and Nasal Polyps (EPOS) [24,25]. Subjects were considered CRS+ if two or more of the following symptoms were reported as present for >8 weeks: (1) nasal blockade/obstruction (2) nasal discharge, (3) facial pain and (4) reduction in or loss of smell. At least one symptom had to be nasal blockade or discharge.

(6) In addition, we quantified the subjects' perception of nasal congestion of each individual nostril by asking them to close one nostril while in the supine position and rate the level of congestion in the free nostril on a scale from 1 to 10, 1 being totally blocked/congested and 10 being totally open/uncongested. The lowest score (denoting greater congestion) of the two self-reported values from the left and right nostril was used for analysis.

(7) Comorbid conditions: Information on comorbid Anxiety/Panic, Depression, GERD and PTSD were obtained from a combination of self-report of physician diagnosis (GERD) obtained in our WTCSNORE questionnaire, standardized questionnaires (Depression, Panic disorder, PTSD) and from the certified conditions listed in WTC Health Program General Responder Data Center (GERD, Depression, Anxiety and Panic Disorder and PTSD) for each subject using the annual visit closest in time to the sleep study. If any of the sources used identified the presence of a co-morbid condition the subject was coded as positive for that condition. Depression was assessed by the patient health questionnaire (PHQ), PTSD (PTSD symptom checklist), panic (PHQ) and anxiety from the GAD-7 [26–29].

Assessment of other relevant variables and Statistical Analysis: Presence/absence of CRS, OSA, PTSD, Anxiety/Depression and GERD were defined as Yes/No (+/−) variables. Summary statistics were calculated and differences were compared using chi-square test for discrete categorical variables and two-sample *t*-test for continuous data. For skewed continuous variables, we used Wilcoxon test instead. Logistic regression analyses, with (i) sleep-related QOL (FOSQ $\geq$ 17 vs <17), (ii) Excessive Daytime Sleepiness (EDS) (Epworth sleepiness score >10 vs $\leq$10), (iii) Poor sleep quality (+/−), (iv) Sleep Onset Insomnia (+/−) and (v) and Sleep Maintenance Insomnia (+/−) as the dependent variables and OSA, CRS, GERD, PTSD, Anxiety/Panic and Depression as the independent variables were used to evaluate the association of sleep parameters and each of the independent variables before and after controlling for age, BMI, gender, sleep duration and the other variables. Statistical significance was defined by $p < 0.05$. All statistical analyses were performed using SAS v9.4 (SAS Institute Inc., Cary, NC, USA).

3. Results

We analyzed data from 626/643 subjects from the parent WTC study (WTCSNORE) in whom CRS data was available. Subjects were predominantly middle-aged men. The demographic data, sleep duration, sleep-related quality of life and sleep complaints are provided in Table 1. 74.8% of subjects had OSA diagnosed by home monitoring, predominantly mild OSA. 47.1% of the subjects were identified as CRS+ by questionnaire, 19.3% had depression, 23.5% had PTSD, 23.5% had anxiety/panic and 52% had GERD.

Table 1. Demographics of the study participants.

Variable	N of Valid Data	Summary
Age (years, Mean ± SD)	626	52.8 ± 8.6
BMI (kg/m², Mean ± SD)	626	29.9 ± 5.5
Female (%)	626	109 (17.3%)
Sleep Duration (h, Mean ± SD)	588	6.4 ± 1.3
≥7 h (%)		42.6%
6–6.99 h (%)		30.9%
<6 h (%)		26.5%
Snoring (Yes, %)	626	312 (49.8%)
Quality of Life (FOSQ) (Mean ± SD)	566	17.4 ± 2.6
Good, ≥17 (%)		62.0%
Poor, <17 (%)		38.0%
Sleepiness (ESS, Mean ± SD)	620	8.3 ± 4.8
Sleepy, >10 (%)		31.3%
Not Sleepy, ≤10 (%)		68.7%
Poor Sleep Quality (Yes, %)	623	441 (70.8%)
Sleep Onset Insomnia (Yes, %)	609	296 (48.6%)
Sleep Maintenance Insomnia (Yes, %)	622	116 (18.7%)
OSA + (%)	592	443 (74.8%)
Mild		274 (46.3%)
Moderate		112 (18.9%)
Severe		57 (9.6%)
CRS + (%)	626	295 (47.1%)
Depression + (%)	612	118 (19.3%)
PTSD + (%)	612	144 (23.5%)
Anxiety and Panic Disorder + (%)	612	144 (23.5%)
GERD + (%)	564	293 (52%)

Notes: BMI-Body Mass Index, ESS- Epworth sleepiness scores, FOSQ- Functional Outcome of Sleep Questionnaire, OSA-Obstructive Sleep Apnea, PSTD-Post Traumatic Stress Disorder, GERD- Gastroesophageal Reflux Disease.

Shorter sleep duration (in hours) was observed in subjects with CRS (CRS+ = 6.3 ± 1.4 vs CRS- = 6.5 ± 1.2, p = 0.03), PTSD (PTSD+ = 6.1 ± 1.5 vs PTSD- = 6.5 ± 1.3, p=0.01), anxiety/panic (anxiety/panic+ =6.0 ± 1.4 vs anxiety/panic- =6.5 ± 1.3, p < 0.0001) and depression (depression+ = 6.0 ± 1.4 vs depression- = 6.5 ± 1.3, p = 0.001) but not GERD (GERD+ = 6.4 ± 1.3 vs GERD- = 6.4 ± 1.3, p = NS) and OSA (OSA+ = 6.4 ± 1.3 vs OSA- = 6.4 ± 1.3, p = NS). Subjects with OSA were older than those without OSA, were predominantly male and had higher BMI, but did not differ in sleep duration, ESS, FOSQ or perception of nasal congestion. Subjects with CRS, PTSD, Anxiety/Panic, Depression and GERD showed greater sleepiness by ESS, worse sleep-related QOL by FOSQ and greater perceived nasal congestion than those without the condition. Of note, subjects with CRS had slightly higher BMI and OSA severity (See Table 2).

Table 2. Comparison of demographic and sleep related variables in subjects with and without OSA, CRS, GERD, PTSD and Anxiety/Panic and Depression.

		Age	Female	BMI kg/m²	Sleep Duration (h)	Sleepiness (ESS)	Quality of Life (FOSQ)	AHI4%/h	RDI/h	Perception of Nasal Congestion at time of Visit
		Mean ± SD	N (%)	Mean ± SD	Mean ± SD	Mean ± SD	Mean ± SD	Median (Q1, Q3)	Median (Q1, Q3)	Mean ± SD
OSA+	N = 443	53.5 ± 8.3 ‡	58 (13.1%) ‡	30.7 ± 5.5 ‡	6.4 ± 1.3	8.4 ± 4.9	17.4 ± 2.7	11 (6, 19) ‡	26 (18, 37) ‡	6.8 ± 2.2
OSA-	N = 149	50.3 ± 8.8	44 (29.5%)	27.5 ± 4.8	6.4 ± 1.3	8.0 ± 4.5	17.6 ± 2.5	2 (1, 3)	9 (8, 12)	6.8 ± 2.2
CRS+	N = 795	52.9 ± 8.9	46 (15.7%)	30.2 ± 5.8 *	6.3 ± 1.4 *	9.2 ± 5.1 †	16.7 ± 3.0 †	9 (4, 17) *	22 (15, 35)	6.2 ± 2.2 †
CRS-	N = 331	52.7 ± 8.4	46 (18.8%)	29.6 ± 5.7	6.5 ± 1.2	7.4 ± 4.5	18.1 ± 2.1	6 (3, 15)	19 (12, 32)	7.3 ± 2.1
GERD+	N = 293	52.6 ± 8.0	45 (15.4%)	30.9 ± 6.1 ‡	6.4 ± 1.3	9.0 ± 5.0 †	16.9 ± 2.9 ‡	8 (4, 17)	22 (15, 34)	6.3 ± 2.2 ‡
GERD-	N = 271	52.9 ± 9.2	54 (20%)	28.8 ± 4.9	6.4 ± 1.3	7.7 ± 4.7	18.0 ± 2.3	7 (3, 14.5)	20 (12, 32)	7.4 ± 2.0
PTSD+	N = 144	51.8 ± 8.0	25 (17.4%)	31.3 ± 6.2 †	6.1 ± 1.5 *	10.8 ± 5.3 ‡	15.3 ± 3.4 ‡	8 (4, 16)	23 (14, 35)	6.0 ± 2.2 ‡
PTSD-	N = 468	53.1 ± 8.8	82 (17.5%)	29.5 ± 5.3	6.5 ± 1.3	7.5 ± 4.4	18.1 ± 2.0	7 (3, 16)	20 (13, 33)	7.0 ± 2.2
Anxiety/Panic+	N = 144	51.9 ± 8.3	24 (16.7%)	30.9 ± 5.8 *	6.0 ± 1.4 ‡	10.6 ± 5.2 ‡	15.6 ± 3.4 ‡	8 (4, 17)	21 (14, 33)	6.2 ± 2.3 †
Anxiety/Panic-	N = 468	53.1 ± 8.7	83 (17.7%)	29.6 ± 5.4	6.5 ± 1.3	7.5 ± 4.4	18.0 ± 2.1	7 (3, 15)	20 (13, 33)	7.0 ± 2.2
Depression+	N = 118	52.9 ± 8.3	22 (18.6%)	31.5 ± 6.8 *	6.0 ± 1.4 †	10.7 ± 5.4 ‡	15.4 ± 3.4 ‡	8 (4, 15)	21 (13, 33)	5.9 ± 2.3 ‡
Depression-	N = 494	52.8 ± 8.7	85 (17.2%)	29.5 ± 5.1	6.5 ± 1.3	7.7 ± 4.5	17.9 ± 2.2	7 (3, 16)	20 (14, 33)	7.0 ± 2.1

Notes: OSA-Obstructive Sleep Apnea, PSTD-Post Traumatic Stress Disorder, GERD- Gastroesophageal Reflux Disease CRS- Chronic Rhinosinusitis. BMI-Body Mass Index, h-hour. Asterisk (*) denotes a p-value of <0.05. Cross (†) denotes a p-value of <0.01. Double dagger (‡) denotes a p-value of <0.0001.

Shorter sleep duration was significantly associated with worse sleep-related quality of life (FOSQ < 17, OR = 0.76 95% CI = 0.63, 0.92, p = 0.004), worse sleep quality (OR = 0.61, 95% CI 0.50, 0.74, p < 0.0001), increased sleepiness (ESS > 10, OR = 0.84, 95% CI 0.72, 0.99, p = 0.03), sleep onset insomnia (OR = 0.63, 95% CI 0.53, 0.74, p < 0.0001) and maintenance insomnia (OR = 0.54, 95% CI 0.43, 0.67, p < 0.0001) using a logistic model controlled for age, BMI, OSA and all comorbidities. In addition, gender was associated with worse sleep-related quality of life (FOSQ) and presence of sleep onset insomnia (p < 0.05). Sleep-related quality of life (FOSQ) and sleepiness (ESS) were significantly negatively correlated (r = −0.62 95% CI −0.67 to −0.57, p < 0.0001) but there was no correlation between sleep disordered breathing indices (SDB, AHI4% or RDI) and FOSQ (r = −0.05 for logAHI4% and r = −0.01 for logRDI, p = NS) or SDB and ESS (r = 0.05, for logAHI4%, r = 0.03, for logRDI, p = NS).

In our dataset, we were unable to demonstrate differences in quality of life, sleepiness, sleep quality, sleep onset insomnia, and sleep maintenance insomnia between subjects with and without OSA. However, presence of the other comorbid conditions (CRS, PTSD, Anxiety/Panic, Depression and GERD) were all significantly associated with worse quality of life, increased sleepiness, worse sleep quality and sleep onset and maintenance insomnia. (Table 3)

Table 3. Proportion of subjects with sleep related complaints in subjects with and without each condition.

		Poor Sleep-Related Quality of Life	Sleepiness	Poor Sleep Quality	Sleep Onset Insomnia	Sleep Maintenance Insomnia
		FOSQ < 17	ESS > 10	Yes	Present	Present
OSA+	N = 443	172 (38.8%)	136 (31.0%)	315 (71.3%)	207 (48.0%)	81 (18.3%)
OSA-	N = 149	52 (34.9%)	45 (30.2%)	99 (66.4%)	71 (48.6%)	25 (16.9%)
CRS +	N = 295	146 (49.5%) ‡	116 (39.9%) ‡	232 (79.5%) ‡	162 (56.8%) ‡	76 (26.0%) ‡
CRS-	N = 331	91 (27.5%)	77 (23.5%)	208 (63.0%)	133 (41.2%)	40 (12.12%)
GERD+	N = 293	132 (45.0%) †	111 (37.9%) †	231 (78.8%) ‡	153 (53.5%) †	60 (20.6%)
GERD-	N = 271	85 (31.4%)	67 (25.1%)	171 (63.3%)	114 (43.2%)	45 (16.7%)
PTSD+	N = 144	92 (63.9%) ‡	73 (51.0%) ‡	123 (85.4%) ‡	110 (78.0%) ‡	52 (36.1%) ‡
PTSD-	N = 468	138 (29.5%)	117 (25.2%)	310 (66.4%)	184 (40.4%)	62 (13.3%)
Anxiety/Panic+	N = 144	85 (59.0%) ‡	68 (47.6%) ‡	123 (86.0%) ‡	93 (66.4%) ‡	47 (32.6%) ‡
Anxiety/Panic-	N = 468	145 (31.0%)	122 (26.2%)	310 (66.2%)	201 (44.0%)	67 (14.4%)
Depression+	N = 118	76 (64.4%) ‡	61 (52.1%) ‡	98 (83.8%) †	83 (72.8%) ‡	39 (33.0%) ‡
Depression-	N = 494	154 (31.2%)	129 (26.3%)	335 (67.8%)	211 (43.7%)	75 (15.2%)

Notes: Asterisk (*) denotes a p-value of <0.05. Cross (†) denotes a p-value of <0.01. Double dagger (‡) denotes a p-value of <0.0001.

Table 4 summarizes the risk of each of the conditions on sleep-related outcomes and shows the associations of quality of life (FOSQ), excessive daytime sleepiness (ESS), sleep quality, sleep onset insomnia and maintenance insomnia with OSA severity, CRS and other co-morbid conditions. Model 1 is the unadjusted data, Model 2 adjusts for age, BMI and sleep duration and Model 3 adjusts for age, BMI, gender, sleep duration and other co-morbid condition. Our data did not show any statistically significant relationship between OSA and any of the sleep-related outcomes. CRS is a significant risk factor for poor quality of life, excessive daytime sleepiness and sleep complaints even in an adjusted model. PTSD was a significant risk factor for poor quality of life, sleep onset insomnia and sleep maintenance insomnia. GERD was a risk factor for poor quality of sleep. Figure 1 is a graphical representation of these odds ratios in Model 3.

Table 4. Odds ratio and 95% CI for presence of poor sleep-related quality of life (FOSQ < 17), sleepiness, poor quality sleep and insomnia in subjects with each condition compared to subjects without this condition.

		Model 1		Model 2		Model 3	
		OR [1]	95% CI	OR [2]	95% CI	OR [3]	95% CI
	OSA Severity						
	Mild OSA vs. No OSA	1.21	(0.80, 1.84)	1.02	(0.65, 1.59)	0.87	(0.51, 1.47)
	Moderate OSA vs. No OSA	1	(0.60, 1.67)	0.8	(0.46, 1.41)	0.73	(0.36, 1.45)
Poor Quality of Life	Severe OSA vs. No OSA	1.46	(0.78, 2.72)	0.98	(0.50,1.95)	1.09	(0.48, 2.49)
(FOSQ < 17)	CRS	2.58 ‡	(1.85, 3.60)	2.44 ‡	(1.72, 3.46)	2.48 ‡	(1.62, 3.80)
	GERD	1.79 †	(1.27, 2.53)	1.80 †	(1.24, 2.60)	1.14	(0.74, 1.76)
	PTSD	4.23 ‡	(2.85, 6.27)	3.93 ‡	(2.60, 5.94)	3.18 †	(1.72, 5.9)
	Anxiety/Panic	3.21 ‡	(2.18, 4.72)	2.87 ‡	(1.91, 4.29)	1.18	(0.66, 2.12)
	Depression	3.99 ‡	(2.62, 6.09)	3.61 ‡	(2.33, 5.59)	1.62	(0.85, 3.11)
	OSA Severity						
	Mild OSA vs. No OSA	1	(0.65, 1.54)	1.07	(0.67, 1.71)	0.9	(0.53, 1.52)
	Moderate OSA vs. No OSA	1.08	(0.63,1.84)	1.2	(0.67, 2.15)	1.07	(0.55, 2.08)
Sleepiness (ESS>10)	Severe OSA vs. No OSA	1.16	(0.60, 2.22)	1.09	(0.53, 2.24)	0.97	(0.42, 2.22)
	CRS	2.16 ‡	(1.53,3.06)	1.93 †	(1.34, 2.77)	1.80 †	(1.17, 2.76)
	GERD	1.82 †	(1.27, 2.62)	1.73 †	(1.18, 2.55)	1.2	(0.78, 1.87)
	PTSD	3.10 ‡	(2.10, 4.58)	2.71 ‡	(1.80, 4.09)	1.64	(0.89, 3.02)
	Anxiety/Panic	2.55 ‡	(1.73, 3.76)	2.03 †	(1.35, 3.06)	1.12	(0.63, 2.01)
	Depression	3.06 ‡	(2.02, 4.63)	2.62 †	(1.70, 4.05)	1.99	(1.05, 3.76)
	OSA Severity						
	Mild OSA vs. No OSA	1.16	(0.75, 1.77)	1.21	(0.75, 1.94)	1.05	(0.62, 1.78)
	Moderate OSA vs. No OSA	1.38	(0.81, 2.37)	1.28	(0.70, 2.36)	1.04	(0.51, 2.13)
Poor Sleep Quality	Severe OSA vs. No OSA	1.55	(0.78,3.10)	1.39	(0.64, 3.04)	1.31	(0.55, 3.15)
	CRS	2.27 ‡	(1.58,3.25)	2.20 ‡	(1.49,3.25)	1.95 †	(1.24, 3.07)
	GERD	2.16 ‡	(1.48,3.14)	2.21 ‡	(1.46, 3.33)	1.67 *	(1.06, 2.64)
	PTSD	2.97 ‡	(1.80,4.90)	2.45 †	(1.44, 4.16)	2.13	(0.96, 4.76)
	Anxiety/Panic	3.13 ‡	(1.88,5.22)	2.38 †	(1.40, 4.06)	1.49	(0.71, 3.13)
	Depression	2.45 †	(1.45, 4.14)	1.96 *	(1.13, 3.42)	0.95	(0.42, 2.14)
	OSA Severity						
	Mild OSA vs. No OSA	0.89	(0.59, 1.33)	0.79	(0.52, 1.20)	0.85	(0.53, 1.38)
	Moderate OSA vs. No OSA	1.13	(0.69,1.86)	0.94	(0.56, 1.57)	0.96	(0.51, 1.79)
Sleep Onset Insomnia	Severe OSA vs. No OSA	1.1	(0.59,2.04)	0.83	(0.43, 1.61)	1.05	(0.49, 2.24)
	CRS	1.88 ‡	(1.36, 2.60)	1.85 †	(1.34, 2.55)	1.63 *	(1.10, 2.41)
	GERD	1.51 *	(1.08, 2.12)	1.44 *	(1.02, 2.02)	0.99	(0.66, 1.47)
	PTSD	5.25 ‡	(3.38, 8.15)	5.22 ‡	(3.34, 8.14)	4.69 †	(2.49, 8.86)
	Anxiety/Panic	2.52 ‡	(1.70, 3.75)	2.48 ‡	(1.66, 3.70)	1.26	(0.71, 2.23)
	Depression	3.45 ‡	(2.20, 5.41)	3.31 ‡	(2.10, 5.20)	0.98	(0.50, 1.92)
	OSA Severity						
	Mild OSA vs. No OSA	1.1	(0.65, 1.87)	0.93	(0.54, 1.60)	0.85	(0.46, 1.56)
	Moderate OSA vs. No OSA	1.07	(0.56, 2.04)	0.8	(0.41, 1.58)	0.56	(0.25, 1.26)
Sleep Maintenance	Severe OSA vs. No OSA	1.18	(0.54, 2.58)	0.78	(0.34, 1.80)	0.75	(0.29, 1.95)
Insomnia	CRS	2.54 ‡	(1.67, 3.87)	2.49 ‡	(1.63, 3.81)	2.41 †	(1.44, 4.04)
	GERD	1.29	(0.84, 1.98)	1.2	(0.77, 1.85)	0.74	(0.44, 1.24)
	PTSD	3.68 ‡	(2.39, 5.68)	3.62 ‡	(2.33, 5.63)	3.53 ‡	(1.82, 6.88)
	Anxiety/Panic	2.89 ‡	(1.87, 4.45)	2.85 ‡	(1.83, 4.42)	1.24	(0.64, 2.37)
	Depression	2.74 ‡	(1.74, 4.33)	2.57 ‡	(1.62, 4.09)	1.06	(0.52, 2.16)

Notes: Asterisk (*) denotes a *p*-value of <0.05. Cross (†) denotes a *p*-value of <0.01. Double dagger (‡) denotes a *p*-value of <0.0001; 1: Unadjusted odds ratio estimates. 2: For responses of 'Poor quality of sleep", "Sleepy" and "FOSQ", the odds ratio estimates are adjusted for age, BMI and sleep duration; for responses of "Sleep onset Insomnia" and "Sleep Maintenance Insomnia", the odds ratio estimates are adjusted for age and BMI. 3 For responses of "Poor quality of sleep", "Sleepy" and "FOSQ", the odds ratio estimates are adjusted for Age, BMI, gender, sleep duration, and all other comorbidities; for response "Sleep onset Insomnia" and "Sleep Maintenance Insomnia", the odds ratio estimates are adjusted for age, BMI, gender and all other comorbidities.

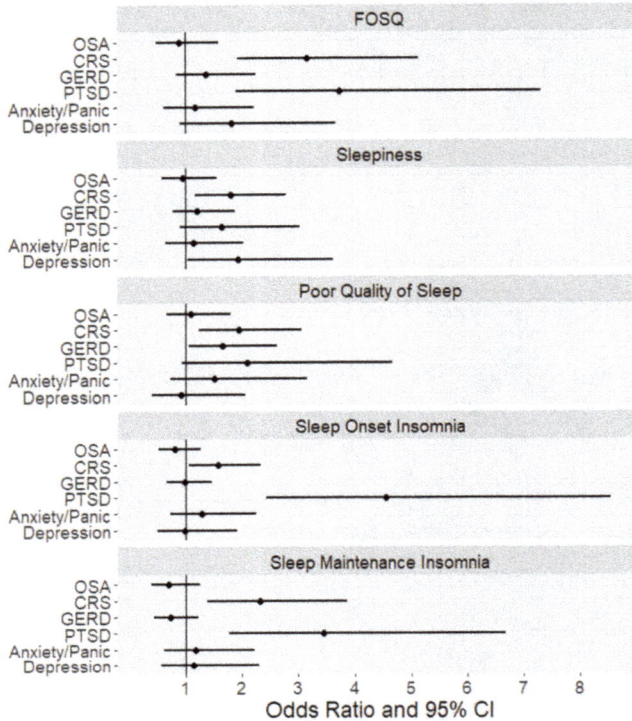

Figure 1. Odds ratio and 95% CI for each comorbid condition as a risk factor for adverse sleep outcomes.

4. Discussion

In this large dataset of WTC responders with and without OSA, CRS and other comorbidities that are known to impact sleep and quality of life, we show a significant relationship of sleep-related quality of life, sleepiness and sleep complaints to CRS and PTSD but little or no relationship to the presence of OSA. In patients with OSA, comorbidities that have typically been emphasized include hypertension, arrhythmias, stroke and other cardiovascular diseases [30–32]. Our data show that it may also be important to assess other comorbidities that directly impact sleep complaints.

The absence of a relationship between OSA and sleep complaints is not entirely unexpected. While sleepiness is one of the main symptoms of OSA, there is significant variability between individuals and the relationship of OSA (or OSA severity) to quality of life (QOL) and sleepiness has been inconsistent, especially in non-clinical populations [7–10]. Our data show that controlling for co-morbid conditions did not help explain the variability in OSA and sleep outcomes. Our dataset has a high prevalence of OSA, but the OSA severity (median AHI4% 11.0/h, median RDI 26.0/h in subjects with OSA) was slightly lower than earlier studies of predominantly moderate-severe OSA subjects [33]. However, OSA severity in our cohort is comparable to recent studies in clinical populations [6]—that also did not show a relationship between OSA severity and sleepiness.

Supporting the validity of our self-reported variables, we show the expected relationship between reduced sleep duration and sleepiness and sleep complaints [6]. Average sleep duration has decreased over the recent decades with over 40% of the U.S. population reporting habitual sleep time below the recommended 7–8 h [34]. The association of reduced sleep duration with poor cardiometabolic outcomes [35,36] highlights the importance of our finding of overall short sleep duration in the entire cohort (average 6.4 h with majority having sleep duration <7h) and suggests the need for further investigation and possible intervention.

Our results are also consistent with recent literature showing that individuals with CRS complain of poor sleep and demonstrate poor QOL related to sleep disruption [11,37,38]. However, these studies did not control for OSA severity or sleep duration. We hypothesized that the sleep complaints in CRS could be due to an increase in OSA, but instead found only a relationship to reduced sleep duration. Subjects with CRS in our study reported greater perception of nasal congestion when awake, suggesting that discomfort from congestion during sleep results in the reduced sleep duration and may account for this finding. However, the relationship of CRS to poor sleep remained even after controlling for sleep duration. We have shown a relationship of CRS to level of WTC exposure [5], and chronic inflammation has also been shown to be part of CRS; it is possible that systemic mediators of inflammation such as cytokines contribute to sleep disruption [37,39].

Poor sleep and sleepiness have also been shown in patients with mental health conditions like PTSD, anxiety and depression [8,40,41]. In our dataset all these conditions were highly correlated with one another, but also correlated with sleep complaints.

Although the relationship of sleep related outcomes to comorbid conditions remained significant despite controlling for BMI in the models, subjects with each of the conditions had a higher BMI than those without (see Table 2). Obesity is associated with short sleep duration [42] and may impact the sleep-related complaints in these subjects.

Strengths of our study include the large well-characterized dataset of subjects naïve to OSA treatment, objective measurement of OSA in all subjects, concurrent assessment of sleep complaints and data on confounders and comorbid conditions.

One potential limitation is that the incidence of both OSA and comorbid conditions was high in our cohort that is comprised mainly of male subjects. However, it has been demonstrated that the severity and type (obstructive vs central) of the OSA in the WTC responders was not different from a general clinic population, suggesting generalizability of our findings, of the correlations and of our causal inferences [43]. Furthermore, other specific groups such as veterans, the elderly [44,45] and some general populations have been shown to have a similarly high prevalence of OSA and these co-morbid conditions, and we suggest that our inferences may apply to these groups also. Another potential limitation is that while OSA was objectively assessed in all subjects, all other variables were based on a combination of self-report diagnoses, questionnaire and certification data from the general WTC database with possibility of being overestimated. However, our prevalence estimates are similar to those reported in WTC rescue and recovery workers [46].

5. Conclusions

Our data highlight the high prevalence of sleep-related complaints and poor quality of sleep in WTC responders. Our results challenge the often accepted clinical practice that in a patient with sleep complaints, the most urgent treatment needs to be directed to any OSA found. While OSA undoubtedly produces sleep symptoms in some, the role of other frequently found comorbid conditions, including CRS, PTSD, Anxiety/Panic, Depression and GERD, should not be underestimated and perhaps pursued more aggressively earlier. Initial interventions in symptomatic patients with both OSA and comorbid conditions may need to be directed at sleep duration, insomnia or the comorbid condition in combination with intervention for OSA.

Author Contributions: Conceptualization, I.A., K.B., D.M.R., S.-E.L. and J.S.; Data curation, I.A., Y.C., N.B., H.S., K.B. and A.T.; Formal analysis, I.A., Y.C., H.S., K.B. and S.-E.L.; Funding acquisition, I.A., D.M.R., S.-E.L. and J.S.; Investigation, N.B., H.S., K.B., and A.T.; Methodology, S.-E.L.; Project administration, I.A., and J.S.; Supervision, I.A., D.M.R., and J.S.; Visualization, Y.C., N.B., H.S., and S.-E.L.; Writing—original draft, I.A., N.B. and H.S.; Writing—review & editing, I.A., Y.C., N.B., H.S., K.B., A.T., D.M.R., S.-E.L. and J.S.

Funding: This study was funded by NIOSH/CDC U01OH010415 and NIH K24 grant HL109156 and in part by the NYU CTSA grant UL1 TR001445 from the National Center for Advancing Translational Sciences, National Institutes of Health, contract and/or grant number(s) U10 OH008232 (DCC), 200-2011-39356 (Mount Sinai

CCE) 200-2011-39385 (Rutgers CCE) and 200-2011-39384 (NYU CCE) from the Centers for Disease Control and Prevention/National Institute for Occupational Safety and Health (CDC/NIOSH). Its contents are solely the responsibility of the authors and do not necessarily represent the official views of CDC/NIOSH.

Acknowledgments: We acknowledge Alan Perez, Jash Vakil, Emma Ducca, Tyler Gumb, Rohan Patel, Clarimel Cepeda, Namrata Kulkarni, Shahnaz Alimokhtari and Marta Hernandez who participated as research assistants, and the subjects who are enrolled in the WTCHP who participated in the study.

Conflicts of Interest: The authors declare no conflict of interest.

Abbreviations

OSA	Obstructive Sleep Apnea
BMI	Body Mass Index
H	Hour/s
CI	Confidence Interval
OR	Odds Ratio
CRS	Chronic Rhinosinusitis
GERD	Gastroesophageal Reflux Disorder
PTSD	Post Traumatic Stress Disorder
WTC	World Trade Center
FOSQ	Functional Outcomes of Sleep Questionnaire
QOL	Quality of Life
AHI4%	Apnea Hypopnea (with 4% O2 desaturation) Index
RDI	Respiratory Disturbance Index
SDB	Sleep Disordered Breathing
PAP	Positive Airway Pressure

References

1. Lioy, P.J.; Georgopoulos, P. The anatomy of the exposures that occurred around the World Trade Center site: 9/11 and beyond. *Ann. N. Y. Acad. Sci.* **2006**, *1076*, 54–79. [CrossRef]
2. Ahuja, S.; Zhu, Z.; Shao, Y.; Berger, K.I.; Reibman, J.; Ahmed, O. Obstructive Sleep Apnea in Community Members Exposed to World Trade Center Dust and Fumes. *J. Clin. Sleep Med.* **2018**, *14*, 735–743. [CrossRef]
3. Weakley, J.; Hall, C.B.; Liu, X.; Zeig-Owens, R.; Webber, M.P.; Schwartz, T.; Prezant, D. The effect of World Trade Center exposure on the latency of chronic rhinosinusitis diagnoses in New York City firefighters: 2001–2011. *Occup. Environ. Med.* **2016**, *73*, 280–283. [CrossRef] [PubMed]
4. Bowler, R.M.; Kornblith, E.S.; Li, J.; Adams, S.W.; Gocheva, V.V.; Schwarzer, R.; Cone, J.E. Police officers who responded to 9/11: Comorbidity of PTSD, depression, and anxiety 10–11 years later. *Am. J. Ind. Med.* **2016**, *59*, 425–436. [CrossRef] [PubMed]
5. Sunderram, J.; Weintraub, M.; Black, K.; Alimokhtari, S.; Twumasi, A.; Sanders, H.; Udasin, I.; Harrison, D.; Chitkara, N.; de la Hoz, R.E.; et al. Chronic Rhinosinusitis Is an Independent Risk Factor for OSA in World Trade Center Responders. *Chest* **2019**, *155*, 375–383. [CrossRef] [PubMed]
6. Prasad, B.; Steffen, A.D.; Van Dongen, H.P.A.; Pack, F.M.; Strakovsky, I.; Staley, B.; Dinges, D.F.; Maislin, G.; Pack, A.I.; Weaver, T.E. Determinants of sleepiness in obstructive sleep apnea. *Sleep* **2018**, *41*. [CrossRef]
7. Budhiraja, R.; Kushida, C.A.; Nichols, D.A.; Walsh, J.K.; Simon, R.D.; Gottlieb, D.J.; Quan, S.F. Predictors of sleepiness in obstructive sleep apnoea at baseline and after 6 months of continuous positive airway pressure therapy. *Eur. Respir. J.* **2017**, *50*, 1700348. [CrossRef] [PubMed]
8. Bixler, E.O.; Vgontzas, A.N.; Lin, H.M.; Calhoun, S.L.; Vela-Bueno, A.; Kales, A. Excessive daytime sleepiness in a general population sample: The role of sleep apnea, age, obesity, diabetes, and depression. *J. Clin. Endocrinol. Metab.* **2005**, *90*, 4510–4515. [CrossRef] [PubMed]
9. Kapur, V.K.; Baldwin, C.M.; Resnick, H.E.; Gottlieb, D.J.; Nieto, F.J. Sleepiness in patients with moderate to severe sleep-disordered breathing. *Sleep* **2005**, *28*, 472–477. [CrossRef]
10. Gottlieb, D.J.; Whitney, C.W.; Bonekat, W.H.; Iber, C.; James, G.D.; Lebowitz, M.; Nieto, F.J.; Rosenberg, C.E. Relation of sleepiness to respiratory disturbance index: The Sleep Heart Health Study. *Am. J. Respir. Crit. Care Med.* **1999**, *159*, 502–507. [CrossRef]

11. Bengtsson, C.; Lindberg, E.; Jonsson, L.; Holmstrom, M.; Sundbom, F.; Hedner, J.; Malinovschi, A.; Middelveld, R.; Forsberg, B.; Janson, C. Chronic Rhinosinusitis Impairs Sleep Quality: Results of the GA2LEN Study. *Sleep* **2017**, *40*. [CrossRef]

12. Gregory, A.M.; Buysse, D.J.; Willis, T.A.; Rijsdijk, F.V.; Maughan, B.; Rowe, R.; Cartwright, S.; Barclay, N.L.; Eley, T.C. Associations between sleep quality and anxiety and depression symptoms in a sample of young adult twins and siblings. *J. Psychosom. Res.* **2011**, *71*, 250–255. [CrossRef] [PubMed]

13. Westermeyer, J.; Khawaja, I.; Freerks, M.; Sutherland, R.J.; Engle, K.; Johnson, D.; Thuras, P.; Rossom, R.; Hurwitz, T. Correlates of daytime sleepiness in patients with posttraumatic stress disorder and sleep disturbance. *Prim. Care Companion J. Clin. Psychiatry* **2010**, *12*. [CrossRef]

14. Lindam, A.; Jansson, C.; Nordenstedt, H.; Pedersen, N.L.; Lagergren, J. A population-based study of gastroesophageal reflux disease and sleep problems in elderly twins. *PLoS ONE* **2012**, *7*, e48602. [CrossRef]

15. Zheng, M.; Wang, X.; Ge, S.; Gu, Y.; Ding, X.; Zhang, Y.; Ye, J.; Zhang, L. Allergic and Non-Allergic Rhinitis Are Common in Obstructive Sleep Apnea but Not Associated With Disease Severity. *J. Clin. Sleep Med.* **2017**, *13*, 959–966. [CrossRef]

16. Pan, M.L.; Tsao, H.M.; Hsu, C.C.; Wu, K.M.; Hsu, T.S.; Wu, Y.T.; Hu, G.C. Bidirectional association between obstructive sleep apnea and depression: A population-based longitudinal study. *Medicine (Baltim.)* **2016**, *95*, e4833. [CrossRef]

17. You, C.R.; Oh, J.H.; Seo, M.; Lee, H.Y.; Joo, H.; Jung, S.H.; Lee, S.H.; Choi, M.G. Association Between Non-erosive Reflux Disease and High Risk of Obstructive Sleep Apnea in Korean Population. *J. Neurogastroenterol. Motil.* **2014**, *20*, 197–204. [CrossRef]

18. Weaver, T.E.; Laizner, A.M.; Evans, L.K.; Maislin, G.; Chugh, D.K.; Lyon, K.; Smith, P.L.; Schwartz, A.R.; Redline, S.; Pack, A.I.; et al. An instrument to measure functional status outcomes for disorders of excessive sleepiness. *Sleep* **1997**, *20*, 835–843.

19. Johns, M.W. A new method for measuring daytime sleepiness: The Epworth sleepiness scale. *Sleep* **1991**, *14*, 540–545. [CrossRef] [PubMed]

20. Ayappa, I.; Norman, R.G.; Seelall, V.; Rapoport, D.M. Validation of a self-applied unattended monitor for sleep disordered breathing. *J. Clin. Sleep Med.* **2008**, *4*, 26–37.

21. Westbrook, P.R.; Levendowski, D.J.; Cvetinovic, M.; Zavora, T.; Velimirovic, V.; Henninger, D.; Nicholson, D. Description and validation of the apnea risk evaluation system: A novel method to diagnose sleep apnea-hypopnea in the home. *Chest* **2005**, *128*, 2166–2175. [CrossRef]

22. Ayappa, I.; Norman, R.G.; Krieger, A.C.; Rosen, A.; O'Malley R, L.; Rapoport, D.M. Non-Invasive detection of respiratory effort-related arousals (RERas) by a nasal cannula/pressure transducer system. *Sleep* **2000**, *23*, 763–771. [CrossRef]

23. American Academy of Sleep Medicine Task Force. Sleep-related breathing disorders in adults: Recommendations for syndrome definition and measurement techniques in clinical research. The Report of an American Academy of Sleep Medicine Task Force. *Sleep* **1999**, *22*, 667–689. [CrossRef]

24. Fokkens, W.J.; Lund, V.J.; Mullol, J.; Bachert, C.; Alobid, I.; Baroody, F.; Cohen, N.; Cervin, A.; Douglas, R.; Gevaert, P.; et al. European Position Paper on Rhinosinusitis and Nasal Polyps 2012. *Rhinol. Suppl.* **2012**, *23*, 1–298.

25. Fokkens, W.J.; Lund, V.J.; Mullol, J.; Bachert, C.; Alobid, I.; Baroody, F.; Cohen, N.; Cervin, A.; Douglas, R.; Gevaert, P.; et al. EPOS 2012: European position paper on rhinosinusitis and nasal polyps 2012. A summary for otorhinolaryngologists. *Rhinology* **2012**, *50*, 1–12. [CrossRef]

26. Kroenke, K.; Spitzer, R.L.; Williams, J.B. The PHQ-9: Validity of a brief depression severity measure. *J. Gen. Intern. Med.* **2001**, *16*, 606–613. [CrossRef]

27. Spitzer, R.L.; Kroenke, K.; Williams, J.B. Validation and utility of a self-report version of PRIME-MD: The PHQ primary care study. Primary Care Evaluation of Mental Disorders. Patient Health Questionnaire. *JAMA* **1999**, *282*, 1737–1744. [CrossRef]

28. Spitzer, R.L.; Kroenke, K.; Williams, J.B.; Lowe, B. A brief measure for assessing generalized anxiety disorder: The GAD-7. *Arch. Intern. Med.* **2006**, *166*, 1092–1097. [CrossRef]

29. Blanchard, E.B.; Jones-Alexander, J.; Buckley, T.C.; Forneris, C.A. Psychometric properties of the PTSD Checklist (PCL). *Behav. Res. Ther.* **1996**, *34*, 669–673. [CrossRef]

30. Peppard, P.E.; Young, T.; Palta, M.; Skatrud, J. Prospective study of the association between sleep-disordered breathing and hypertension. *N. Engl. J. Med.* **2000**, *342*, 1378–1384. [CrossRef]

31. Yaggi, H.K.; Concato, J.; Kernan, W.N.; Lichtman, J.H.; Brass, L.M.; Mohsenin, V. Obstructive sleep apnea as a risk factor for stroke and death. *N. Engl. J. Med.* **2005**, *353*, 2034–2041. [CrossRef] [PubMed]
32. Mehra, R.; Benjamin, E.J.; Shahar, E.; Gottlieb, D.J.; Nawabit, R.; Kirchner, H.L.; Sahadevan, J.; Redline, S. Association of nocturnal arrhythmias with sleep-disordered breathing: The Sleep Heart Health Study. *Am. J. Respir. Crit. Care Med.* **2006**, *173*, 910–916. [CrossRef] [PubMed]
33. Quan, S.F.; Chan, C.S.; Dement, W.C.; Gevins, A.; Goodwin, J.L.; Gottlieb, D.J.; Green, S.; Guilleminault, C.; Hirshkowitz, M.; Hyde, P.R.; et al. The association between obstructive sleep apnea and neurocognitive performance—The Apnea Positive Pressure Long-term Efficacy Study (APPLES). *Sleep* **2011**, *34*, 303–314. [CrossRef]
34. Hirshkowitz, M.; Whiton, K.; Albert, S.M.; Alessi, C.; Bruni, O.; DonCarlos, L.; Hazen, N.; Herman, J.; Adams Hillard, P.J.; Katz, E.S.; et al. National Sleep Foundation's updated sleep duration recommendations: Final report. *Sleep Health* **2015**, *1*, 233–243. [CrossRef] [PubMed]
35. St-Onge, M.P.; Grandner, M.A.; Brown, D.; Conroy, M.B.; Jean-Louis, G.; Coons, M.; Bhatt, D.L. Sleep Duration and Quality: Impact on Lifestyle Behaviors and Cardiometabolic Health: A Scientific Statement From the American Heart Association. *Circulation* **2016**, *134*, e367–e386. [CrossRef]
36. Cappuccio, F.P.; Cooper, D.; D'Elia, L.; Strazzullo, P.; Miller, M.A. Sleep duration predicts cardiovascular outcomes: A systematic review and meta-analysis of prospective studies. *Eur. Heart J* **2011**, *32*, 1484–1492. [CrossRef]
37. Alt, J.A.; Smith, T.L. Chronic rhinosinusitis and sleep: A contemporary review. *Int. Forum Allergy Rhinol.* **2013**, *3*, 941–949. [CrossRef]
38. Alt, J.A.; Smith, T.L.; Mace, J.C.; Soler, Z.M. Sleep quality and disease severity in patients with chronic rhinosinusitis. *Laryngoscope* **2013**, *123*, 2364–2370. [CrossRef]
39. Mahdavinia, M.; Schleimer, R.P.; Keshavarzian, A. Sleep disruption in chronic rhinosinusitis. *Expert Rev. Anti-Infect. Ther.* **2017**, *15*, 457–465. [CrossRef]
40. Ohayon, M.M.; Shapiro, C.M. Sleep disturbances and psychiatric disorders associated with posttraumatic stress disorder in the general population. *Compr. Psychiatry* **2000**, *41*, 469–478. [CrossRef]
41. Jenkins, M.M.; Colvonen, P.J.; Norman, S.B.; Afari, N.; Allard, C.B.; Drummond, S.P. Prevalence and Mental Health Correlates of Insomnia in First-Encounter Veterans with and without Military Sexual Trauma. *Sleep* **2015**, *38*, 1547–1554. [CrossRef] [PubMed]
42. Cappuccio, F.P.; Taggart, F.M.; Kandala, N.B.; Currie, A.; Peile, E.; Stranges, S.; Miller, M.A. Meta-analysis of short sleep duration and obesity in children and adults. *Sleep* **2008**, *31*, 619–626. [CrossRef] [PubMed]
43. de la Hoz, R.E.; Aurora, R.N.; Landsbergis, P.; Bienenfeld, L.A.; Afilaka, A.A.; Herbert, R. Snoring and obstructive sleep apnea among former World Trade Center rescue workers and volunteers. *J. Occup. Environ. Med.* **2010**, *52*, 29–32. [CrossRef]
44. Haba-Rubio, J.; Marques-Vidal, P.; Andries, D.; Tobback, N.; Preisig, M.; Vollenweider, P.; Waeber, G.; Luca, G.; Tafti, M.; Heinzer, R. Objective sleep structure and cardiovascular risk factors in the general population: The HypnoLaus Study. *Sleep* **2015**, *38*, 391–400. [CrossRef] [PubMed]
45. Heinzer, R.; Vat, S.; Marques-Vidal, P.; Marti-Soler, H.; Andries, D.; Tobback, N.; Mooser, V.; Preisig, M.; Malhotra, A.; Waeber, G.; et al. Prevalence of sleep-disordered breathing in the general population: The HypnoLaus study. *Lancet Respir. Med.* **2015**, *3*, 310–318. [CrossRef]
46. Wisnivesky, J.P.; Teitelbaum, S.L.; Todd, A.C.; Boffetta, P.; Crane, M.; Crowley, L.; de la Hoz, R.E.; Dellenbaugh, C.; Harrison, D.; Herbert, R.; et al. Persistence of multiple illnesses in World Trade Center rescue and recovery workers: A cohort study. *Lancet* **2011**, *378*, 888–897. [CrossRef]

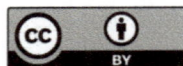

International Journal of
Environmental Research and Public Health

MDPI

Article

Increased Incidence of Thyroid Cancer among World Trade Center First Responders: A Descriptive Epidemiological Assessment

Stephanie Tuminello [1], Maaike A. G. van Gerwen [1], Eric Genden [2], Michael Crane [3], Wil Lieberman-Cribbin [1] and Emanuela Taioli [1,4,5,*]

1   Institute for Translational Epidemiology and Department of Population Health Science and Policy, Icahn School of Medicine at Mount Sinai, New York, NY 10029, USA; Stephanie.Tuminello@mssm.edu (S.T.); maaike.vangerwen@icahn.mssm.edu (M.A.G.v.G.); wil.lieberman-cribbin@icahn.mssm.edu (W.L.-C.)
2   Department of Otolaryngology-Head and Neck Surgery, Icahn School of Medicine at Mount Sinai, New York, NY 10029, USA; Eric.Genden@mountsinai.org
3   Division of Occupational and Environmental Medicine, Department of Environmental Medicine and Public Health, Icahn School of Medicine at Mount Sinai, New York, NY 10029, USA; michael.crane@mssm.edu
4   Department of Thoracic Surgery, Icahn School of Medicine at Mount Sinai, New York, NY 10029, USA
5   Tisch Cancer Institute, Icahn School of Medicine at Mount Sinai, New York, NY 10029, USA
*   Correspondence: emanuela.taioli@mountsinai.org; Tel.: +1-212-659-9590

Received: 20 February 2019; Accepted: 4 April 2019; Published: 9 April 2019

Abstract: An increased incidence of thyroid cancer among 9/11 rescue workers has been reported, the etiology of which remains unclear but which may, at least partly, be the result of the increased medical surveillance this group undergoes. This study aimed to investigate thyroid cancer in World Trade Center (WTC) responders by looking at the demographic data and questionnaire responses of thyroid cancer cases from the Mount Sinai WTC Health Program (WTCHP). WTCHP thyroid cancer tumors were of a similar size ($p = 0.4$), and were diagnosed at a similar age ($p = 0.2$) compared to a subset of thyroid cancer cases treated at Mount Sinai without WTC exposure. These results do not support the surveillance bias hypothesis, under which smaller tumors are expected to be diagnosed at earlier ages. WTCHP thyroid cancer cases also reported a past history of radiation exposure and a family history of thyroid conditions at lower rates than expected, with higher than expected rates of previous cancer diagnoses, family histories of other cancers, and high Body Mass Indexes (BMIs). Further research is needed to better understand the underlying risk factors that may play a role in the development of thyroid cancer in this group.

Keywords: thyroid cancer; 9/11 disaster; World Trade Center; surveillance bias

1. Introduction

An increased incidence of thyroid cancer has been reported in the Mount Sinai World Trade Center (WTC) responders [1], WTC-exposed fire fighters [2], and the New York City (NYC) Department of Health exposed residents [3] with an excess risk in the range of two to three times the incidence reported by New York City, New York State, and other national reference populations. This is despite the fact that established risk factors for thyroid cancer, such as exposure to radiation or iodine-131 [4,5], have not been reported in connection to Ground Zero [6]. The 9/11 attack did result in residents and responders being acutely exposed to several carcinogens mixed with dust and particles [1,7–9], although the direct link with WTC exposure and increased risk of cancer in WTC first responders remains unclear. Moreover, while the time and length of exposure of these responders have been reconstructed from questionnaires, this measure is clearly imprecise as recall bias is an important factor in a situation of extreme stress [10].

A possible explanation for the excess number of thyroid cancers observed in the responders cohort is over-diagnosis of thyroid cancer because of increased surveillance [11]. The large number of respiratory health issues developed by responders after their exposure to WTC dust has prompted a higher rate of diagnostic imaging of the chest, thus increasing the possibility of a chance thyroid nodule discovery [12,13]. Preliminary evidence, however, examining the thyroid nodules of WTC first responders found that all tissue samples tested were positive for biomarkers of malignancy, suggesting that while surveillance bias may be occurring, over-diagnosis of false-positives cannot sufficiently explain the excess risk of thyroid cancer observed in this group [14].

Disentangling the roles of various contributors to this excess risk of thyroid cancer would have major clinical and preventive consequences for the WTC responders. The aims of this study were to (a) examine non-modifiable demographic factors such as age, sex, race or ethnicity, as well as other contributing exposures predating thyroid cancer diagnosis; and (b) to better describe these WTC cancers and the similarities and differences of WTC thyroid cancers to non-WTC thyroid cancers.

2. Methods

2.1. Participant Selection and Enrollment

One of the cohorts in which excess thyroid cancer risk has been observed [1] is the Mount Sinai World Trade Center Health Program (WTCHP). Responders who participated (as employees or volunteers) in the rescue, recovery, and cleanup efforts at the WTC sites have been enrolled at Mount Sinai in the WTCHP, which is funded under the James Zadroga 9/11 Health and Compensation Act of 2010, on the basis of eligibility criteria including type of duties, site location, and dates and hours worked [15]. The medical protocol for the monitoring program includes self-administered physical and mental health questionnaires, as well as a physical examination, laboratory tests, spirometry, and a chest radiograph [15,16]. Over 27,000 responders have had a least one monitoring visit in the WTCHP and have consented for their data to be aggregated, of which a total of 20,984 have consented for their records to be used for medical research [15].

Cancer cases were identified through periodical linkage with the cancer registries of New York, New Jersey, Pennsylvania, and Connecticut, as these states account for 98% of the responders' residencies at time of WTCHP enrollment. The full linkage methodology has been described elsewhere [15]. Only thyroid cancer cases validated by a cancer registry, and only those whose enrollment into the WTCHP pre-dated their cancer diagnosis, were considered eligible to participate in this study. Between 2002 and 2013 there were 73 eligible first responders who had developed thyroid cancer.

Eligible participants were contacted by phone, and those interested in participating were mailed an initial letter further explaining the research project, along with a consent form and brief questionnaire. This questionnaire was sectioned, with questions asking about past exposure to radiation, family medical history, personal medical history, smoking history, and other demographic information. Participants filled out the questionnaire at home and returned it by mail using a pre-stamped and pre-addressed return envelope. Participants had the contact information of the research assistant working on the project if they had any questions. In one case the questionnaire was filled out over the phone as the participant had trouble reading and writing. A signed copy of their study consents was mailed back to each participant. Of the 73 participants in the WTCHP cohort of responders who were eligible to be contacted, four had to be excluded because they did not speak English or because they had no viable contact information. Of the remaining 69 WTC thyroid cancer cases, 35 (51%) consented to completing the questionnaire. The study protocol was approved by the Icahn School of Medicine at Mount Sinai's Institutional Review Board (IRB-17-01323).

2.2. Data Processing and Statistical Analysis

Upon return of the questionnaires, the data were input into excel to create a database of questionnaire responses, and this database was uploaded into SAS for statistical analysis. Some questionnaire responses were collapsed to make results more interpretable. If a participant reported having had an X-ray of their head or neck, a computed tomography (CT) scan of their head, neck or chest, or having had radiation therapy in the head or neck region predating their thyroid cancer diagnosis they were considered as having had some sort of radiation exposure. A diagnosis of another cancer was recorded and specified if that cancer diagnosis predated or postdated their diagnosis of thyroid cancer. BMI was calculated using the self-reported height and weight of the study participants, and with the cutoffs used for underweight, overweight and obese were <25, 25–30 and >30 kg/m^2, respectively, as suggested by the Center for Disease Control and Prevention [17].

The data obtained from the questionnaires, as well as the initial data reported by the WTCHP (age at diagnosis, race, gender, histology, marital status, education and smoking status) were compared to a sample of thyroid cancer from the Mount Sinai Cancer Registry generated by an official from the Cancer Registry. This sample was limited to those diagnosed with thyroid cancer and treated at Mount Sinai between 2002 and 2013, in order to cover a comparable time-frame.

Chi-square test, or Fisher's exact test for small sample size were used to compare WTC and Sinai Registry data for categorical variables. Wilcoxon Rank Sum Test was used for continuous variables not normally distributed. All statistical analysis was conducted using SAS version 9.4 (SAS Institute Inc., Cary, NC, USA).

3. Results

There were 73 thyroid cancer cases from the WTCHP cohort and these were compared to 949 thyroid cancer cases from the Mount Sinai Cancer Registry. The majority of thyroid cancer cases were white, both in the WTCHP group (71.9%) and in the Mount Sinai Cancer Registry (70.2%) ($p = 0.8$). There was, however, a statistically significant difference in gender ($p < 0.0001$), with WTCHP cases more likely to be male (78.1%). There was no significant difference between the two groups in terms of tumor size ($p = 0.4$), and the mean tumor size was small in both the WTCHP and the Mount Sinai group, 1.4 cm and 1.8 cm, respectively. Age at diagnosis was also similar between the two groups ($p = 0.2$); the mean age for those diagnosed after WTC exposure was 48.9 years while the Mount Sinai Registry mean diagnosis age was 51 years old. There was a statistically significant difference in terms of histology ($p = 0.04$), with those in the WTCHP cohort more likely to be diagnosed with a subtype of papillary carcinoma. There was also a statistically significant difference between the WTCHP and Mount Sinai group in terms of smoking ($p = 0.0385$), whereby those in the WTCHP group were more likely to be current smokers, and in terms of marital status ($p < 0.0001$), with those in the WTCHP cohort being more likely to be married (Table 1).

Out of the 69 eligible WTC thyroid cancer cases, 35 (51%) consented to complete the questionnaire. Those who consented and completed the questionnaire did not differ significantly in terms of race, gender, age at diagnosis or histology than those who did not participate in the study (data not shown). A total of 23% of cases reported some sort of radiation exposure. While only 9% reported a family history of thyroid health issues (either a benign goiter or thyroid cancer), 67% reported a family history of other cancer types. Additionally, 21% reported a previous history of cancer before the diagnosis of thyroid cancer. The majority of the study cohort had a BMI between 25 and 30 Kg/m^2 (44%) or >30 kg/m^2 (44%). Most participants (62%) reported that their thyroid cancer was diagnosed as a consequence of routine or incidental medical surveillance, and not because they went to a doctor with symptoms consistent with thyroid cancer (Table 2).

Table 1. Description of World Trade Center Health Program (WTCHP) and Mount Sinai Registry thyroid cancer cases.

Demographic and Clinical Characteristics *	WTCHP (n = 73)		Sinai Cancer Registry (n = 949)		p Value
	n	%	n	%	
Race/Ethnicity					0.8177
White	41	71.9	634	70.2	
Black	3	5.3	68	7.5	
Other	13	22.8	201	22.3	
Gender					<0.0001
Female	16	21.9	695	73.3	
Male	57	78.1	253	26.7	
Tumor Size (cm)	Mean (1.4)	SD (1.2)	Mean (1.8)	SD (1.9)	0.4053
Age at Diagnosis	Mean (48.9)	SD (8.0)	Mean (51.0)	SD (16.2)	0.2252
Histology ^					0.0363
Papillary Carcinoma	66	90.4	792	83.5	
Papillary Adenocarcinoma NOS	(63.6%)		(58.7%)		
Papillary Carcinoma Follicular Variant	(28.8%)		(22.0%)		
Papillary Microcarcinoma	(3.0%)		(17.7%)		
Papillary Carcinoma Columnar Cell	(4.5%)		(1.6%)		
Other Adenocarcinoma	5	6.9	41	4.3	
Oxyphilic Adenocarcinoma	(60.0%)		(46.3%)		
Follicular Adenocarcinoma	(40.0%)		(53.7%)		
Other	2	2.7	116	12.2	
Smoking Status					0.0385
Current Smoker	3	5.1	14	1.5	
Former or Never Smoker	56	94.9	925	98.5	
Marital Status					<0.0001
Married or Partnered	42	70.0	519	59.7	
Separated or Divorced	12	20.0	56	6.4	
Single	3	5.0	241	27.7	
Widowed	3	5.0	53	6.1	

* Race n_{WTC} = 57, $n_{registry}$ = 903; gender n_{WTC} = 73, $n_{registry}$ = 948; tumor size n_{WTC} = 27, $n_{registry}$ = 753; age at diagnosis n_{WTC} = 73, $n_{registry}$ = 949; histology n_{WTC} = 73, $n_{registry}$ = 94, marital status n_{WTC} = 60, $n_{registry}$ = 869. ^ Histology is based on International Classification of Diseases for Oncology (ICD-O-3) coding: Papillary adenocarcinoma NOS = 8260, oxyphilic adenocarcinoma = 8290, follicular adenocarcinoma NOS = 8330, papillary carcinoma follicular variant = 8340, papillary microcarcinoma = 8341, papillary carcinoma columnar cell = 8344.

Table 2. WTC thyroid cases questionnaire responses (n = 35).

Exposures and Medical History *	n	%
Radiation Exposure		
Yes	8	22.9
No	27	77.1
Family History of Thyroid Issues		
Yes	3	8.8
No	31	91.2
Family History Other Cancer		
Yes	22	66.7
No	11	33.3
Personal History of Another Cancer		
Before Thyroid Cancer	7	20.6
After Thyroid Cancer or Unknown dx Date	8	23.5
No Other Cancer	19	55.9
BMI (kg/m^2)		
<25	4	11.8
25–30	15	44.1
>30	15	44.1
Diagnosis Method		
Because of Symptoms	21	61.8
Due to Routine Screening or Unrelated Medical Event	13	38.2

* Missing data for family history of other cancer (1), family history of other cancer (2), personal history of other cancer (1), smoking history (1), BMI (1), diagnosis method (1).

4. Discussion

Whether or not surveillance bias is occurring in the WTCHP cohort, and the extent to which this bias may be contributing to the increased incidence of thyroid cancer among first responders, remains unclear. The similar clinical characteristics observed between the WTCHP responders and those in the Mount Sinai Registry suggest that the excess risk of thyroid cancer in first responders cannot be adequately explained by surveillance bias alone. Under the surveillance bias hypothesis, we would expect increased detection of small thyroid nodules [11,18], yet there was no statistical difference between the average tumor size of the WTCHP and Mount Sinai Registry groups. Moreover, the average age at diagnosis was similar between the two groups, while if surveillance bias was introduced then smaller cancers should have been detected at an earlier age in the WTC cohort. It is important to consider how surveillance bias may be occurring across the US as a whole; previous research has found that much of the national increase in thyroid cancer incidence can be attributed to an increase in small (<1 cm) tumors, unlikely to be found in the absence of routine or incidental surveillance [11]. Moreover, the majority of WTC participants reported that their cancers were diagnosed due to routine or incidental screening, which may be higher than the expected rate of asymptomatic thyroid cancer detection [19].

The WTCHP and Mount Sinai thyroid cancer groups statistically differed in terms of gender, histology, smoking history and marital status; they were not statistically different in terms of race. Comparison of gender between the two groups, however, is difficult to interpret, since the WTCHP is composed predominantly of males [20]. WTCHP thyroid cancer cases were more likely to be papillary histology, which tend to have a favorable prognosis [21]. Moreover, those in the WTCHP cohort were more likely to be current smokers when compared to the Mount Sinai Registry group, though the number of reported current smokers was small for both groups. It remains controversial what affect smoking has on thyroid cancer risk; a decrease in risk of thyroid cancer in men who are current smokers has actually been observed, although there is no known biological justification for this [22,23]. WTCHP responderts with thyroid cancer were also more likely to be married or have a partner; data indicate reduced mortality from cancer associated with being married as opposed to being single, possibly because of increased social support [24].

While WTCHP thyroid cancer cases do not appear to be clinically distinct, their reported risk factors and carcinogenic exposure history may be uncommon. Only about 23% reported having had some sort of previous diagnostic radiation exposure before their thyroid cancer diagnosis, while other studies have found that this number could be as high as 85%, even suggesting this type of radiation exposure contributes to the carcinogenic process [25].

Increased BMI is also associated with increased risk of thyroid cancer [26] and 44.1% of WTCHP responders reported a BMI 25–29 km/m^2, with an additional 44.1% reporting a BMI >30 km/m^2. Neta et al. reported 15.9% and 12% of the thyroid cancer cases having a BMI of 25–29, and ≥30 km/m^2, respectively, which is lower than what was observed in the WTCHP cohort. However, these percentages seem to be in keeping with what has been reported for the overall WTCHP general responder cohort, suggesting that the thyroid cancer cases represent a random subset of the total group in terms of BMI [25].

Moreover, few WTCHP responders (8.8%) reported in their questionnaire that they had a family history of thyroid cancer or benign thyroid issues. Having a first-degree relative with thyroid cancer is known to increase thyroid cancer risk [27]. Other studies have found that as high as 15.6% of thyroid cancer cases report a family history of thyroid cancer [25,28]. A family history of another malignant disease has also been shown to be associated with thyroid cancer [29], and having a family history of cancer was reported by 66.7% of WTCHP respondents. This is higher than reported by past research, which found that 49% of thyroid cancer cases reported a family history of cancer in first-degree relative [29]. It is possible that some WTC respondents may have reported past cancers of relatives more distant than first-degree relatives, thus inflating the statistic.

Having a previous cancer diagnosis has also been shown to be associated with thyroid cancer [30], and 20.6% of WTCHP respondents reported having had another cancer before being diagnosed with thyroid cancer. This is higher than what was reported in the SEER database [31], where only 10.9% of thyroid cancer cases had another cancer predating thyroid cancer diagnosis. It is possible that this is related to the fact that WTC responders are at an increased risk for several types of cancer, including prostate cancer [1]; an alternative explanation could be an increased familial risk among WTCHP responders.

The WTCHP responders were also likely (23.5%) to develop a second primary cancer after thyroid cancer, which is in keeping with the observed increase in risk of secondary cancers associated with a primary thyroid cancer [32]. This number is higher, however, than what would be expected based on SEER registry data, whereby just 8% of thyroid cancer cases developed a second type of tumor. Again, it remains unclear if this increased risk of multiple primary cancers is because of WTC dust and debris exposure having a carcinogenic effect on 9/11 first responders or because of other genetic or environmental factors.

This study had some limitations, which includes a small sample size that may have been affected by recall bias, since participants were asked about past exposure and family history. Although selection bias could have been possible, an attempt was made to verify that those who participated were not statistically different from those who chose not to.

Among the strengths, this study represents an important contribution to the literature by helping to fill the gap in understanding why 9/11 first responders experience an increased risk of thyroid cancer. The descriptive epidemiology presented here will hopefully inform future, more in-depth studies that may explain this phenomenon. Future research on germline and somatic tumor alterations of these cancers may help to shed light on the possibility of a WTC-related carcinogenic mechanism.

5. Conclusions

Cancer surveillance of WTC first responders should continue, and specifically thyroid health should be part of regular screening procedures. Ultrasound techniques instead of radiation-based diagnostic procedures might be a more appropriate first step approach.

Author Contributions: S.T., M.A.G.v.G. and W.L.-C. collected data; S.T. also performed data analysis. E.G., M.C. and E.T. conceptualized the study design and provided expertise for interpreting the results. All authors helped in writing the manuscript and have read the final version.

Funding: This research was funded by National Institute for Occupational Safety and Health (1U01OH010984-01A1).

Acknowledgments: We would like to acknowledge the contributions of Chanda Williams, who prepared the Mount Sinai Registry data, and Naomi Alpert, who generated the numbers from SEER used for comparison to the WTCHP cohort.

Conflicts of Interest: The authors declare no conflict of interest.

References

1. Solan, S.; Wallenstein, S.; Shapiro, M.; Teitelbaum, S.L.; Stevenson, L.; Kochman, A.; Kaplan, J.; Dellenbaugh, C.; Kahn, A.; Biro, F.N.; et al. Cancer Incidence in World Trade Center Rescue and Recovery Workers, 2001–2008. *Environ. Health Perspect.* **2013**, *121*, 699–704. [CrossRef]
2. Zeig-Owens, R.; Webber, M.P.; Hall, C.B.; Schwartz, T.; Jaber, N.; Weakley, J.; Rohan, T.E.; Cohen, H.W.; Derman, O.; Aldrich, T.K.; et al. Early assessment of cancer outcomes in New York City firefighters after the 9/11 attacks: An observational cohort study. *Lancet* **2011**, *378*, 898–905.
3. Jordan, H.T.; Brackbill, R.M.; Cone, J.E.; Debchoudhury, I.; Farfel, M.R.; Greene, C.M.; Hadler, J.L.; Kennedy, J.; Li, J.; Liff, J.; et al. Mortality among survivors of the 11 September 2001, World Trade Center disaster: Results from the World Trade Center Health Registry cohort. *Lancet* **2011**, *378*, 879–887. [CrossRef]
4. Zimmermann, M.B.; Galetti, V. Iodine intake as a risk factor for thyroid cancer: A comprehensive review of animal and human studies. *Thyroid Res.* **2015**, *8*, 8. [CrossRef]

5. Nikiforov, Y.E. Radiation-induced thyroid cancer: What we have learned from Chernobyl. *Endocr. Pathol.* **2006**, *17*, 307–318. [CrossRef] [PubMed]
6. Siemiatycki, J.; Richardson, L.; Straif, K.; Latreille, B.; Lakhani, R.; Campbell, S.; Rousseau, M.-C.; Boffetta, P. Listing Occupational Carcinogens. *Environ. Health Perspect.* **2004**, *112*, 1447–1459. [CrossRef] [PubMed]
7. Lioy, P.J.; Georgopoulos, P. The Anatomy of the Exposures That Occurred around the World Trade Center Site. *Ann. N. Y. Acad. Sci.* **2006**, *1076*, 54–79. [CrossRef]
8. McGee, J.K.; Chen, L.C.; Cohen, M.D.; Chee, G.R.; Prophete, C.M.; Haykal-Coates, N.; Wasson, S.J.; Conner, T.L.; Costa, D.L.; Gavett, S.H. Chemical analysis of World Trade Center fine particulate matter for use in toxicologic assessment. *Environ. Health Perspect.* **2003**, *111*, 972–980. [CrossRef] [PubMed]
9. Offenberg, J.H.; Eisenreich, S.J.; Gigliotti, C.L.; Chen, L.C.; Xiong, J.Q.; Quan, C.; Lou, X.; Zhong, M.; Gorczynski, J.; Yiin, L.-M.; et al. Persistent organic pollutants in dusts that settled indoors in lower Manhattan after September 11, 2001. *J. Expo. Sci. Environ. Epidemiol.* **2004**, *14*, 164–172.
10. Kuan, P.-F.; Mi, Z.; Georgopoulos, P.; Hashim, D.; Luft, B.J.; Boffetta, P. Enhanced exposure assessment and genome-wide DNA methylation in World Trade Center disaster responders. *Eur. J. Cancer Prev.* **2018**, *28*, 225–233. [CrossRef]
11. Davies, L.; Welch, H.G. Increasing incidence of thyroid cancer in the United States, 1973–2002. *JAMA* **2006**, *295*, 2164–2167. [CrossRef]
12. Wisnivesky, J.F.; Teitelbaum, S.L.; Todd, A.C.; Boffetta, P.; Crane, M.; Crowley, L.; de la Hoz, R.E.; Dellenbaugh, C.; Harrison, D.; Herbert, R.; et al. Persistence of multiple illnesses in World Trade Center rescue and recovery workers: A cohort study. *Lancet* **2011**, *378*, 888–897. [CrossRef]
13. Swensen, S.J.; Jett, J.R.; Hartman, T.E.; Midthun, D.E.; Sloan, J.A.; Sykes, A.-M.; Aughenbaugh, G.L.; Clemens, M.A. Lung Cancer Screening with CT: Mayo Clinic Experience. *Radiology* **2003**, *226*, 756–761. [CrossRef]
14. van Gerwen, M.; Tuminello, S.; Riggins, G.; Mendes, T.; Donovan, M.; Benn, E.; Genden, E.; Cerutti, J.; Taioli, E. Investigating the increased incidence in thyroid cancer among World Trade Center responders. **2019**, under review.
15. Lieberman-Cribbin, W.; Tuminello, S.; Gillezeau, C.; van Gerwen, M.; Brody, R.; Donovan, M.; Taioli, E. The development of a Biobank of cancer tissue samples from World Trade Center responders. *J. Transl. Med.* **2018**, *16*, 280. [CrossRef]
16. Icitovic, N.; Onyebeke, L.C.; Wallenstein, S.; Dasaro, C.R.; Harrison, D.; Jiang, J.; Kaplan, J.R.; Lucchini, R.G.; Luft, B.J.; Moline, J.M.; et al. The association between body mass index and gastroesophageal reflux disease in the World Trade Center Health Program General Responder Cohort. *Am. J. Ind. Med.* **2016**, *59*, 761–766. [CrossRef] [PubMed]
17. About Adult BMI | Healthy Weight | CDC. Available online: https://www.cdc.gov/healthyweight/assessing/bmi/adult_bmi/index.html (accessed on 15 February 2019).
18. Kent, W.D.T.; Hall, S.F.; Isotalo, P.A.; Houlden, R.L.; George, R.L.; Groome, P.A. Increased incidence of differentiated thyroid carcinoma and detection of subclinical disease. *CMAJ* **2007**, *177*, 1357–1361. [CrossRef]
19. Davies, L.; Ouellette, M.; Hunter, M.; Welch, H.G. The increasing incidence of small thyroid cancers: Where are the cases coming from? *Laryngoscope* **2010**, *120*, 2446–2451. [CrossRef] [PubMed]
20. Rahbari, R.; Zhang, L.; Kebebew, E. Thyroid cancer gender disparity. *Future Oncol.* **2010**, *6*, 1771–1779. [CrossRef] [PubMed]
21. Yu, X.-M.; Schneider, D.F.; Leverson, G.; Chen, H.; Sippel, R.S. Follicular Variant of Papillary Thyroid Carcinoma is a Unique Clinical Entity: A Population-Based Study of 10,740 Cases. *Thyroid* **2013**, *23*, 1263–1268. [CrossRef]
22. Kreiger, N.; Parkes, R. Cigarette smoking and the risk of thyroid cancer. *Eur. J. Cancer* **2000**, *36*, 1969–1973. [CrossRef]
23. Cho, A.; Chang, Y.; Ahn, J.; Shin, H.; Ryu, S. Cigarette smoking and thyroid cancer risk: A cohort study. *Br. J. Cancer* **2018**, *119*, 638–645. [CrossRef]
24. Martínez, M.E.; Unkart, J.T.; Tao, L.; Kroenke, C.H.; Schwab, R.; Komenaka, I.; Gomez, S.L. Prognostic significance of marital status in breast cancer survival: A population-based study. *PLoS ONE* **2017**, *12*. [CrossRef]

25. Zhang, Y.; Chen, Y.; Huang, H.; Sandler, J.; Dai, M.; Ma, S.; Udelsman, R. Diagnostic radiography exposure increases the risk for thyroid microcarcinoma: A population-based case-control study. *Eur. J. Cancer Prev.* **2015**, *24*, 439–446. [CrossRef]

26. Sado, J.; Kitamura, T.; Sobue, T.; Sawada, N.; Iwasaki, M.; Sasazuki, S.; Yamaji, T.; Shimazu, T.; Tsugane, S. Risk of thyroid cancer in relation to height, weight, and body mass index in Japanese individuals: A population-based cohort study. *Cancer Med.* **2018**, *7*, 2200–2210. [CrossRef]

27. Thyroid Cancer Risk Factors. Available online: https://www.cancer.org/cancer/thyroid-cancer/causes-risks-prevention/risk-factors.html (accessed on 4 February 2019).

28. Neta, G.; Rajaraman, P.; Berrington de Gonzalez, A.; Doody, M.M.; Alexander, B.H.; Preston, D.; Simon, S.L.; Melo, D.; Miller, J.; Freedman, D.M.; et al. A prospective study of medical diagnostic radiography and risk of thyroid cancer. *Am. J. Epidemiol.* **2013**, *177*, 800–809. [CrossRef]

29. Xu, L.; Li, G.; Wei, Q.; El-Naggar, A.K.; Sturgis, E.M. Family history of cancer and risk of sporadic differentiated thyroid carcinoma. *Cancer* **2012**, *118*, 1228–1235. [CrossRef]

30. Hallquist, A.; Hardell, L.; Degerman, A.; Boquist, L. Thyroid cancer: Reproductive factors, previous diseases, drug intake, family history and diet. A case-control study. *J. Cancer Prev.* **1994**, *3*, 481–488. [CrossRef]

31. Surveillance, Epidemiology, and End Results Program. Available online: https://seer.cancer.gov/index.html (accessed on 13 February 2019).

32. Kim, C.; Bi, X.; Pan, D.; Chen, Y.; Carling, T.; Ma, S.; Udelsman, R.; Zhang, Y. The Risk of Second Cancers After Diagnosis of Primary Thyroid Cancer Is Elevated in Thyroid Microcarcinomas. *Thyroid* **2013**, *23*, 575–582. [CrossRef]

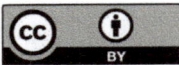

International Journal of
Environmental Research and Public Health

MDPI

Article

Clinical Evaluation of Sarcoidosis in Community Members with World Trade Center Dust Exposure

Kerry M. Hena [1,*], Scarlett Murphy [1], Yian Zhang [2], Yongzhao Shao [2], Angeliki Kazeros [1] and Joan Reibman [1,2]

[1] Department of Medicine, New York University, New York, NY 10016, USA;
scarlett.murphy@nyulangone.org (S.M.); angeliki.kazeros@nyulangone.org (A.K.);
joan.reibman@nyulangone.org (J.R.)

[2] Department of Population Health and Environmental Medicine, New York University, New York, NY 10016, USA; yian.zhang@nyulangone.org (Y.Z.); yongzhao.shao@nyulangone.org (Y.S.)

[*] Correspondence: kerry.hena@nyulangone.org

Received: 28 February 2019; Accepted: 4 April 2019; Published: 10 April 2019

Abstract: *Background*: Sarcoidosis is a granulomatous disease involving intrathoracic and extrathoracic organs. Genetic and environmental factors, such as exposure to World-Trade Center (WTC) dust after 9/11, may play a role in clinical presentation. Characterization of sarcoidosis in community members with exposure to the WTC dust can provide further insight into the relationship between environmental exposure and sarcoidosis. *Methods*: Patients with documented sarcoidosis were identified in the WTC Environmental Health Center (EHC), a treatment program for community members. Demographic and clinical data were collected from standardized questionnaires and chart review. Organ involvement was assessed with a standard instrument. *Results*: Among patients in the WTC EHC, 87 were identified with sarcoidosis after 9/11. Sarcoidosis cases were more likely African-American, local workers, and had more respiratory symptoms, compared with non-sarcoidosis WTC EHC patients. Many (46%) had ≥ Scadding stage 3 on chest imaging, and had reduced lung function measures. Extrathoracic involvement was identified in 33/87 (38%) with a diversity of organs involved. *Conclusions*: WTC-exposed sarcoidosis in community members is often characterized by severe pulmonary disease and a high rate of diverse extrathoracic involvement. Further analysis is required to characterize the course of disease progression or resolution.

Keywords: sarcoidosis; World Trade Center (WTC); Scadding stage; lung function; severe lung disease; extrathoracic sarcoidosis; cardiac sarcoidosis

---

1. Introduction

Sarcoidosis is a multisystem granulomatous disease of unknown etiology that is currently considered a genetically primed abnormal immune response to an antigenic exposure or trigger [1]. Rather than a single disease entity, sarcoidosis may be a constellation of "sarcoidoses," with a characteristic pattern of organ involvement, depending upon the underlying genotype and triggering exposure. Exposure to the dust and fumes from the destruction of the World Trade Center (WTC) on 11 September 2001 (9/11) has been suggested to be one such trigger with sarcoidosis diagnoses described in WTC-exposed members of the Fire Department of the City of New York (FDNY), those involved in rescue and recovery efforts (responders), and community members ("survivors") with WTC dust exposure [2–7]. Increased incidence rates have been reported for the firefighters and responders [2,3,6].

Whereas sarcoidosis can affect nearly all organs and tissues, intrathoracic involvement including hilar and mediastinal lymph nodes and/or lungs is the most common presentation [8,9]. However, extrathoracic involvement often distinguishes sarcoidosis from other granulomatous diseases and contributes to its diagnosis [9]. Indeed, in a large survey of sarcoidosis patients (A Case Control

Etiologic Study of Sarcoidosis; ACCESS) 95% of the population had intrathoracic involvement and 50% extrathoracic involvement [8]. The presence of extrathoracic involvement was associated with age, race and sex [8]. In addition, differences in progression of intrathoracic and extrathoracic organ involvement were noted; intrathoracic involvement improved or remained stable whereas extrathoracic involvement typically increased over time [10,11]. Development of new organ involvement was more common in African-Americans [10]. The characteristics of sarcoidosis associated with WTC exposure, particularly those in community members, are less well described. A recent study of the clinical course of WTC-related sarcoidosis in the WTC-exposed Fire Department of the City of New York (FDNY) suggested a phenotype with a high rate of cardiac and rheumatologic (bone/joint) involvement, suggesting a unique response to their environmental exposure [7].

The WTC Environmental Health Center (WTC EHC) is a treatment program for self-referred community members, or "survivors," with medical and mental health conditions secondary to acute exposure to the WTC dust on 9/11 (dust cloud) and/or chronic exposure to the WTC dust and fumes in their homes and/or workplaces over the ensuing days and months [12]. These community members include local residents, local workers, students, those involved in clean-up activities, and those who were passing by on 9/11. In contrast to the firefighter and responder populations, nearly 50% of the community members are women, and are of diverse race/ethnicity [13]. This heterogeneity and diversity of exposure to the WTC dust and fumes distinguishes them from the WTC-exposed responders, and their unique exposure sets them apart from the non-exposed general population. Characteristics of community members with sarcoidosis have been incompletely described. Exploration of their clinical presentation in comparison to other sarcoid variants may help us to better understand the relationship between exposure and sarcoidosis phenotype, providing further insight into sarcoidosis etiology. We now report a case series of community members in the WTC EHC with a diagnoses of post 9/11 sarcoidosis to further characterize the clinical presentation of sarcoidosis in this unique population. We describe similarities and differences between this population and other WTC and non-WTC sarcoidosis.

2. Materials and Methods

2.1. Study Population

2.1.1. Inclusion-Exclusion Criteria

Patients were included for review if they were enrolled in the Bellevue Hospital WTC EHC with a "certified" diagnosis as defined by the Centers of Disease Control (https://www.cdc.gov/wtc/handbook.html#certifications) and signed consent to have their data analyzed. By federal rules, WTC-exposed sarcoidosis cases allowed to enroll in the WTC EHC must have intrathoracic involvement presumed secondary to their relevant WTC exposure. The Institutional Review Board of New York University School of Medicine approved the research database (NCT00404898), and only data from patients who provided informed consent were used for analysis. Patients were included for analysis if they had biopsy proven sarcoidosis or chest imaging with characteristic findings of sarcoidosis defined as bilateral symmetrical mediastinal and/or hilar adenopathy, perilymphatic nodules, or fibrosis with bronchial distortion, at time of diagnosis or initial evaluation and without alternative etiology [9]. Signs or symptoms suggesting extrathoracic involvement such as confirmed uveitis or characteristic rash with concomitant elevated ACE level, were also used to establish a diagnosis [9]. Patients with a sarcoidosis diagnosis that predated 9/11 were excluded from analysis.

2.1.2. "Non-Sarcoidosis" Comparison Population

Study cases were compared to WTC exposed community members without sarcoidosis. In addition to WTC exposure, their entry into the WTC EHC required a physical complaint and diagnosis (e.g., lower or upper airway disease, GERD, other interstitial lung disease and/or cancer).

2.2. Clinical Evaluation

Pathology reports were reviewed for all patients with available information to confirm histologic culture-negative, noncaseating granulomas. For those without a biopsy, imaging reports were reviewed to confirm characteristic findings. Information on demographic and clinical characteristics, including WTC and other exposures, were obtained from a standardized questionnaire completed upon entry into the WTC EHC [13]. Information in this questionnaire included direct exposures to the WTC dust clouds, potential for exposure in the home or workplace, and duration of exposure in the home or workplace prior to cleanup. The Modified Medical Research Council (mMRC) questionnaire was used to assess dyspnea. Additional clinical information obtained at entry into the WTC EHC included complete blood count, metabolic panel, and liver enzyme levels. Lung function measurements performed as routine screening were assessed. Chart reviews were performed to obtain additional information including CXR, computed tomography (CT) scans, ophthalmologic findings, EKG and advanced cardiac imaging. Additional diagnostic studies, e.g., serum angiotensin-converting enzyme (ACE) and serum vitamin D (25-hydroxy and 1,25 dihydroxy) levels obtained in the WTC EHC at time of entry into the program or during subsequent evaluation, were also reviewed.

2.3. Assessment of Disease Severity and Organ Involvement

Sarcoidosis cases were staged for pulmonary disease by both CXR and/or CT scan using Scadding staging: stage 0: no adenopathy or infiltrates; stage 1: hilar and mediastinal adenopathy alone; stage 2: adenopathy and pulmonary infiltrates; stage 3: pulmonary infiltrates alone; and stage 4: pulmonary fibrosis [14]. Radiographic studies were selected for review based on temporality to disease onset with images used that were closest to date of diagnosis.

The World Association of Sarcoidosis and Other Granulomatous Diseases (WASOG) organ assessment instrument was used to categorize sarcoidosis involvement of each organ system at time of initial evaluation [15]. A finding of "highly probable" or "at least probable" was considered diagnostic for organ involvement. Positive findings on cardiac MRI (cMRI) were required to confirm a diagnosis of cardiac sarcoidosis, "at least probable" criteria by WASOG [15]. Other cardiac imaging modalities obtained after time of initial visit included electrocardiograms, echocardiograms, and continuous ambulatory ECG monitoring. These were reviewed for findings suggestive of possible cardiac involvement. Determination of ocular involvement required documentation of an ophthalmology visit in which fundoscopic findings confirming sarcoidosis were described. Patients with a brain MRI demonstrating characteristic abnormal enhancement after initial WTC clinic visit were identified as having neurologic involvement of sarcoidosis. Abnormal electromyography (EMG) findings were considered "suggestive but not diagnostic;" a field of "no consensus" in the WASOG organ assessment instrument [15]. Patients were identified as having cutaneous manifestations if biopsies showed pathognomonic granulomas and/or a dermatologist documented rashes with characteristic morphology "at least probable" or "highly probable" by WASOG [15]. Liver, spleen or gastrointestinal involvement was identified from available pathology, CT or MRI imaging.

2.4. Statistics

Descriptive statistics were used to summarize the study cohort. We used count and percentage for categorical variables and median and IQR (Q1, Q3) for continuous variables. Univariate analyses were performed to compare the demographic characteristics, clinical characteristics, laboratory values and pulmonary function metrics between sarcoidosis patients and non-sarcoidosis patients and also between sarcoidosis patients who had lung disease at Scadding stage 1–2 and those who had stage 3–4 disease. The comparison tests include χ^2 test for categorical variables and Mann-Whitney U test for continuous factors. Fisher exact test was performed in place of χ^2 test if the expected count of a category was less than 5. All statistical analyses were accomplished using SAS 9.4 software (SAS Institute Inc., Gary, NC, USA). *p*-Values < 0.05 were considered statistically significant.

3. Results

3.1. Demographic Characteristics

Among 5849 community members at Bellevue Hospital enrolled between 17 August 2005 and 30 March 2018 with signed consents for analysis, 98 were identified with WTC-related sarcoidosis as per defined federal rules. Patients with a sarcoidosis diagnoses that predated 9/11 ($n = 11$) were excluded from analysis. This resulted in 87 individuals with sarcoidosis available for analysis. Biopsy-proven sarcoidosis was identified in 77, and an imaging diagnosis was obtained for 10. Sarcoidosis diagnosis occurred on average 7 years (SD = 4.5) after 9/11/2001 and 3 years (SD = 4.8) before enrollment in the WTC EHC, with mean time to enrollment being 10 years (SD = 4.4) after 9/11/2001.

As far as the 5751 non-sarcoidosis community members, patients without lung function values ($n = 607$) were excluded to allow meaningful comparison of pulmonary physiology. For these non-sarcoidosis patients ($n = 5144$), time to enrollment in the WTC EHC occurred on average 9 years (SD = 3.8) after 9/11/2001.

Basic exposure and demographic characteristics are shown (Table 1). Many (51%) of the WTC-exposed community members with sarcoidosis were caught in the dust cloud on 9/11/2001, and most were local workers (73%). Almost half were female (48%) and the majority were never smokers (67%). Patients with sarcoidosis had a median age of 40 years on 9/11. Race/ethnicity was diverse with 44% reporting as black/African-American, 36% white and 18% Hispanic. We did not identify a statistically significant association between WTC dust cloud exposure and sarcoidosis status in WTC EHC. Those with sarcoidosis were more likely to be African-American and local workers compared with patients without sarcoidosis.

Table 1. Basic demographic characteristics.

Characteristic	Non-Sarcoidosis (N = 5144)	Sarcoidosis (N = 87)	p-Value
Age on 9/11/2001, *yr*, median (Q1, Q3)	43 (35, 50)	40 (33, 45)	0.015 *
Age on Initial Visit, *yr*, median (Q1, Q3)	59.7 (52, 67)	57.5 (51, 62)	0.017 *
Gender, *n* (%)			0.8
Female	2551 (50)	42 (48)	
Male	2593 (50)	45 (52)	
Race/Ethnicity, *n* (%)			<0.0001 ***
Asian	427 (8)	2 (2)	
Hispanic	1483 (29)	15 (18)	
NH-Black	942 (19)	38 (44)	
NH-White	2176 (43)	31 (36)	
Native American	11 (0.2)	-	
Other	51 (1)	-	
Ever smoke cigarettes, *n* (%)			0.2
Yes	2032 (40)	29 (33)	
No	3087 (60)	58 (67)	
WTC Exposure Category, *n* (%)			<0.0001 ***
Local worker	2751 (53)	63 (73)	
Resident	1163 (23)	8 (9)	
Rescue/Recovery/Other	603 (12)	15 (17)	
Clean-up worker	613 (12)	1 (1)	
WTC Dust Cloud Exposure, *n* (%)			0.6
Yes	2711 (53)	44 (51)	
No	2388 (47)	43 (49)	

p-Value: *** < 0.0001; * < 0.05.

3.2. Clinical Characteristics

Entry into the WTC EHC required a physical complaint and diagnosis, and most patients entered with respiratory symptoms and diagnoses consistent with asthma, chronic obstructive pulmonary disease or interstitial lung disease. Despite the frequency of these diagnoses, those with sarcoidosis were more likely to report dyspnea, cough and wheeze ≥ two times/week within 4 weeks of entry into the clinic, as well as a decreased exercise tolerance after 9/11 (Table 2). Many reported comorbid nasal drip or sinus congestion (57%) and heartburn (49%) while some endorsed rash (38%).

Table 2. Respiratory symptoms at time of enrollment.

Symptom, n (%)	Non-Sarcoidosis ($N = 5144$)	Sarcoidosis ($N = 87$)	p-Value
Cough	3278 (64)	67 (78)	0.009 **
Wheezing	2608 (51)	58 (67)	0.004 **
Dyspnea with exercise	3929 (77)	76 (89)	0.009 **
Dyspnea at rest	1731 (34)	49 (56)	<0.0001 ***
MMRC			0.03 *
<3	3509 (79)	56 (69)	
≥3	928 (21)	25 (31)	

p-Value: *** < 0.0001; ** < 0.01; * < 0.05.

Lung function measurements including pre and post bronchodilator (bd) spirometry, lung volume and diffusion capacity measures were evaluated in patients with sarcoidosis compared with the non-sarcoidosis patients (Table 3). Sarcoidosis patients had a reduced FEV_1 and pre-bronchodilator FEV_1/FVC compared with non-sarcoidosis patients. Sarcoidosis patients were also characterized according to Scadding stage based on chest imaging. Thirty-six of 79 (46%) sarcoidosis patients with available chest imaging had severe lung disease defined as Scadding stage 3 or 4. Patients with more severe radiographic disease had reduced FEV_1, FVC and D_LCO compared with patients with milder radiographic changes (Table 3).

Table 3. Lung function: Stage 1–2 vs. Stage 3–4 pulmonary sarcoidosis.

	Non-Sarcoidosis ($N = 5144$)	Sarcoidosis ($N = 79$)		Non-Sarcoidosis vs. Sarcoidosis p-Value	Stage 1–2 vs. Stage 3–4 p-Value
		Lung Disease Stage 1–2 ($N = 43$)	Lung Disease Stage 3–4 ($N = 36$)		
FEV_1, L, median (%[†])					
Pre bd	2.69 (90)	2.86 (88)	2.10 (75)	0.03 *	0.002 **
Post bd	2.80 (94)	3.01 (89)	2.06 (77)	0.02 *	0.0004 **
FVC, L, median (%[†])					
Pre bd	3.51 (92)	3.55 (92)	3.02 (83)	0.25	0.03 *
Post bd	3.56 (93)	3.68 (89)	2.78 (81)	0.13	0.008 **
FEV_1/FVC, %[†]					
Pre bd	78	76	75	0.04 *	0.65
Post bd	80	79	79	0.27	0.42
TLC, L, median (%)	5.15 (91)	4.83 (90)	4.39 (67)	0.22	0.22
DLCO, $mmHg$, median (%)	19.15 (87)	19.50 (84)	15.10 (60)	0.11	0.013 *

FEV_1: forced expiratory volume in one second; FVC: forced vital capacity; TLC: total lung capacity; DLCO: diffusing capacity of the lungs for carbon monoxide; bd: bronchodilator; %[†]: National Health and Nutrition Examination Survey (NHANES) III reference values [16]; p-Value: *** < 0.0001; ** < 0.01; * < 0.05.

3.3. Organ Involvement

Thirty-three (38%) of the sarcoidosis patients had evidence of extrathoracic involvement: 19 (22%) had two organs involved, 10 (12%) had three organs involved, and 5 (6%) had ≥ four. Diverse organ involvement was identified; however, ocular involvement (15%) was the most common extrathoracic manifestation followed by skin (13%). Fewer had confirmed nervous system (3%) or cardiac (6%) involvement (Table 4). There were no significant differences in demographic or

WTC exposure characteristics for isolated intrathoracic ($n = 54$) versus extrathoracic disease, severe lung disease (Scadding Stage 3 or 4; $n = 36$), or extent of extrathoracic organ involvement (3 or more organ systems involved; $n = 15$). Few patients (9/62; 15%) had elevated ACE levels. Median neutrophil-to-lymphocyte ratio (NLR) was 2.4, compared to a reported mean of 1.65 in an adult, non-geriatric, healthy population [17].

Table 4. Organ involvement.

Organ System, n (%)		Sarcoidosis ($N = 87$)
Intrathoracic *	Stage 1	18 (23)
	Stage 2	25 (32)
	Stage 3	17 (22)
	Stage 4	19 (24)
Cardiac		5 (6)
Eyes		13 (15)
ENT		3 (3)
Bone-Joints		1 (1)
Bone marrow		2 (2)
Skin		11 (13)
Nervous System		3 (3)
Liver		3 (3)
Spleen		3 (3)
Kidney		1 (1)
Calcium		3 (3)
Extrathoracic lymph nodes		2 (2)
Thyroid		1 (1)
Gastrointestinal		2 (2)
Appendix		1 (1)

* All with certified pulmonary involvement; eight without readily available chest imaging for review ($n = 79$).

3.4. Cardiac Sarcoidosis: Screening and Diagnosis

Electrocardiograms were available for review in 75 individuals; 10 had abnormalities suggestive of potential cardiac sarcoidosis, including left or right bundle branch block, left anterior fascicular block or other interventricular conduction delay. Subsequent transthoracic echocardiogram was performed in 7/10 of these patients. The majority (86%) had normal left ventricular ejection fraction without any associated wall motion abnormalities.

A total of 14 patients were referred for advanced cardiac imaging (either cMRI or PET). 6/14 were referred due to abnormal ECG, echocardiogram, and/or continuous ambulatory ECG monitoring; the remaining eight were referred due to concerning cardiac symptoms alone (e.g., atypical chest pain, palpitations, dizziness/syncope). Cardiac involvement was confirmed in 5/14 patients, one with a supporting myocardial biopsy and two with an unremarkable screening study. Many patients were awaiting advanced cardiac imaging at the time of this publication, including 7 patients with an abnormal EKG and 6 with abnormal continuous ambulatory ECG monitoring.

4. Discussion

We described the clinical characteristics of a heterogeneous cohort of WTC-exposed community members, or "survivors," with post-9/11 sarcoidosis. The demographic characteristics of the WTC EHC population with sarcoidosis differed from the FDNY, with many more patients who were female or who identified as African American or Hispanic. These characteristics were more similar to the general population described in ACCESS and the cohort from Medical University of South Carolina (MUSC) [8,10,11].

By definition, WTC-exposed sarcoidosis cases must have intrathoracic involvement (100%). However, the WTC-exposed survivors with sarcoidosis differed from other sarcoidosis variants—the

WTC-exposed FDNY cohort as well as previously reported non-exposed general population(s)—in terms of severity of their intrathoracic disease [7,8,10,11]. Forty-six percent had Scadding stage 3 or 4 on initial evaluation chest imaging, indicating advanced pulmonary involvement, which was associated with reduced lung function measures. This frequency of severe disease is higher than that described in the initial ACCESS study (15% with stage 3 or 4) and even greater than that described in the FDNY cohort (7%) [7,8]. Importantly, the MUSC study, which evaluated the last available radiograph allowing for progression of Scadding stage, still described lower rates (27%) of stage 3 or 4 disease than that identified in the WTC EHC cohort (46%). The severity of intrathoracic disease is consistent with the respiratory symptoms reported at time of enrollment (Table 2). However, it is unknown whether our cohort represents those with more symptomatic, severe disease rather than sarcoidosis all-comers given the distinct self-referral entry into the WTC-EHC.

The frequency of extrathoracic involvement (38%) was slightly less than that reported in ACCESS (50%) [8]. However, the extrathoracic involvement in the WTC-EHC was distinguished by its variety and extent of extrathoracic organs involved. Similar to general population studies with comparable race/ethnic distribution, ocular and skin involvement were most common [8,10,11]. This is in contrast to the predominantly Caucasian male FDNY cohort, for which eye and skin involvement were relatively rare (5% and 2% respectively) [7]. Rare, but unique organ involvement included thyroid (1%), gastrointestinal (2%) and the appendix (1%). The extent of organ involvement (17% with three or more organs involved), was similar to that reported in the general population (20%) [8]. However, unlike the ACCESS and MUSC studies where African Americans tended to have more organs involved, we detected no significant differences in demographic variables for intrathoracic versus extrathoracic disease or extent of extrathoracic organ involvement [8,10,11].

Cardiac sarcoidosis remains a challenging diagnosis with current guidelines recommending advance cardiac imaging only in patients with symptoms, abnormal (ECG), or abnormal echocardiogram [18,19]. However, screening modalities have limited sensitivity; a study on predictors of cardiac sarcoidosis cited a sensitivity of 58% for ECGs and 62% for echocardiograms [20]. While continuous ambulatory ECG monitoring for 24 hours or more has higher sensitivity (89%), it has low specificity (21%) [20]. The rate of confirmed cardiac sarcoidosis (6%) in the survivor cohort is consistent with that of non-WTC general population studies, with clinically evident cardiac sarcoidosis manifested by conduction abnormalities, ventricular arrhythmias, and/or heart failure evident in only 2–7% of sarcoidosis patients [8,10,11]. Although cardiac sarcoidosis was clinically detected in 16% (19/57) of the WTC-exposed FDNY cohort at follow-up, this may have been due to increased screening in relatively asymptomatic patients [7]. A lower threshold for advanced cardiac imaging in the survivor population might result in higher rates of detection, beyond those already awaiting confirmatory diagnostics.

This study has several limitations. Complete analyses of all patients were not possible due to missing data. Many patients referred to the WTC EHC also receive care at outside institutions, including some critical components of sarcoidosis screening for extrathoracic disease. Thus data from other institutions may not have been captured by our study, leading to potential underreporting of extrathoracic organ involvement. Furthermore, although a standardized approach to diagnosis and evaluation was recommended at the WTC EHC, diagnostic studies were varied. Patients shared a common WTC exposure; however, the degree and extent of that exposure, including differences among the WTC dust characteristics, is known to vary, complicating the environmental exposure analysis. Patients had ranging dates of initial sarcoidosis diagnosis. Given the tendency of sarcoidosis organ involvement to increase per year, it is likely that patients in our cohort with more recent dates of diagnosis will continue to develop extrathoracic involvement as time progresses. In addition, longitudinal analysis was confounded by irregular follow-up by many patients, and visit incongruity made it difficult to compare number of organs involved per equivalent time period. Additional analyses are needed to further characterize clinical course.

5. Conclusions

Our data suggest a WTC-exposed sarcoidosis phenotype in community members or "survivors" often characterized by severe pulmonary disease and diverse extrathoracic involvement. These characteristics differ from those described for the FDNY. Similarities to general population studies are likely secondary to comparable gender and race/ethnicity distribution with differences in severity of pulmonary disease and rare organ involvement potentially explained by WTC exposure. Further analysis is required to characterize the course of disease progression or resolution.

Author Contributions: Conceptualization, K.M.H., A.K. and J.R.; methodology, K.M.H., S.M., Y.Z.; software, Y.Z. and Y.S.; validation, Y.Z. and Y.S.; formal analysis, K.M.H., S.M., J.R., Y.Z. and Y.S.; investigation, K.M.H., S.M. and Y.Z.; resources, A.K., Y.Z. and Y.S.; data curation, K.M.H., S.M., Y.Z. and Y.S.; writing—original draft preparation, K.M.H. and S.M.; writing—review and editing, K.M.H., A.K., J.R., Y.Z. and Y.S.; visualization, Y.Z.; supervision, K.M.H., Y.S. and J.R.; project administration, Y.S. and J.R.; funding acquisition, Y.S. and J.R.

Funding: This research was supported by the City of New York, US Centers for Disease Prevention and Control (CDC) and the National Institute of Occupational Safety and Health (NIOSH) contracts 200–2017–93327 and 200–2017–93427, as well as the National Institute of Environmental Health Sciences grant 5P30ES000260.

Conflicts of Interest: The authors declare no conflict of interest. The funders had no role in the design of the study; in the collection, analyses, or interpretation of data; in the writing of the manuscript, or in the decision to publish the results.

References

1. Valeyre, D.; Prasse, A.; Nunes, H.; Uzunhan, Y.; Brillet, P.-Y.; Müller-Quernheim, J. Sarcoidosis. *Lancet* **2014**, *383*, 1155–1167. [CrossRef]
2. Izbicki, G.; Chavko, R.; Banauch, G.I.; Weiden, M.D.; Berger, K.I.; Aldrich, T.K.; Hall, C.; Kelly, K.J.; Prezant, D.J. World Trade Center "Sarcoid-Like" Granulomatous Pulmonary Disease in New York City Fire Department Rescue Workers. *Chest* **2007**, *131*, 1414–1423. [CrossRef] [PubMed]
3. Crowley, L.E.; Herbert, R.; Moline, J.M.; Wallenstein, S.; Shukla, G.; Schechter, C.; Skloot, G.S.; Udasin, I.; Luft, B.J.; Harrison, D.; et al. "Sarcoid like" granulomatous pulmonary disease in World Trade Center disaster responders. *Am. J. Ind. Med.* **2010**, *54*, 175–184. [CrossRef] [PubMed]
4. Jordan, H.T.; Stellman, S.D.; Prezant, D.; Teirstein, A.; Osahan, S.S.; Cone, J.E. Sarcoidosis Diagnosed After September 11, 2001, Among Adults Exposed to the World Trade Center Disaster. *J. Occup. Environ. Med.* **2011**, *53*, 966–974. [CrossRef] [PubMed]
5. Parsia, S.S.; Yee, H.; Young, S.; Turetz, M.L.; Marmor, M.; Wilkenfeld, M.; Kazeros, A.; Caplan-Shaw, C.E.; Reibman, J. Characteristics of Sarcoidosis in Residents and Workers Exposed to World Trade Center (WTC) Dust, Gas and Fumes Presenting for Medical Care. *Am. Thorac. Soc.* **2010**, A1740. [CrossRef]
6. Webber, M.P.; Yip, J.; Zeig-Owens, R.; Moir, W.; Ungprasert, P.; Crowson, C.S.; Hall, C.B.; Jaber, N.; Weiden, M.D.; Matteson, E.L.; et al. Post-9/11 Sarcoidosis in WTC-Exposed Firefighters and Emergency Medical Service Workers. *Respir. Med.* **2017**, *132*, 232–237. [CrossRef] [PubMed]
7. Hena, K.M.; Yip, J.; Jaber, N.; Goldfarb, D.; Fullam, K.; Cleven, K.; Moir, W.; Zeig-Owens, R.; Webber, M.P.; Spevack, D.M.; et al. Clinical Course of Sarcoidosis in World Trade Center-Exposed Firefighters. *Chest* **2017**, *153*, 114–123. [CrossRef] [PubMed]
8. Baughman, R.P.; Teirstein, A.S.; Judson, M.A.; Rossman, M.D.; Yeager, H.; Bresnitz, E.A.; DePalo, L.; Hunninghake, G.; Iannuzzi, M.C.; Johns, C.J.; et al. Clinical Characteristics of Patients in a Case Control Study of Sarcoidosis. *Am. J. Respir. Crit. Care Med.* **2001**, *164*, 1885–1889. [CrossRef] [PubMed]
9. Valeyre, D.; Bernaudin, J.-F.; Uzunhan, Y.; Kambouchner, M.; Brillet, P.-Y.; Soussan, M.; Nunes, H. Clinical Presentation of Sarcoidosis and Diagnostic Work-Up. *Semin. Respir. Crit. Care Med.* **2014**, *35*, 336–351. [PubMed]
10. Judson, M.A.; Baughman, R.P.; Thompson, B.W.; Teirstein, A.S.; Terrin, M.L.; Rossman, M.D.; Yeager, H.; McLennan, G.; Bresnitz, E.A.; DePalo, L.; et al. Two year prognosis of sarcoidosis: the ACCESS experience. *Sarcoidosis Vasc. Diffus. Lung Dis.* **2003**, *20*, 204–211.
11. Judson, M.A.; Boan, A.D.; Lackland, D.T. The clinical course of sarcoidosis: presentation, diagnosis, and treatment in a large white and black cohort in the United States. *Sarcoidosis Vasc. Diffus. Lung Dis.* **2012**, *29*, 119–127.

12. Reibman, J.; Levy-Carrick, N.; Miles, T.; Flynn, K.; Hughes, C.; Crane, M.; Lucchini, R.G. Destruction of the World Trade Center Towers. Lessons Learned from an Environmental Health Disaster. *Ann. Am. Thorac. Soc.* **2016**, *13*, 577–583. [CrossRef] [PubMed]

13. Reibman, J.; Liu, M.; Cheng, Q.; Liautaud, S.; Rogers, L.; Lau, S.; Berger, K.I.; Goldring, R.M.; Marmor, M.; Fernandez-Beros, M.E.; et al. Characteristics of a Residential and Working Community with Diverse Exposure to World Trade Center Dust, Gas, and Fumes. *J. Occup. Environ. Med.* **2009**, *51*, 534–541. [CrossRef] [PubMed]

14. Scadding, J.G. Prognosis of Intrathoracic Sarcoidosis in England. *BMJ* **1961**, *2*, 1165–1172. [CrossRef] [PubMed]

15. Judson, M.A.; Costabel, U.; Drent, M.; Wells, A.; Maier, L.; Koth, L.; Shigemitsu, H.; Culver, D.A.; Gelfand, J.; Valeyre, D.; et al. The WASOG Sarcoidosis Organ Assessment Instrument: An update of a previous clinical tool. *Sarcoidosis Vasc. Diffus. Lung Dis.* **2014**, *31*, 19–27.

16. Hankinson, J.L.; Odencrantz, J.R.; Fedan, K.B. Spirometric Reference Values from a Sample of the General U.S. Population. *Am. J. Respir. Crit. Care Med.* **1999**, *159*, 179–187. [CrossRef] [PubMed]

17. Forget, P.; Khalifa, C.; Defour, J.-P.; Latinne, D.; Van Pel, M.-C.; De Kock, M. What is the normal value of the neutrophil-to-lymphocyte ratio? *BMC Res. Notes* **2017**, *10*, 995. [CrossRef] [PubMed]

18. Mehta, D.; Lubitz, S.A.; Frankel, Z.; Wisnivesky, J.P.; Einstein, A.J.; Goldman, M.; Machac, J.; Teirstein, A. Cardiac Involvement in Patients with Sarcoidosis. *Chest* **2008**, *133*, 1426–1435. [CrossRef] [PubMed]

19. Hulten, E.; Aslam, S.; Osborne, M.; Abbasi, S.; Bittencourt, M.S.; Blankstein, R. Cardiac sarcoidosis—State of the art review. *Cardiovasc. Diagn. Ther.* **2016**, *6*, 50–63. [PubMed]

20. Freeman, A.M.; Curran-Everett, D.; Weinberger, H.D.; Fenster, B.E.; Buckner, J.K.; Gottschall, E.B.; Sauer, W.H.; Maier, L.A.; Hamzeh, N.Y. Predictors of Cardiac Sarcoidosis Using Commonly Available Cardiac Studies. *Am. J. Cardiol.* **2013**, *112*, 280–285. [CrossRef] [PubMed]

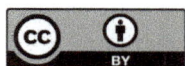

International Journal of
*Environmental Research
and Public Health*

MDPI

Article

Unmet Mental Health Care Needs among Asian Americans 10–11 Years After Exposure to the World Trade Center Attack

Winnie W. Kung [1,*], Xiaoran Wang [1], Xinhua Liu [2], Emily Goldmann [3] and Debbie Huang [2]

1   Fordham University, Graduate School of Social Service, 113 West 60th Street, New York, NY 11375, USA;
    xwang150@fordham.edu
2   Columbia University, Mailman School of Public Health, 722 W 168th Street, New York, NY 10032, USA;
    xl26@cumc.columbia.edu (X.L.); dh2652@cumc.columbia.edu (D.H.)
3   New York University, College of Global Public Health, 715/719 Broadway, 10th floor, New York,
    NY 10003, USA; esg236@nyu.edu
*   Correspondence: kung@fordham.edu

Received: 28 February 2019; Accepted: 5 April 2019; Published: 11 April 2019

Abstract: This study investigated the prevalence of unmet mental health care needs (UMHCN) and their associated factors among 2344 Asian Americans directly exposed to the World Trade Center (WTC) attack 10–11 years afterwards. Given the pervasive underutilization of mental health services among Asians, their subjective evaluation of unmet needs could provide more nuanced information on disparities of service. We used the WTC Health Registry data and found that 12% of Asian Americans indicated UMHCN: 69% attributing it to attitudinal barriers, 36% to cost barriers, and 29% to access barriers. Among all the factors significantly related to UMHCN in the logistic model, disruption of health insurance in the past year had the largest odds ratio (OR = 2.37, 95% confidence interval: 1.61–3.48), though similar to functional impairment due to mental disorders. Post-9/11 mental health diagnosis, probable mental disorder and ≥14 poor mental health days in the past month were also associated with greater odds of UMHCN, while greater social support was associated with lower odds. Results suggest that continued outreach efforts to provide mental health education to Asian communities to increase knowledge about mental illness and treatment options, reduce stigmatization of mental illness, and offer free mental health services are crucial to address UMHCN.

Keywords: unmet mental health care needs; Asian Americans; World Trade Center attack; disaster; mental health conditions; mental health service use; health insurance; social support; stressful life events

1. Introduction

Numerous studies have examined the mental health impact of the September 11, 2001 attack at the World Trade Center (WTC) on those who were directly exposed to the disaster, but fewer have investigated these individuals' use of mental health services [1,2]. While Asian Americans constituted a sizeable number of those affected by the disaster [3] and there has been a well-documented history of underutilization of mental health services within this population [4], our team was the first to study this group's mental health service use and its associated factors (the authors, in press). In this study, we further investigate the unmet mental health care needs (UMHCN) of Asian Americans affected by the WTC attack and correlates of having unmet needs.

Mental health service utilization is a typical measure of whether mental health care needs are met among persons with potential mental health issues [5]. It has been used as an objective measure to detect systemic disparities in service provision and access across sociodemographic groups [6].

However, we cannot assume that receiving services is equivalent to having mental health needs met [5,7]. Individuals' subjective perception of UMHCN is an important measure to complement the objective information on treatment use and reveals the "actual demand for service" [7] or treatment gap. According to the National Comorbidity Survey-Replication, help seeking for mental health treatment is often delayed; for example, studies have noted a median lag of 12 years between the onset of posttraumatic stress disorder (PTSD) and the initial treatment contact [8]. Together with the often delayed symptom manifestation and worsening of symptoms with time [9], investigation of UMHCN some years after the WTC attack is important. This study examines the UMHCN of Asian Americans 10–11 years after the disaster. We aimed to better understand the extent of such unmet needs and their associated factors to inform outreach efforts in this underserved population and to find ways to provide more effective services to meet their needs. This is especially relevant given the provision of public funds to monitor and provide needed health and mental health treatment to eligible individuals affected by the WTC attack through the James Zadroga 9/11 Health and Compensation Act being extended until 2090 [10]. Meeting such unmet mental health needs may not only reduce human suffering but also ameliorate economic loss that incurs to society due to compromised productivity and increased future treatment costs when untreated conditions deteriorate [11].

UMHCN may be more common among individuals with specific clinical, sociodemographic, and behavioral characteristics. Individuals who have more mental health issues, including those with formal diagnoses or symptoms of probable mental disorder, may have more mental health care needs and are thus more likely to feel such needs not being met. However, since UMHCN captures the subjective perception of these needs, those who do not have a formal or probable diagnosis but feel that their needs have not been met should also be considered [5]. Furthermore, many individuals without apparent mental disorders also consume services [12]. The fact that the majority of ethnic and racial minorities with a diagnosable mental disorder did not receive pertinent treatment despite contacts with the health care system in the previous year [12] and the questionable validity and reliability of mental health assessment tools for minority groups [13] increase the need to examine Asian Americans without formal clinical evaluation to understand their subjective UMHCN. Poorer perception of mental well-being and greater subsequent impaired functioning in work, family or social life may also cause them to recognize that their mental health needs are not being met. Functional impairment may be even more important than mental health symptoms themselves among Asians, who tend to minimize their psychological distress [14], particularly for those who have fewer resources to sustain themselves and their families when they cannot perform their expected roles, especially work role, which is highly valued among Asians [15].

Limited economic resources such as low or unreliable income and the lack or disruption of health insurance coverage may also be practical barriers that could result in UMHCN [6]. Likewise, access barriers such as unavailability of culturally-relevant and linguistically-appropriate mental health services, lack of knowledge of available services, or inconvenience in service use like distance and long waiting periods may also lead to UMHCN [16]. These practical barriers may have a particularly strong impact on Asian Americans given their lower prevalence of English proficiency (76.5%) [17] and shortage of bilingual mental health services [18,19].

In addition to practical barriers, UMHCN can also be a result of "subjective chosen unmet needs" [6], in which individuals with mental health issues refuse to seek help due to beliefs such as the fear of stigma associated with being identified as mentally ill or needing psychiatric help [20,21]. These attitudinal or emotional barriers may be aggravated among Asians due to their cultural tendency to link mental illness to moral failure such as punishment by God or ancestors for one's past transgressions [22] and weakness in spiritual strength, causing shame and disgrace to family [23]. As a result, the need to seek treatment could pose a threat to one's self-esteem [24,25].

Social support resources may also determine UMHCN. Social networks can provide emotional support, which may buffer the psychological impact of trauma [26] and subsequently reduce the need for professional help [27]. These networks can also provide practical support through sharing of information about available mental health services and alleviating access barriers, such as providing child care [5]. Asians' tendency to handle personal issues within close circles of family and friends may reduce their perceived need for help from outsiders, especially professionals [13,28]. Moreover, the social network's attitude towards mental health issues and treatment could also aggravate the fear of stigma associated with using external help [25]. Further, those who have mental health issues but are unaware of such a need would understate their unmet need [6,29]. It was noted that minorities, including Asians, with limited English proficiency tend to be less likely to identify mental health care needs [30].

Not only could individuals who have received mental health treatment still find their needs unmet, prior studies, including those on the WTC attack, consistently find that individuals who have used services in the past are more likely to report UMHCN [2,5,7,27]. It is suggested that those who have received treatment before are more aware of the range of potential help to which they have no access, or they may better recognize the limitations of these services [5]. Those with prior experience with mental health services may also express greater dissatisfaction with the quality of treatment they receive [7]. Minority populations, in particular, may be more likely to receive inconsistent diagnoses or inappropriate medication, or be offered treatments that are not evidence-based [13,31]. Service users may also judge treatments to be inadequate when their expectations are not met. If their expectations are unrealistic, such as a quick fix, they can be corrected through good communication between service providers and consumers. However, for many minorities, including Asians, this is harder to attain due to the different socioeconomic, cultural, and linguistic backgrounds between consumers and service providers [32–34]. Studies indicate that minorities often find that their service providers do not listen to or understand them [35,36]. For mental health treatment to be effective, verbal communication between recipients and providers is of paramount importance so that consumers' subjective experience can be understood and providers can effectively monitor and provide treatment. This applies not only to counseling where a therapeutic alliance is the vehicle for change [37,38] but also for pharmacological treatment, in which trust is often tied to medication compliance [39]. When discrimination is experienced by minority service recipients, including Asians [26,40], such negative encounters can leave them feeling that their mental health needs have not been met.

The underutilization of mental health service among Asian Americans has been well documented for decades [4] and was noted to have persisted in more recent reviews [34]. However, it is possible that the widely publicized and acknowledged trauma of the WTC attack could reduce the stigma of mental illness, thereby normalizing the need for mental health service and increasing awareness of unmet needs. This study aimed to examine the prevalence and factors associated with UMHCN among this understudied and marginalized Asian American population 10–11 years after the disaster.

2. Methods

2.1. Study Participants

The World Trade Center Health Registry: The current study used data collected from the WTC Health Registry (hereafter referred to as the Registry). Funded by the US Federal Emergency Management Agency (FEMA), the Registry was developed in 2002 through the collaboration of the New York City Department of Health and Mental Hygiene and the Agency for Toxic Substances and Disease Registry to monitor the long-term health effects of the 9/11 attacks. Eligible participants included rescue and recovery workers, workers in the WTC and nearby buildings, passersby, and residents in lower Manhattan. Data were collected in 2003–2004 (wave 1), 2006–2007 (wave 2), 2011–2012 (wave 3), and 2015–2016 (wave 4). At wave 1, 71,437 participants age 18 or above were recruited. Full details of the recruitment and data collection processes have been described elsewhere [41,42].

Current Study Participants: To understand longer-term UMHCN among Asian American participants in the Registry, this study employed wave 3 data collected 10–11 years after the disaster. We included all adult participants (aged 18 or older) at wave 3 who self-identified as Asian American

(N = 2538). We then excluded those with missing values for UMHCN and those with pre-9/11 mental health diagnosis. A total of 2344 Asians were included in the final analytic sample. Institutional Review Board approvals were obtained from the first and second authors' affiliated institution, the Centers for Disease Control and Prevention, and the New York City Department of Health and Mental Hygiene.

2.2. Measures

Unmet mental health care needs (UMHCN) were the outcome of interest and were captured by asking if, in the past 12 months, the respondent "needed mental health care or counseling but didn't receive it". Attributions for UMHCN were divided into *attitudinal barriers*, which included endorsement of any one or more of the statements: "preferred to manage myself", "didn't think anything could help", "afraid to ask for help or of what others would think" or "didn't get around to it or didn't bother."; *cost barriers*, which included endorsement of "couldn't afford to pay" or "no insurance or not covered by insurance."; and *access barriers*, which included endorsement of any one or more of the statements: "did not know where to go or what kind of doctor to go to for care", "problems with transportation, scheduling, childcare, or other family responsibilities", or "was unable to find a provider who could diagnose or treat my condition." Participants could check all that applied; thus, the three categories were not mutually exclusive. Sociodemographic variables included gender (female or male), education (college graduate or college graduate/higher, collected at wave 1), age (18–24, 25–44, 45–64, 65+, calculated at wave 3), marital status (married/living with partner, divorced/separated/widowed, or never married, collected at wave 3), household income, nativity, and employment status (collected at wave 3). WTC attack exposure quantified direct disaster exposure and was measured as the number of distinct disaster experiences endorsed (collected in waves 1 and 2), including having been in a damaged/collapsed building during the attack, witnessing three or more horrific events (e.g., saw a plane hit a tower), experiencing intense dust cloud, sustaining any injury (excluding eye irritation), fearing being injured/killed, having a relative die in 9/11, having a friend die in 9/11, having a co-worker die in 9/11, being a rescue/recovery worker, losing possessions due to damage, being evacuated from one's home for at least 48 hours after the attack, and losing a job because of 9/11 [2]. The total number of exposures was then divided into three categories: 0, 1–3, more than 3 exposures.

Mental health conditions included four factors. (1) *Post-9/11 mental health diagnosis* was measured as a dichotomous variable, indicating whether or not participants reported being diagnosed with depression, PTSD, or anxiety disorder other than PTSD by a doctor or other mental health professional after 2001, the year of the attack. If the participant reported any diagnoses having occurred in 2001, we considered the diagnoses to have happened after 9/11 if the respondent did not report any traumatic event other than the WTC attack experienced before 9/11. We used respondents' wave 2 data to supplement their answers in wave 3 to reduce recall bias. (2) *Number of probable mental disorders*, which indicated symptom severity, was defined as the number of current probable mental disorders in the past 30 days for which respondents met criteria as measured by the PTSD Checklist, Civilian Version (PCL-C, score $\geq$44) [43], Patient Health Questionnaire Depression Scale (PHQ-8, score $\geq$10) [44], and Generalized Anxiety Disorder scale (GAD-7, score $\geq$10) [45]. Within each of the measures, if a certain item was missing, it was coded as "0"; item scores were then summed to see if the respondent met the criteria for the probable disorders based on the cutoff scores indicated above. A variable was then created to indicate the total number of distinct probable disorders present (range 0–3). Individuals who had no response for a certain measure altogether were categorized as not having that disorder. It should be noted that these measures indicated probable PTSD, depression, and generalized anxiety disorder, and were not clinical diagnoses. (3) *Functional impairment* captured the level of difficulty associated with working, taking care of things at home or getting along with others due to PTSD or depression symptoms in the last 30 days from "not difficult at all" to "extremely difficult". We derived a composite score using the highest level of functional impairment associated with either disorder. Based on the frequency distribution, we dichotomized the variable into "not difficult at all" as not impaired, and "at least somewhat difficult" or higher as impaired. (4) *Poor mental health days* was measured by asking respondents to report the number of days in the past 30 days when their mental health was not good, which was dichotomized as <14 days and ≥14 days. The number of probable mental health diagnoses and the number of poor mental health days were measured within the same time frame and were moderately correlated (Spearman correlation coefficient $r = 0.46$, $p < 0.0001$). We included both in the analyses—the former as an indication of distinct probable disorders and the latter as a more general subjective measure of mental health.

Social support was measured using five items related to perceived social support received in the past 12 months, including how often someone was available to take the respondent to the doctor, have a good time with them, hug them, prepare meals if they are unable to do it themselves, and understand their problems. Each item was rated on a Likert scale from 1 (none of the time) to 5 (all of the time) (recoded as 0–4). Item scores (Cronbach's alpha = 0.92) were summed to create a total score and divided into quartiles (0–6, 7–11, 12–15, and 16–20). Stress events was defined as experiencing one of the following in the last 12 months: Could not pay for food, housing, or other basic necessities for a period of 3 months or longer; serious family problems involving spouse, child, or parent; took care of a close family member or friend with a serious or life-threatening illness; serious legal problem; and/or lost someone close due to accidental death, murder, or suicide.

Mental health service use was defined as having seen a doctor or health professional or taken any prescription medication for depression, PTSD, anxiety disorder, or nerves, emotions, or other mental health problems or having sought treatment for PTSD symptoms in the past 12 months.

Lacking or disrupted health insurance refers to not having health care insurance at any point in the past 12 months.

2.3. Statistical Analyses

To avoid bias due to exclusion of all missing data and to preserve sample size, we used a "missing" category for all factors with missing values. We examined the distribution of participant characteristics using frequencies and percentages and calculated the prevalence of UMHCN within categories of each factor. We used Chi-square tests to assess bivariate associations between each factor and UMHCN. We also conducted logistic regression analyses, with the outcome of UMHCN, to examine its associations with predictors of interest, adjusting for sets of covariates hierarchically. Mental health condition variables were the main predictors in Model 1, controlling for age, gender, and other sociodemographic as well as WTC exposure variables. Covariates no longer associated with the outcome in the model were removed, with the exception of age and gender, which are important demographic variables in their own right. Model 1 included pre-9/11 mental health diagnosis, number of probable mental disorders, functional impairment due to PTSD or depression, and poor mental health days, as well as the covariates of age, gender, and income. Model 2 included an additional set of predictors related to social support and stressful events. Model 3 extended Model 1 by adding mental health service use and health insurance, since their unique contribution is of interest based on the literature. Model 4 included both social support and stressful events as well as health insurance and service use, controlling for all variables in Model 1. We derived covariate-adjusted odds ratios (aOR) and 95% confidence intervals (CI) from the estimated model parameters to aid interpretation. All analyses were conducted using SAS 9.4 [46].

3. Results

Characteristics of the study sample are described in Table 1. The majority of the sample was 25–44 or 45–64 years (79.48%), male (51.54%), had a college degree or higher (57.04%), had a household income of $50,000 or more (55.50%), was employed (64.33%), married or cohabitating (66.60%), and was foreign-born or did not report nativity (70.05%). Close to two-thirds of the participants experienced 1–3 WTC-related exposures (64.29%).

Table 1. UMHCN of Asian American Participants and their Characteristics (*N* = 2344).

Factors		N	%	UMHCN N	UMHCN %	*p*-Value
UMHCN (DV)	Yes	281	11.99			
Reasons for UMHCN by type	Attitudinal	193	68.68			
	Cost	102	36.30			
	Access	80	28.47			
Demographics						
Age (years)	18–24	78	3.33	8	10.26	
	25–44	736	31.40	98	13.32	0.17
	45–64	1127	48.08	119	10.56	
	65+	403	17.19	56	13.90	
Gender	Male	1208	51.54	140	11.59	
	Female	1076	45.90	136	12.64	0.442
	Missing	60	2.56	5	8.33	
Education	<College graduate	902	38.48	133	14.75	
	≥College graduate	1337	57.04	136	10.17	0.001
	Missing	105	4.48	12	11.43	
Income	<$50,000	915	39.04	171	18.69	
	≥$50,000	1301	55.50	95	7.30	<0.001
	Missing	128	5.46	15	11.72	
Employment status	Employed	1508	64.33	149	9.88	
	Unemployed	815	34.77	121	14.85	<0.001
	Missing	21	0.90	11	52.38	
Marital status	Married/cohabiting	1561	66.60	159	10.19	
	Divorced/separated/widowed	324	13.82	54	16.67	<0.001
	Never married	439	18.73	63	14.35	
	Missing	20	0.85	5	25.00	
Nativity	US born	702	29.95	77	10.97	0.002
	Foreign-born/unreported	1642	70.05	204	12.42	
WTC Attack Exposure						
WTC Exposure	0	452	19.28	40	8.85	
	1–3	1507	64.29	167	11.08	<0.001
	≥4	385	16.42	74	19.22	
Mental Health Condition						
Post-9/11 mental health diagnosis	No	2103	89.72	212	10.08	<0.001
	Yes	241	10.28	69	28.60	
No. of probable mental disorders (PCL, PHQ-8, GAD-7)	0	1807	77.09	129	7.14	
	1	243	10.37	49	20.16	
	2	129	5.50	39	30.23	<0.001
	3	145	6.19	60	41.38	
	Missing	20	0.85	4	20.00	
Functional impairment due to PTSD/depression	Not impaired	1008	43.00	45	4.46	
	Some impairment	1043	44.50	222	21.28	<0.001
	Missing	293	12.50	14	4.78	
Poor mental health days	<14	1874	79.95	155	8.27	
	≥14	415	17.70	117	28.19	<0.001
	Missing	55	2.35	9	16.36	
Social Support and Stress						
Social support (Cronbach coefficient alpha=0.92)	0-6	504	21.50	121	24.01	
	7-11	481	20.52	71	14.76	
	12-15	527	22.48	39	7.40	<0.001
	16-20	742	31.66	29	3.90	
	Missing	90	3.84	21	23.33	
Stressful events in the last 12 months	No	1793	76.49	163	9.09	<0.001
	Yes	551	23.51	118	21.42	

Table 1. *Cont.*

Factors		N	%	UMHCN N	UMHCN %	*p*-Value
Mental Health Service Use and Health Care Resources						
No health insurance at any point within 12 months	No	2031	86.65	189	9.31	<0.001
	Yes	227	9.68	67	29.52	
	Missing	86	3.67	25	29.07	
Service use in past 12 months	No	1562	66.64	158	10.12	<0.001
	Yes	369	15.74	99	26.83	
	Missing	413	17.62	24	5.81	

UMHCN = unmet mental health care need, DV = dependent variable, WTC = World Trade Center, PCL = PTSD checklist, PHQ-8 = Patient Health Questionnaire, GAD-7 = generalized anxiety disorder, PTSD = posttraumatic stress disorder. All *p*-values were from Chi-square tests using data with missing category excluded.

Over 10% had a post-9/11 mental health diagnosis, 22.91% had at least one probable mental disorder, 44.50% had at least some functional impairment due to PTSD or depression symptoms, and 17.70% reported 14 or more poor mental health days in the past 30 days. Over 15% used mental health services in the past 12 months, and approximately 12% had UMHCN in the past 12 months. Among the 281 participants with UMHCN, attitudinal barriers were the most attributed cause for unmet need (68.68%), followed by cost barriers (36.30%) and access barriers (28.47%).

Having UMHCN was significantly associated with several demographic, WTC attack exposure, psychosocial, and clinical factors (Table 1). Higher prevalence of unmet mental health needs was present among those with lower education, lower household income, those who were unemployed, divorced/separated/widowed, and were foreign-born or had unreported nativity. Greater proportion of unmet needs was also noted among those who experienced >3 WTC-related exposures, at least one past year stressful event, and among those with less social support. UMHCN was also more prevalent among those with post-9/11 mental health diagnosis, those with current mental health disorders/impairment, those lacking or having interrupted health insurance, and those who used mental health services in the past 12 months.

In covariate-adjusted regression analysis, mental health and demographic factors other than gender were associated with greater odds of UMHCN across all four models, although several of these associations were attenuated in models with additional covariates (Table 2). Among the sociodemographic variables, income was significantly associated with UMHCN in all models. Participants younger than 45 years of age had higher odds of unmet needs than those that were older. Adjusting for age, gender, and income, the four variables representing mental health conditions were all significantly associated with UMHCN. Specifically, participants having post-9/11 mental health diagnosis; functional impairment due to PTSD or depression; 14 or more poor mental health days in the past month; and greater number of probable mental disorders had higher odds of unmet mental health needs. Model 2 showed additional effects of stress and social support; the odds of UMHCN were greater among those who experienced at least one stressful event in the past year but lower among those with greater social support. Inclusion of these two factors seemed to slightly attenuate the associations between the outcome and some Model 1 variables, such as income, comorbidity, and functional impairment, but strengthened the effect of age and post-9/11 mental health diagnosis. When controlling for age, gender, income, and mental health conditions in Model 3, the odds of UMHCN greatly increased with the lack of or disrupted health insurance in the past year but were not associated with mental health service use in the past year. The addition of the factors for disrupted health insurance and mental health service use slightly attenuated the associations of all factors in Model 1 with the outcome.

Table 2. Covariate-adjusted odds ratio (aOR) and 95% confidence interval (CI) derived from logistic models for UMHCN (N = 2344).

Factors		Model 1	Model 2	Model 3	Model 4
		aOR (CI)	aOR (CI)	aOR (CI)	aOR (CI)
		Demographics			
Age (years)	18–24	2.08 (0.63–6.90)	2.95 (0.85–10.23)	1.75 (0.52–5.91)	2.47 (0.70–8.68)
	25–44	1.70 (1.12–2.57)	1.91 (1.25–2.93)	1.41 (0.92–2.18)	1.67 (1.07–2.60)
	45–64	0.90 (0.62–1.32)	0.88 (0.59–1.29)	0.79 (0.53–1.17)	0.78 (0.52–1.17)
	65+	1	1	1	1
Income	≥$50,000	1	1	1	1
	<$50,000	2.61 (1.92–3.54)	2.03 (1.48–2.79)	2.03 (1.47–2.80)	1.61 (1.15–2.25)
		Mental Health Conditions			
Post-9/11 mental health diagnosis	No	1	1	1	1
	Yes	1.73 (1.21–2.49)	2.49 (1.84–1.27)	1.52 (1.04–2.23)	1.61 (1.08–2.38)
No. of probable mental disorders (PCL, PHQ-8, GAD-7)	0	1	1	1	1
	1	1.79 (1.21–2.66)	1.68 (1.12–2.51)	1.70 (1.14–2.55)	1.59 (1.05–2.39)
	2	2.18 (1.36–3.48)	1.85 (1.14–2.98)	2.08 (1.29–3.35)	1.76 (1.08–2.86)
	3	2.88 (1.81–4.59)	2.46 (1.52–3.98)	2.71 (1.68–4.38)	2.33 (1.42–3.81)
Functional impairment due to PTSD or depression	Not impaired	1	1	1	1
	Some impairment	3.04 (2.09–4.43)	2.40 (1.64–3.53)	2.94 (2.01–4.30)	2.36 (1.60–3.48)
Poor mental health days	<14	1	1	1	1
	≥14	1.68 (1.21–2.34)	1.63 (1.16–2.27)	1.57 (1.12–2.20)	1.53 (1.09–2.16)
		Social Support and Stress			
Social support	0–6		1		1
	7–11		0.58 (0.41–0.83)		0.55 (0.38–0.79)
	12–15		0.38 (0.25–0.57)		0.37 (0.24–0.57)
	16–20		0.25 (0.16–0.40)		0.25 (0.16–0.41)
Stressful events in the last 12 months	No		1		1
	Yes		1.44 (1.06–1.96)		1.32 (0.96–1.81)
		Mental Health Service Use and Health Care Resources			
No health insurance at any point within 12 months	No			1	1
	Yes			2.47 (1.69–3.61)	2.37 (1.61–3.48)
Service use in past 12 months	No			1	1
	Yes			1.26 (0.89–1.77)	1.31 (0.92–1.86)

PCL = PTSD Checklist, PHQ = Patient Health Questionnaire, GAD = Generalized Anxiety Disorder, PTSD = posttraumatic stress disorder. Each model includes variables for which there are estimates provided in that column.

Model 4 included all factors of interest. Greater odds of UMHCN were noted with an increase in number of probable mental disorder (meeting criteria for one vs. no disorder , aOR = 1.59, 95% CI: 1.05–2.39; 2 vs. 0 disorder, aOR = 1.76, 95% CI: 1.08–2.86; 3 vs. 0 disorder, aOR = 2.33, 95% CI: 1.42–3.81), among those with a post-9/11 mental health diagnosis (aOR = 1.61, 95% CI: 1.08–2.38), functional impairment (aOR = 2.36, 95% CI: 1.60–3.48), and having 14 or more poor mental health days (aOR = 1.53, 95% CI: 1.09–2.16). Being aged 25–44 vs. 65 or older (aOR = 1.67, 95% CI: 1.07–2.60) and having a lower vs. higher income (aOR = 1.61, 95% CI: 1.15–2.25) were also associated with greater odds of unmet needs. In Model 4, greater social support was associated with lower odds of unmet need (45–75% reduction), while having experienced stressful events (aOR = 1.32, 95% CI: 0.96–1.81, $p = 0.08$) and lacking or disrupted health insurance in the past year (aOR = 2.37, 95% CI: 1.61–3.48) were both associated with greater odds of UMHCN. Compared to results in Model 2, further controlling for health insurance and service use attenuated the effect of stressful event but had no impact on the association between social support and UMHCN. Similarly, compared to results in Model 3, the addition of social support and stressful events slightly attenuated the effect of health insurance on odds of UMHCN.

4. Discussion

A sizeable proportion of Asian Americans had UMHCN 10–11 years after direct exposure to the WTC attack (12%), which is much higher than that reported in other community samples (e.g.,

4.5%) [5], indicating greater unmet needs in those affected by this mass trauma more than a decade later. The prevalence of UMHCN is also higher than that reported among the Asian group at wave 2 of the Registry, which was 5–6 years after the disaster (4.4%) [2]. This may be related to delayed manifestation of PTSD symptoms and deferred mental health service use [8]. This high prevalence of UMHCN may also be attributed to dwindling of resources for free services provided by governmental and nongovernmental organizations after the attack (e.g., Project Liberty and American Red Cross 9/11 Fund) [47,48]. This is consistent with our finding that lack or disruption of health insurance had the strongest association with UMHCN among all other factors.

Among those who reported UMHCN, attitudinal barriers were most common, followed by cost and access barriers. This is in line with other studies that have reported attitudinal barriers (e.g., acceptability) as more likely causes of unmet needs compared to other tangible barriers, such as accessibility and availability of mental health services [5]. Within those who attributed their unmet need to attitudinal barriers, "prefer to manage myself" was the most endorsed item (62.1%, not shown in tables), which may indicate the desire to keep the issue private and potentially related to being "afraid to ask for help/of what others would think" (25.4%). Both may be manifestations of fear of stigma. Other common reasons like "didn't get around to it/didn't bother" (37.8%), and "don't think anything could help" (34.2%) may reflect the tendency to undervalue treatment due to the lack of knowledge about mental illness and its treatment. These figures are disconcerting since these Asian Americans had been directly exposed to the WTC attack and should have heard of its mental health impact from the media. It is possible that they no longer relate their mental health need to the disaster a decade later.

In terms of factors associated with UMHCN, it is noteworthy that those who lacked or had disrupted insurance in the past year had more than twice the odds of having unmet needs than those who did not. However, this was consistent with greater odds of UMHCN for individuals from household income of <$50,000 than those of higher income, and the significant association persisted throughout the hierarchical regression models. Close to 40% of Asian participants reported household income below $50,000, and 15% were unemployed; thus, they may not be able to afford or willing to pay for services to meet their mental health needs. This is consistent with cost being the second most common reason for UMHCN after attitudinal barriers. Asians at the prime years of their lives (25–44) had significantly higher odds of having UMHCN, which may reflect the challenges of financial and family-related responsibilities [49,50].

The association between mental health conditions and UMHCN noted in this study is expected, since less favorable mental health conditions would increase mental health care needs and thus lead to a higher chance that the need is not being met. The finding is consistent with reports from previous studies based on the Registry across race [27] and other data [7]. These mental health factors were all significant in their association with the outcome throughout the four models. It is of interest to note that among the mental health factors, functional impairment from PTSD or depression had the strongest association with UMHCN, with even higher odds compared to having comorbidity of three probable mental disorders, which indicated severe symptomatology. This may reflect Asians' tendency to dismiss their mental health need unless it interferes with their daily functioning [14]. Further, those with a low income and those who were unemployed may also be less able to compensate for their inability to perform expected roles at work and at home to sustain themselves and their families, which may cause them to recognize their UMHCN. The association between post-9/11 mental health diagnosis and UMHCN suggests that Asian Americans who had previous contact with mental health professionals may have been more aware of their mental health needs and when those needs were not met, whether or not they continued treatment.

Asian Americans with stressful life events in the past year, including financial and health challenges to themselves or families, could tax their coping resources and thus increase mental health issues and thereby heighten the awareness of their UMHCN. However, social support may have alleviated unmet needs by reducing access barriers to mental health care by providing practical assistance [5] such as child care or meal preparation when individuals sought mental health care, or accompanying them to see the doctor. At the same time, the relatively higher mental health stigma noted among Asian Americans in general [51] may have attenuated the positive impact of social support on UMHCN in this study. The fact that attitudinal barriers were the most common reasons for UMHCN among Asians may also indicate fear of stigma within the social network should they seek mental health services. Thus, exploration of the perception of stigma within the community or within social networks and its relation to unmet needs is an important area of future inquiry in disaster-affected Asian communities.

The lack of association between previous mental health service use and UMHCN found in this study contrasts with findings from most studies in which previous consumers were more likely to indicate unmet needs [5,27], potentially due to dissatisfaction with the quality of treatment, recognition of potential help that they cannot access, or limitations of services in providing desired help after being exposed to the formal mental health care system [5]. This nonsignificant finding was unexpected also because it contradicts with our expectation that there would be higher dissatisfaction with mental health treatment among Asians due to poorer quality of service [4] and lower therapeutic alliance due to cultural and linguistic barriers [34,35]. It is possible that the smaller proportion of Asian Americans having received mental health services (e.g., compared to the non-Hispanic white group, 15.7% vs. 26.6%; the authors, in press) limited statistical power. However, the tendency of Asian Americans to terminate treatment prematurely [13] suggests that they may be less exposed to the mental health care system, hence less likely to recognize the range of available treatment that is inaccessible to them, and therefore less likely to indicate UMHCN [5]. Moreover, lower mental health literacy could also prevent them from recognizing an unmet need [25], also called "unperceived unmet need" [6]. Furthermore, their mental health need might have been satisfied through effective mental health services such as those provided by the WTC Health Program [52], or the use of alternative healing methods such as traditional Chinese medicine [53] or other folk healing within their unique communities [54].

4.1. Study Limitations and Strengths

The findings of this study should be considered in light of the study's limitations. The study was unable to capture ethnic diversity among Asian Americans in the sample. While there are similarities among Asian ethnic groups, it is possible that the various factors we examined may be associated with UMHCN differentially among the Asian subgroups [55–57]. Further, since UMHCN is captured by self-report without any clinical record for confirmation, which could indicate individuals' mental health care needs and premature termination; when individuals are unaware of their mental health need, this could cause underestimation of its prevalence. This is particularly an issue for many Asian Americans who have limited mental health knowledge and the tendency to ignore their psychological distress [13,14]. The prevalence of unmet needs may also be underestimated due to social desirability bias, in which participants avoided reporting mental health care needs to avoid stigma [25]. The lack of information on the duration of previous treatment, number of visits to mental health service, type of providers seen, or satisfaction with services also limited our ability to assess the impact of previous mental health service use on UMHCN. Due to sample size limitations, we were also unable to assess specific factors associated with UMHCN due to attitudinal, cost, and access barriers separately. Further inquiry in this regard could better inform strategies to ameliorate the effects of these specific barriers. Finally, since the investigation is based mainly on cross-sectional data from wave 3, causal relationships could not be established.

Despite these limitations, this study is the single largest investigation of UMHCN among Asian Americans who were directly exposed to the WTC attack, and the first large-scale study examining Asians' subjective perception of their UMHCN after a massive trauma. The direct assessment of individuals' subjective perception of unmet needs has the advantage of capturing a potential service gap without assuming that a mental health service need is satisfied with service use alone.

The comprehensive recruitment and follow-up efforts of the Registry through the use of Asian-language interviewers and outreach efforts [42] enabled the inclusion of individuals who were not proficient in English, which constituted a large proportion of the Asian American population (75%) [17]. The longitudinal design of the study allows for examination of longer term unmet needs, which is critical in light of the often delayed manifestation of PTSD symptoms and service use [8].

4.2. Study Implications

Our finding suggests that a substantial proportion of Asian Americans have UMHCN a decade after the WTC attack, which was even greater than that noted 5 years prior in another study [2]. This may indicate that continued outreach efforts to this community are necessary to provide treatment options. During the years after the disaster, with heightened awareness of its impact through media coverage and outreach efforts from government and nongovernmental organizations, mental health services were made more readily available. However, with time, the number of organizations providing free services and public awareness of some continued programs declined, potentially increasing practical barriers such as accessibility and cost. Thus, programs such as the Registry's Treatment Referral Program which reaches out to enrollees who lived or worked near the disaster area and reported a physical and/or mental health symptom should be continued long term [58]. Since those with worse current mental health conditions and previous diagnoses have higher odds of UMHCN, they should also be targeted for interventions that bring them to treatment and to improve treatment adherence. To ensure that culturally competent mental health service providers are available is also important [21] to increase continuation and satisfaction with services in fully meeting their needs.

Since the largest proportion of UMHCN among Asian Americans exposed to the WTC attack was attributed to attitude about mental illness and its treatment, a "subjective chosen unmet need" [6], public mental health education may well be key to address unmet needs with this population. Increasing knowledge about the cause, manifestation, and course of mental illness could help to reduce stigma, increase awareness of individuals' mental health needs, and promote appropriate expectations of the treatment process so as to encourage service use and reduce dropout. These public education efforts should be tailored to the languages, needs, and cultures of the various minority communities [21]. The importance of post-disaster large-scale public mental health education and outreach efforts is also relevant for future disasters.

Another important implication of this study's findings is the strong role of health insurance, income, and employment in unmet needs. This suggests that free mental health care related to the WTC attack should be continued. The WTC Health Program under the WTCHR has provided health and mental health services to individuals directly exposed to the disaster, and outreach efforts to affected individuals through the Treatment Referral Program continues to date. Enrollees who lived or worked in the 9/11 disaster area and reported a physical and/or mental health symptom were encouraged to seek care from 9/11-specialty providers [52]. This program should be continued given the considerable UMHCN noted in this study among the Asians, who may not be able to afford needed services. Although the James Zadroga 9/11 Health and Compensation Act enacted in 2010 was extended through 2090 [10], the recent report on the September 11th Victim Compensation Fund released in February 2019 is concerning, which revealed funding insufficiency and needs for reduced awards due to greater claim than anticipated [59]. Congress would need to consider providing more resources for free services through adequate compensation of treatment expenses. Given the long-term nature of mental illnesses, especially PTSD, this is an important consideration.

With the persistent and striking underutilization of mental health services among Asian Americans, the value of the subjective account of UMHCN to better understand the actual demand for mental health services and the perceived adequacy and quality of treatment [7] becomes more important, and research along this line is necessary. In future studies, ethnicity within the Asian American population should be disaggregated to gain a more nuanced understanding of unique unmet needs and their specific barriers so that improvement in outreach efforts and mental health treatment could be made to ameliorate the disparities in mental health services [6]. Further, for those who have used mental health services before and still find their needs unmet, we need to understand in greater depth the "dosage" of services received, whether or not it was premature termination, and reasons for their dissatisfaction. More detailed exploration of the stigma Asians ascribe to mental health problems and treatment should be explored so that relevant community mental health education can more effectively address any misunderstanding.

5. Conclusions

The prevalence of UMHCN among Asian Americans directly exposed to the WTC attack remained sizeable a decade after the attack, and the cause of unmet need was attributed most frequently to attitudinal barriers, followed by cost and access barriers. Thus, continued outreach efforts to Asian communities through public mental health education to increase knowledge about mental illness and the value of and options for mental health treatment, and to destigmatize the illness and treatment, is of paramount importance. Free and convenient access to mental health services to eligible individuals through adequate allocation of public funding is crucial to ensure that issues of cost and access will also not prevent individuals from addressing their mental health needs. Further exploration of subjective perception of UMHCN to provide information on the actual demand for mental health services and ways to improve treatment among Asian Americans is also warranted.

Author Contributions: Conceptualization, W.W.K. and E.G.; Methodology, all authors contributed; Data analyses: X.W., X.L., W.W.K., D.H.; Writing, review, and editing: all authors contributed.

Funding: This research was funded by the Center for Disease Control and Prevention, National Institute of Occupational Safety and Health, Grant Number 1U01OH010516-01A1.The study was also supported by the Fordham-New York University Research Fellowship and National Institute of Mental Health training grant, T32 MH013043. The contents of the study are solely the responsibility of the authors and do not necessarily represent the official views of the funders.

Acknowledgments: We would also like to express our sincere gratitude to the World Trade Center Health Registry for sharing their data for our study.

Conflicts of Interest: All authors declare no competing interests.

References

1. Boscarino, J.A.; Adams, R.E.; Stuber, J.; Galea, S. Disparities in mental health treatment following the World Trade Center Disaster: Implications for mental health care and health services research. *J. Trauma. Stress* **2005**, *18*, 287–297. [CrossRef]
2. Brackbill, R.M.; Stellman, S.D.; Perlman, S.E.; Walker, D.J.; Farfel, M.R. Mental health of those directly exposed to the World Trade Center disaster: Unmet mental health care need, mental health treatment service use, and quality of life. *Soc. Sci. Med.* **2013**, *81*, 110–114. [CrossRef]
3. Asian American Federation of New York. Asian American Mental Health: A Post-September 11th Needs Assessment. Available online: http://www.aafny.org/doc/AsianAmericanMentalHealth.pdf (accessed on 26 February 2019).
4. U.S. Department of Health and Human Services. *Mental Health: Culture, Race, and Ethnicity—A Supplement to Mental Health: A Report of the Surgeon General*; U.S. Department of Health and Human Services: Washington, DC, USA, 2001.
5. Nelson, C.H.; Park, J. The nature and correlates of unmet health care needs in Ontario, Canada. *Soc. Sci. Med.* **2006**, *62*, 2291–2300. [CrossRef]
6. Allin, S.; Grignon, M.; Le Grand, J. Subjective unmet need and utilization of health care services in Canada: What are the equity implications? *Soc. Sci. Med.* **2010**, *70*, 465–472. [CrossRef] [PubMed]
7. Mojtabai, R. Unmet need for treatment of major depression in the United States. *Psychiatr. Serv.* **2009**, *60*, 297–305. [CrossRef]
8. Wang, P.S.; Berglund, P.; Olfson, M.; Pincus, H.A.; Wells, K.B.; Kessler, R.C. Failure and delay in initial treatment contact after first onset of mental disorders in the National Comorbidity Survey Replication. *Arch. Gen. Psychiatry* **2005**, *62*, 603–613. [CrossRef] [PubMed]

9.   Bowler, R.M.; Harris, M.; Li, J.; Gocheva, V.; Stellman, S.D.; Wilson, K.; Alper, H.; Schwarzer, R.; Cone, J.E. Longitudinal mental health impact among police responders to the 9/11 terrorist attack. *Am. J. Ind. Med.* **2012**, *55*, 297–312. [CrossRef]

10.   114th U.S. Congress. H.R.1786—James Zadroga 9/11 Health and Compensation Reauthorization Act. Available online: https://www.congress.gov/bill/114th-congress/house-bill/1786 (accessed on 26 February 2019).

11.   Insel, T.R. Assessing the economic costs of serious mental illness. *Am. J. Psychiatry* **2008**, *165*, 663–665. [CrossRef]

12.   Wang, P.S.; Lane, M.; Olfson, M.; Pincus, H.A.; Wells, K.B.; Kessler, R.C. Twelve-month use of mental health services in the United States: Results from the National Comorbidity Survey Replication. *Arch. Gen. Psychiatry* **2005**, *62*, 629–640. [CrossRef]

13.   Leong, F.T.; Lau, A.S. Barriers to providing effective mental health services to Asian Americans. *Ment. Health Serv. Res.* **2001**, *3*, 201–214. [CrossRef] [PubMed]

14.   Kung, W.W.; Lu, P.C. How symptom manifestations affect help seeking for mental health problems among Chinese Americans. *J. Nerv. Ment. Dis.* **2008**, *196*, 46–54. [CrossRef]

15.   Yang, L.H.; Chen, F.P.; Sia, K.J.; Lam, J.; Lam, K.; Ngo, H.; Lee, S.; Kleinman, A.; Good, B. "What matters most:" A cultural mechanism moderating structural vulnerability and moral experience of mental illness stigma. *Soc. Sci. Med.* **2014**, *103*, 84–93. [CrossRef] [PubMed]

16.   Kung, W.W. Cultural and practical barriers to seeking mental health treatment for Chinese Americans. *J. Community Psychol.* **2004**, *32*, 27–43. [CrossRef]

17.   U.S. Census Bureau. 2010–2014 American Community Survey 5-Year Estimates. Available online: https://factfinder.census.gov/faces/nav/jsf/pages/index.xhtml (accessed on 26 February 2019).

18.   Kung, W. Tangible needs and external stressors faced by Chinese American families with a member having schizophrenia. *Soc. Work Res.* **2016**, *40*, 53–63. [CrossRef]

19.   Alegría, M.; Chatterji, P.; Wells, K.; Cao, Z.; Chen, C.-N.; Takeuchi, D.; Jackson, J.; Meng, X.-L. Disparity in depression treatment among racial and ethnic minority populations in the United States. *Psychiatr. Serv.* **2008**, *59*, 1264–1272. [CrossRef] [PubMed]

20.   Clement, S.; Schauman, O.; Graham, T.; Maggioni, F.; Evans-Lacko, S.; Bezborodovs, N.; Morgan, C.; Rusch, N.; Brown, J.S.; Thornicroft, G. What is the impact of mental health-related stigma on help-seeking? A systematic review of quantitative and qualitative studies. *Psychol. Med.* **2015**, *45*, 11–27. [CrossRef]

21.   Norris, F.H.; Alegria, M. Mental health care for ethnic minority individuals and communities in the aftermath of disasters and mass violence. *CNS Spectr.* **2005**, *10*, 132–140. [CrossRef]

22.   Tung, W.-C. Cultural barriers to mental health services among Asian Americans. *Home Health Care Manag. Pract.* **2011**, *23*, 303–305. [CrossRef]

23.   Geaney, J. Guarding moral boundaries: Shame in early Confucianism. *Philos. East West* **2004**, *54*, 113–142. [CrossRef]

24.   Link, B.G.; Struening, E.L.; Neese-Todd, S.; Asmussen, S.; Phelan, J.C. Stigma as a barrier to recovery: The consequences of stigma for the self-esteem of people with mental illnesses. *Psychiatr. Serv.* **2001**, *52*, 1621–1626. [CrossRef]

25.   Yang, L.H.; Kleinman, A.; Link, B.G.; Phelan, J.C.; Lee, S.; Good, B. Culture and stigma: Adding moral experience to stigma theory. *Soc. Sci. Med.* **2007**, *64*, 1524–1535. [CrossRef]

26.   Inman, A.G.; Yeh, C.J.; Madan-Bahel, A.; Nath, S. Bereavement and coping of South Asian families post 9/11. *J. Multicult. Couns. Dev.* **2007**, *35*, 101–115. [CrossRef]

27.   Ghuman, S.J.; Brackbill, R.M.; Stellman, S.D.; Farfel, M.R.; Cone, J.E. Unmet mental health care need 10–11 years after the 9/11 terrorist attacks: 2011–2012 results from the World Trade Center Health Registry. *BMC Public Health* **2014**, *14*, 684–699. [CrossRef]

28.   Kung, W.W. Chinese Americans' help seeking for emotional distress. *Soc. Serv. Rev.* **2003**, *77*, 110–134. [CrossRef]

29.   Mojtabai, R.O.M.; Mechanic, D. Perceived need and help-seeking in adults with mood, anxiety, or substance use disorders. *Arch. Gen. Psychiatry* **2002**, *59*, 77–84. [CrossRef]

30.   Bauer, A.M.; Chen, C.N.; Alegría, M. English language proficiency and mental health service use among Latino and Asian Americans with mental disorders. *Med. Care* **2010**, *48*, 1097–1104. [CrossRef]

31. Primm, A.B.; Vasquez, M.J.; Mays, R.A.; Sammons-Posey, D.; McKnight-Eily, L.R.; Presley-Cantrell, L.R.; McGuire, L.C.; Chapman, D.P.; Perry, G.S. The role of public health in addressing racial and ethnic disparities in mental health and mental illness. *Prev. Chronic Dis.* **2010**, *7*, A20.

32. Balsa, A.I.; McGuire, T.G. Statistical discrimination in health care. *J. Health Econ.* **2001**, *20*, 881–907. [CrossRef]

33. Balsa, A.I.; McGuire, T.G. Prejudice, clinical uncertainty and stereotyping as sources of health disparities. *J. Health Econ.* **2003**, *22*, 89–116. [CrossRef]

34. Sue, S.; Yan Cheng, J.K.; Saad, C.S.; Chu, J.P. Asian American mental health: A call to action. *Am. Psychol.* **2012**, *67*, 532–544. [CrossRef]

35. Okazaki, S.; Kassem, A.M.; Tu, M.C. Addressing Asian American mental health disparities: Putting community-based research principles to work. *Asian Am. J. Psychol.* **2014**, *5*, 4–12. [CrossRef]

36. Kouyoumdjian, H.; Zamboanga, B.L.; Hansen, D.J. Barriers to community mental health services for Latinos: Treatment considerations. *Clin. Psychol. Sci. Pract.* **2003**, *10*, 394–422. [CrossRef]

37. Horvath, A.O.; Del Re, A.; Flückiger, C.; Symonds, D. Alliance in individual psychotherapy. *Psychotherapy* **2011**, *48*, 9–16. [CrossRef]

38. Martin, D.J.; Garske, J.P.; Davis, M.K. Relation of the therapeutic alliance with outcome and other variables: A meta-analytic review. *J. Consult. Clin. Psychol.* **2000**, *68*, 438–450. [CrossRef]

39. McCabe, R.; Bullenkamp, J.; Hansson, L.; Lauber, C.; Martinez-Leal, R.; Rössler, W.; Salize, H.J.; Svensson, B.; Torres-Gonzalez, F.; van den Brink, R. The therapeutic relationship and adherence to antipsychotic medication in schizophrenia. *PLoS ONE* **2012**, *7*, e36080. [CrossRef]

40. Burgess, D.J.; Ding, Y.; Hargreaves, M.; van Ryn, M.; Phelan, S. The association between perceived discrimination and underutilization of needed medical and mental health care in a multi-ethnic community sample. *J. Health Care Poor Underserved* **2008**, *19*, 894–911. [CrossRef]

41. Brackbill, R.; Thorpe, L.; DeGrande, L.; Perrin, M.; Sapp, J.H.; Wu, D.; Campolucci, S.; Walker, D.J.; Cone, J.; Thalji, L.; et al. Surveillance for World Trade Center disaster health effects among survivors of collapsed and damaged buildings. *Morb. Mortal. Wkly. Rep.* **2006**, *55*, 1–18.

42. Farfel, M.; DiGrande, L.; Brackbill, R.; Prann, A.; Cone, J.; Friedman, S.; Walker, D.J.; Pezeshki, G.; Thomas, P.; Galea, S. An overview of 9/11 experiences and respiratory and mental health conditions among World Trade Center Health Registry enrollees. *J. Urban Health* **2008**, *85*, 880–909. [CrossRef]

43. Weathers, F.W.; Litz, B.T.; Herman, D.S.; Huska, J.A.; Keane, T.M. The PTSD Checklist (PCL): Reliability, validity, and diagnostic utility. In Proceedings of the Annual Convention of the International Society for Traumatic Stress Studies, San Antonio, TX, USA, 25 October 1993.

44. Kroenke, K.; Spitzer, R.L.; Williams, J.B.; Löwe, B. An ultra-brief screening scale for anxiety and depression: The PHQ-4. *Psychosomatics* **2009**, *50*, 613–621.

45. Spitzer, R.L.; Kroenke, K.; Williams, J.B.; Löwe, B. A brief measure for assessing generalized anxiety disorder: The GAD-7. *Arch. Intern. Med.* **2006**, *166*, 1092–1097. [CrossRef]

46. SAS Institute Inc. *SAS 9.4 [Computer Software]*; SAS Institute Inc.: Cary, NC, USA, 2014.

47. Felton, C.J. Project liberty: A public health response to new yorkers' mental health needs arising from the world trade center terrorist attacks. *J. Urban Health* **2002**, *79*, 429–433. [CrossRef]

48. Kapucu, N. Non-profit response to catastrophic disasters. *Disaster Prev. Manag. Int. J.* **2007**, *16*, 551–561. [CrossRef]

49. Soldo, B.J. Cross pressures on middle-aged adults: A broader view. *J. Gerontol. Soc. Sci.* **1996**, *51B*, S271–S273. [CrossRef]

50. Härenstam, A.; Bejerot, E. Combining professional work with family responsibilities—A burden or a blessing? *Int. J. Soc. Welf.* **2001**, *10*, 202–214. [CrossRef]

51. Ryder, A.G.; Bean, G.; Dion, K.L. Caregiver responses to symptoms of first-onset psychosis: A comparative study of Chinese-and Euro-Canadian families. *Transcult. Psychiatry* **2000**, *37*, 255–266. [CrossRef]

52. Welch, A.E.; Caramanica, K.; Debchoudhury, I.; Pulizzi, A.; Farfel, M.R.; Stellman, S.D.; Cone, J.E. A qualitative examination of health and health care utilization after the September 11th terror attacks among World Trade Center Health Registry enrollees. *BMC Public Health* **2012**, *12*, 721. [CrossRef]

53. Yang, L.H.; Phelan, J.C.; Link, B.G. Stigma and beliefs of efficacy towards traditional Chinese medicine and Western psychiatric treatment among Chinese-Americans. *Cult. Divers. Ethn. Minority Psychol.* **2008**, *14*, 10. [CrossRef]

54. Abe, J. A community ecology approach to cultural competence in mental health service delivery: The case of Asian Americans. *Asian Am. J. Psychol.* **2012**, *3*, 168–180. [CrossRef]

55. Barreto, R.M.; Segal, S.P. Use of Mental Health Services by Asian Americans. *Psychiatr. Serv.* **2005**, *56*, 746–748. [CrossRef]

56. Abe-Kim, J.; Takeuchi, D.T.; Hong, S.; Zane, N.; Sue, S.; Spencer, M.S.; Appel, H.; Nicdao, E.; Alegría, M. Use of mental health-related services among immigrant and US-Born Asian Americans: Results from the National Latino and Asian American Study. *Am. J. Public Health* **2007**, *97*, 91–98. [CrossRef]

57. Cho, H.; Kim, I.; Velez-Ortiz, D. Factors associated with mental health service use among Latino and Asian Americans. *Community Ment. Health J.* **2014**, *50*, 960–967. [CrossRef]

58. Welch, A.E.; Caramanica, K.; Maslow, C.B.; Brackbill, R.M.; Stellman, S.D.; Farfel, M.R. Trajectories of PTSD among lower Manhattan residents and area workers following the 2001 World Trade Center Disaster, 2003–2012. *J. Trauma. Stress* **2016**, *29*, 158–166. [CrossRef]

59. Bhattacharyya, R. Seventh Annual Status Report and Third Annual Reassessment of Policy and Procedures, September 11th Victim Compensation Fund. Available online: https://www.vcf.gov/pdf/VCFStatusReportFeb2019.pdf (accessed on 26 February 2019).

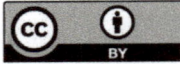

International Journal of
Environmental Research and Public Health

MDPI

Article

A Cognitive Reserve and Social Support-Focused Latent Class Analysis to Predict Self-Reported Confusion or Memory Loss among Middle-Aged World Trade Center Health Registry Enrollees

Kacie Seil *, Shengchao Yu and Howard Alper

New York City Department of Health and Mental Hygiene, World Trade Center Health Registry, 125 Worth
Street, New York, NY 10013, USA; syu@health.nyc.gov (S.Y.); halper@health.nyc.gov (H.A.)
* Correspondence: kseil@health.nyc.gov; Tel.: +1-646-632-6215

Received: 25 February 2019; Accepted: 13 April 2019; Published: 18 April 2019

Abstract: The World Trade Center Health Registry includes 9/11 survivors who have been surveyed about their health conditions over time. The prevalence of posttraumatic stress disorder (PTSD) remains high among the cohort and is a risk factor for cognitive impairment or dementia. We thus sought to examine the degree to which confusion or memory loss (CML)—potential symptoms of cognitive decline—are occurring among enrollees aged 35–64 years. Cognitive reserve theory suggests that higher levels of education and engaging in cognitively challenging activities can create stronger neural connections, offering protection against cognitive decline. We hypothesized that enrollees with less cognitive reserve would be more likely to report CML. In this study, we: (1) estimated the incidence of CML in our study sample; (2) identified indicators of cognitive reserve (e.g., indicators of educational attainment, social support); and (3) determined whether CML is associated with cognitive reserve level, stratified by PSTD status. First, we described demographics of the study sample (n = 14,574) and probable PTSD status, also stratifying by CML. Next, we conducted a latent class analysis on two groups: those with probable PTSD and those without probable PTSD, creating classes with varying cognitive reserve levels. Finally, using adjusted log binomial models, we predicted risk of CML based on cognitive reserve level. The probable PTSD group (n = 1213) and not probable PTSD group (n = 13,252) each had four latent classes: low, medium-low, medium-high, and high cognitive reserve. In the probable PTSD model, compared to the high cognitive reserve class, those with medium-low cognitive reserve were 35% more likely to report CML (relative risk (RR) = 1.4, 95% confidence interval (CI): 1.1, 1.7). Among the not probable PTSD group, those with low and medium levels of cognitive reserve were significantly more likely to report CML (RR = 1.8 and 1.4, respectively). Overall, those with less cognitive reserve were more likely to report CML regardless of PTSD status.

Keywords: cognitive reserve; cognitive decline; latent class analysis; disaster epidemiology; PTSD

1. Introduction

The terrorist attacks on the World Trade Center (WTC) in New York City (NYC) on 11 September 2001 resulted in thousands of deaths and non-fatal injuries. Survivors of the attacks also witnessed traumatic events and were exposed to dust and debris related to the towers' collapse, the health effects of which include posttraumatic stress disorder (PTSD), asthma, cancer, and other conditions [1–3]. Seventeen years after the event, survivors continue to exhibit effects. As the cohort ages, the prevalence of chronic conditions associated with older age will likely increase. Mild to severe forms of cognitive decline affect a large number of Americans, particularly those over the age of 65 years, though they can affect younger individuals as well [4,5].

Co-morbid health conditions can put one at greater risk for cognitive decline; PTSD is associated with greater likelihood of developing cognitive impairment or various forms of dementia [6–12]. It is possible that 9/11-related exposures and resulting health conditions may put enrollees at greater risk for cognitive decline than the general population [11,13]. Research has shown elevated levels of PTSD among the WTC Health Registry (WTCHR) cohort in the years following the disaster [1,14]. Research by Clouston et al. (2017) examined WTC responders from the WTC Health Program and found that 14.8% of responders had cognitive dysfunction identified via a battery of tests. This proportion was larger than expected compared to normative data from age-matched healthy adults. Cognitive dysfunction was also associated with PTSD symptom severity and working at the 9/11 site for more than five weeks [11].

People who are less socially isolated (i.e., engaging in more social activities and having larger social networks) are less likely to have cognitive problems later in their lives [15,16]. Research has also shown that increases in "out of home" activities and walking duration can be protective against cognitive impairment as well [17]. Similarly, social interaction and cognitive control skills specific to certain kinds of occupations appear to be protective against neurodegeneration [18–22]. Engaging in cognitively stimulating activities is also positively associated with cognition [22,23]. Research shows that greater levels of cognitive reserve may help to stave off the symptoms of early forms of cognitive decline, leading to more time spent in good health [24,25]. Cognitive reserve theory suggests that higher levels of education, as well as engaging in cognitively challenging activities, can create stronger neural connections, which may offer protection against cognitive decline symptoms [5,20,22,25–28]. The more cognitive reserve a person has, the more plastic and adaptable their brain is; a brain with more plasticity can handle damage more effectively before showing clinical symptoms [25,29–31].

Questions about confusion and memory loss were included on the two most recent WTCHR major surveys, allowing researchers to better understand the degree to which early signs of cognitive decline may be occurring among this population. Rather than assessing the direct link between 9/11-related health conditions, such as PTSD and cognitive decline, this study focused on identifying certain individual-level factors that may be protective against confusion or memory loss among WTCHR enrollees. In this study, self-reported confusion or memory loss is a surrogate measure for potential cognitive issues. It is not intended to be a substitute for cognitive testing or a clinical diagnosis.

The goals of this study were to: (1) estimate the degree of self-reported confusion or memory loss among those exposed to the WTC attacks; (2) identify indicators of cognitive reserve (with a particular focus on social support) that can be created from survey variables (i.e., indicators of educational attainment, marital status, employment status, social support, social integration, and physical activity); and (3) determine whether confusion or memory loss is associated with differing levels of cognitive reserve. We hypothesized that groups with less cognitive reserve would be more likely to report confusion or memory loss.

2. Materials and Methods

2.1. Study Population and Sample

The WTCHR maintains a longitudinal cohort of over 71,000 enrollees who were exposed to the terrorist attacks on 11 September 2001. Enrollees in the registry have been surveyed about their exposures to the disaster as well as their short- and long-term health effects in four major surveys: wave 1 (2003–2004), wave 2 (2006–2007), wave 3 (2011–2012), and wave 4 (2015–2016). Health effects will continue to be monitored for years to come. Enrollees include rescue/recovery workers, residents, area workers, passers-by, and students and staff from local schools. The WTCHR was approved by the institutional review boards of the Centers for Disease Control and Prevention (CDC) (3793) and the NYC Department of Health and Mental Hygiene (02-058).

The study sample consisted of enrollees in the WTCHR who met certain criteria (see Figure 1). Individuals in the study had to have completed the wave 3 and wave 4 surveys, both of which contained the self-reported confusion or memory loss questions. Because we were interested in the earlier/milder forms of cognitive decline, we limited our sample to enrollees who were between the ages of 35 and 64 years at the time of the wave 4 survey. We excluded those with a history of stroke [11]. Finally, individuals who reported confusion or memory loss at wave 3 were excluded from the study sample, as we wanted the majority of the predictor variables used in the analysis to precede the outcome of interest, which was confusion or memory loss at wave 4. This also allowed for a better approximation of cognitive decline, as the outcome was measuring a change in self-reported confusion or memory loss between wave 3 and wave 4. The total study sample included 14,574 enrollees.

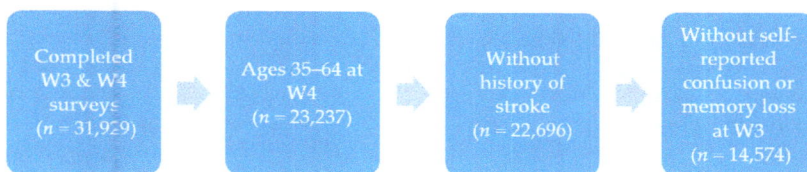

Figure 1. Study sample inclusion criteria.

2.2. Study Variables

The outcome of interest was confusion or memory loss measured by the wave 4 question as follows: "During the last 12 months, have you experienced confusion or memory loss, other than occasionally forgetting the name of someone you recently met?" Cognitive reserve was measured by seven dichotomized indicators: educational attainment, marital status, employment status, number of close friends, communication with friends in last 30 days, people who understand your problems, and general physical activity. PTSD status at wave 3 was classified using the total score from the Post-Traumatic Stress Disorder Checklist (PCL) scale [1,32]. The scale includes measures of re-experiencing, avoidance, and arousal symptoms, and a score of 44 or greater indicates probable PTSD. Demographic factors and other covariates used in this study included gender, age group, race/ethnicity, history of depression, history of anxiety disorder, history of drug or alcohol use problems, and smoking status.

2.3. Data Analysis

First, we described the study sample by basic demographics, probable PTSD status, and the seven indicators that measured cognitive reserve. Then, we performed a latent class analysis and identified a latent class membership, or cognitive reserve level in this case, for each individual in the study sample based on the seven indicators mentioned above. Latent class analysis is a process through which distinct classes are created using a set of chosen variables wherein each record gets assigned to one latent class [33]. We used SAS PROC LCA [34], a statistical procedure for latent class analysis, and reviewed the outputted statistics to assess model fit, comparing the fit for 2, 3, 4, and 5 classes [33,35]. Determining that four classes provided the optimal fit, we then grouped the classes by probable PTSD status, as we knew it was likely to be a risk factor for confusion or memory loss. Latent class composition differed by probable PTSD status, so we conducted two separate latent class analyses: one for those with probable PTSD and one for those without probable PTSD. Those analyses resulted in four latent classes for each group. Next, we predicted the risk of confusion or memory loss in wave 4 by latent class membership (i.e., cognitive reserve level) using log binomial modeling. We chose this method because it produces an unbiased estimate of the relative risk whether the disease is rare or common, whereas logistic regression produces odds ratios, which approximate the relative risk for only rare diseases [36]. We ran adjusted models on the probable PTSD group and not probable PTSD group, adjusting for most of the covariates described above. We did not include age group in the models because we did not expect it to be a major predictor of the outcome, largely due to our study sample being limited to middle-aged enrollees. All analyses were completed with SAS 9.4 software.

3. Results

Self-reported confusion or memory loss was common among the study sample, despite the age group being limited to middle-aged individuals—those between the ages of 35 and 64 years (see Table 1). A total of 3262 out of 14,574 (22%) enrollees in the study sample reported confusion or memory loss at wave 4. About 8% of enrollees had probable PTSD at wave 3, and the majority of the study sample was male (62%). There were twice as many enrollees between the ages of 55 and 64 years in this study compared to those between the ages of 35 and 44 years (43% vs. 19%, respectively). In the total study sample, 60% of enrollees had at least a bachelor's degree. Most enrollees were married or living with a partner in wave 3: 72%. More than four out of five enrollees (84%) were currently employed at the time of the wave 3 survey. Overall level of social integration was high among the study sample; nearly all respondents reported having at least three close friends and having visited, talked, or emailed with friends at least twice in the past 30 days (87% and 94%, respectively). Two-thirds of enrollees reported high levels of social support—specifically, that someone was available to understand their problems most or all of the time. Over three-quarters of the study sample reported being very or somewhat physically active in general.

When stratifying these factors by confusion or memory loss status, there were some proportional differences. The proportion of probable PTSD was much greater among those with confusion or memory loss compared to those without confusion or memory loss (17% vs. 6%, respectively). Among those with confusion or memory loss, 50% had a bachelor's degree or higher level of education; 62% of those without confusion or memory loss had at least a bachelor's degree. Higher levels of social support were reported by those without confusion or memory loss: 71% of them had people available to understand their problems compared to 58% of those who reported having confusion or memory loss. Similarly, a larger proportion of those without confusion or memory loss reported being very or somewhat physically active compared to those with confusion or memory loss (81% vs. 70%, respectively).

The initial latent class analysis on the total study sample indicated that class membership differed significantly based on probable PTSD status at wave 3 (results not shown). However, for both the probable PTSD group and the not probable PTSD group, four classes were determined to be optimal based on the model fit statistics from the latent class analysis. The four classes were assigned as follows in both groups: low cognitive reserve, medium-low cognitive reserve, medium-high cognitive reserve, and high cognitive reserve (referent).

Among those with probable PTSD, class 1, the low cognitive reserve class, constituted about 15% of the group (see Table 2). This group had low levels of social integration and social support (e.g., only 8% of class 1 members reported that someone was available to understand their problems most or all of the time); members were also characterized by overall lower levels of educational attainment, being less likely to be married, having medium levels of current employment, and having lower levels of physical activity. Notable differences between class 2 (8%, medium-low cognitive reserve) and class 3 (37%, medium-high cognitive reserve) are that class 2 had low levels of educational attainment, and class 3 had low levels of social support. Class 4 (40%, high cognitive reserve) was the referent group: having medium levels of educational attainment, being very likely to be married, reporting high levels of social integration and support, having medium levels of current employment, and reporting medium levels of physical activity.

Similar results were presented in Table 2 for those who did not have probable PTSD. Class 4 (high cognitive reserve) made up the majority of the not probable PTSD group: 61%. This group was the referent due to the high proportion of the cognitive reserve indicators therein:, with 73% having at least a bachelor's degree, 79% married or living with a partner, 90% being currently employed, 97% having three or more close friends, 100% who visited/talked/emailed with friends at least twice in last 30 days, 93% having someone available to understand your problems most or all of the time, and 86% being very or somewhat physically active in general.

Table 1. Description of study sample demographics and cognitive reserve indicators.

Sample Characteristics	Total Study Sample (n = 14,574) [1,2] n (%)	Confusion or Memory Loss at W4 (n = 3262, 22%) [1,2] n (%)	No Confusion or Memory Loss at W4 (n = 11,312, 78%) [1,2] n (%)
Probable PTSD			
Yes	1213 (8.3%)	550 (16.7%)	663 (5.9%)
No	13,252 (90.9%)	2675 (82.0%)	10,577 (93.5%)
Gender			
Male	8975 (61.6%)	2016 (61.8%)	6959 (61.5%)
Female	5599 (38.4%)	1246 (38.2%)	4353 (38.5%)
Age group			
35–44 years	2827 (19.4%)	570 (17.5%)	2257 (20.0%)
45–54 years	5526 (37.9%)	1277 (39.2%)	4249 (37.6%)
55–64 years	6221 (42.7%)	1415 (43.4%)	4806 (42.5%)
Educational attainment			
Bachelor's degree or more	8693 (59.7%)	1666 (51.1%)	7027 (62.1%)
Less than a bachelor's degree	5820 (39.9%)	1576 (48.3%)	4244 (37.5%)
Marital status			
Married or living with partner	10,482 (71.9%)	2269 (69.6%)	8213 (72.6%)
Divorced/separated, widowed, or never married	4033 (27.7%)	979 (30.0%)	3054 (27.0%)
Employment status			
Currently employed	12,193 (83.7%)	2671 (81.9%)	9522 (84.2%)
Not currently employed	2335 (16.0%)	579 (17.8%)	1756 (15.5%)
Number of close friends			
Have 3 or more close friends	12,719 (87.3%)	2720 (83.4%)	9999 (88.4%)
Have 0–2 close friends	1452 (10.0%)	448 (13.7%)	1004 (8.9%)
Communicate with friends			
Visited/talked/emailed with friends at least twice in last 30 days	13,681 (93.9%)	2950 (90.4%)	10,731 (94.9%)
Did not visit/talk/email with friends at least twice in last 30 days	729 (5.0%)	265 (8.1%)	464 (4.1%)
People who understand your problems			
Someone is available to understand your problems most or all of the time	9952 (68.3%)	1888 (57.9%)	8064 (71.3%)
Someone is available to understand your problems none to some of the time	4401 (30.2%)	1311 (40.2%)	3090 (27.3%)
Physical activity			
Very or somewhat physically active in general	11,413 (78.3%)	2287 (70.1%)	9126 (80.7%)
Not or not very physically active in general	3096 (21.2%)	951 (29.2%)	2145 (19.0%)

[1] Column percentages may sum to <100% due to missing data. [2] Column percentages may sum to >100% due to rounding. PTSD: posttraumatic stress disorder; W4: wave 4.

Using the latent class groups as predictors for confusion or memory loss at wave 4, we ran separate log binomial models for those with probable PTSD and those without probable PTSD, controlling for relevant covariates (see Table 4). The medium-low cognitive reserve group was significantly more likely to report confusion or memory loss compared to the high cognitive reserve group among the probable PTSD group (relative risk (RR) = 1.35, 95% confidence interval (CI): 1.08, 1.69). Significant covariates in the probable PTSD model included female gender (RR = 0.84, 95% CI: 0.72, 0.97) and history of drug or alcohol use problems (RR = 1.26, 95% CI: 1.03, 1.53). Other covariates approached statistical significance, as did the relative risks for the low cognitive reserve and medium-high cognitive reserve groups. Among the non-probable PTSD group, however, every cognitive reserve group was at significantly greater risk of confusion or memory loss compared to the referent. The low cognitive reserve group was 81% more likely than the high cognitive reserve group to report confusion or memory loss at wave 4. The medium-low and medium-high groups were approximately 40% more likely to report confusion or memory loss compared to the referent. Significant covariates in the not probable PTSD group model included black non-Hispanic race (RR = 1.16, 95% CI: 1.02, 1.31), other race (RR = 1.19, 95% CI: 1.04, 1.35), history of depression (RR = 1.26, 95% CI: 1.14, 1.39), history of anxiety disorder (RR = 1.13, 95% CI: 1.00, 1.27), history of drug or alcohol use problems (RR = 1.40, 95% CI: 1.20, 1.65), being a former smoker (RR = 1.20, 95% CI: 1.11, 1.29), and being a current smoker (RR = 1.18, 95% CI: 1.05, 1.33).

Table 2. Latent class membership by probable PTSD status based on cognitive reserve indicators.

Cognitive Reserve Indicators	Probable PTSD (*n* = 1,213) [1,2]				Not Probable PTSD (*n* = 13,252) [1,2]			
	Class 1 (14.5%)	Class 2 (8.3%)	Class 3 (36.9%)	Class 4 (40.3%)	Class 1 (5.1%)	Class 2 (15.6%)	Class 3 (18.4%)	Class 4 (60.9%)
Proportion in each latent class								
Bachelor's degree or more	0.345	0.050	0.588	0.504	0.331	0.183	0.673	0.725
Married or living with partner	0.572	0.665	0.466	0.797	0.772	0.817	0.445	0.792
Currently employed	0.747	0.080	0.768	0.809	0.778	0.697	0.850	0.895
Have three or more close friends	0.398	0.728	0.742	0.901	0.421	0.955	0.818	0.969
Visited/talked/emailed with friends at least twice in last 30 days	0.245	0.766	0.998	0.966	0.527	0.939	0.978	0.995
Someone is available to understand your problems most or all of the time	0.083	0.432	0.036	0.866	0.266	0.880	0.005	0.933
Very or somewhat physically active in general	0.491	0.255	0.662	0.730	0.627	0.724	0.725	0.859

[1] 109 records did not have valid Post-Traumatic Stress Disorder Checklist (PCL) scores at wave 3 (W3), so the total does not sum to *n* = 14,574; [2] Numbers presented are probability of indicator among that class.

Table 3. Adjusted log binomial model to predict confusion or memory loss by probable PTSD status.

Sample Characteristics	Probable PTSD *n* = 1213		Not Probable PTSD *n* = 13,252	
	RR (95% CI)	p-Value	RR (95% CI)	p-Value
Latent class				
Class 1: low cognitive reserve	1.13 (0.90, 1.47)	0.292	1.81 (1.55, 2.11)	<0.0001
Class 2: medium-low cognitive reserve	1.35 (1.08, 1.69)	0.008	1.36 (1.21, 1.52)	<0.0001
Class 3: medium-high cognitive reserve	1.15 (0.98, 1.34)	0.080	1.44 (1.33, 1.56)	<0.0001
Class 4: high cognitive reserve	Referent	–	Referent	–
Gender				
Female	0.84 (0.72, 0.97)	0.017	0.93 (0.86, 1.00)	0.055
Male	Referent	–	Referent	–
Race/ethnicity				
White non-Hispanic	Referent	–	Referent	–
Black non-Hispanic	1.06 (0.84, 1.34)	0.609	1.16 (1.02, 1.31)	0.020
Hispanic	1.09 (0.90, 1.32)	0.376	1.06 (0.95, 1.20)	0.304
Other races	0.89 (0.67, 1.20)	0.451	1.19 (1.04, 1.35)	0.010

Table 4. *Cont.*

Sample Characteristics	Probable PTSD n = 1213		Not Probable PTSD n = 13,252	
	RR (95% CI)	p-Value	RR (95% CI)	p-Value
Health conditions				
History of depression	1.15 (0.99, 1.33)	0.074	1.26 (1.14, 1.39)	<0.0001
History of anxiety	1.01 (0.86, 1.18)	0.908	1.13 (1.00, 1.27)	0.050
History of drug or alcohol use problems	1.26 (1.03, 1.53)	0.024	1.40 (1.20, 1.65)	<0.0001
Smoking status				
Never smoker	Referent	–	Referent	–
Former smoker	1.11 (0.95, 1.29)	0.187	1.20 (1.11, 1.29)	<0.0001
Current smoker	1.16 (0.98, 1.38)	0.087	1.18 (1.05, 1.33)	0.005

4. Discussion

Our hypothesis was that enrollees with greater levels of cognitive reserve would be less likely to report confusion or memory loss, and our results support this. The relationship between cognitive reserve and confusion or memory loss was similar regardless of PTSD status. For both the probable PTSD and not probable PTSD groups, we found that groups with greater cognitive reserve were less likely to report confusion or memory loss, although the association was more significant and stronger for the group without probable PTSD. This finding suggested that for those who did not have probable PTSD, cognitive reserve factors may play an even more important role in modifying or delaying cognitive decline processes among 9/11 survivors.

Cognitive reserve indicators in this study included educational attainment, social integration, social support, marital status, current employment status, and physical activity. For simplicity, the four classes for both groups (probable PTSD and not probable PTSD) were assigned equivalent names (i.e., low, medium-low, medium-high, or high cognitive reserve) despite their composition differing somewhat between the two groups. Generally, the medium-high, medium-low, and low cognitive reserve groups were at greater risk of having confusion or memory loss at wave 4 compared to the high cognitive reserve groups. There was an interesting discrepancy among the probable PTSD group in that the medium-low cognitive reserve group actually had the greatest relative risk, suggesting that it was the true low cognitive reserve group. In looking at the composition of the medium-low group, we posit that the very low probability of individuals having a bachelor's degree or higher is the factor driving the increased risk for confusion or memory loss.

Theories on cognitive reserve are rooted in research showing that neural connections can change throughout an individual's life [37]—often described as brain plasticity [25,37]. Individuals with greater cognitive reserve are able to process cognitive information more efficiently or use different strategies to reason through issues [27], even using additional brain regions related to memory task performance [38–40]. Even later in life, positive behaviors that increase one's cognitive reserve can have an effect. For instance, cognitive training that promotes memory control and strategies for real-life memory challenges has been shown to be beneficial among older adults [41]. Although educational attainment is often the simplest and most direct proxy for cognitive reserve, our results show that other modifiable factors may be instrumental in protecting against confusion or memory loss as well. People who are active (physically and mentally) and those who engage or feel supported by others have better cognitive outcomes than those who are most isolated. Being socially engaged with others can be cognitively demanding, helping to boost one's level of cognitive reserve [15].

A healthy lifestyle and better cognitive functioning are protective against countless other negative health outcomes as well [42–44]. Maximizing time lived in good health has a positive impact on the individual and societal levels. Greater life expectancy typically involves more years lived with cognitive impairment. However, greater educational attainment (and presumably, greater cognitive reserve) has proven to be associated with increased life expectancy and fewer years of cognitive impairment [25].

Gender, race/ethnicity, history of depression, history of drug or alcohol use problems, and smoking status were also associated with the outcome in our models. Existing literature has suggested that memory issues are correlated with anxiety and depression [45]. The nature of psychiatric comorbidities is complex, and multiple studies have concluded that risk of cognitive decline is greater among those with comorbid PTSD and depression [8,46], though depression on its own may not increase risk [46]. In fact, cognitive reserve may exert more influence than depression; Lee et al. determined that among those with greater levels of educational attainment, better memory function was seen regardless of depressive mood [28]. Ambient air pollutants or fine particulate matter may be associated with declines in domain-specific cognitive functions or development of mild cognitive impairment [13,47], but the composition of the dust cloud resulting from the attacks of 11 September 2001 differed from these exposures in composition and duration [48]. For these reasons, we did not include this type of exposure as a covariate.

Limitations of this study include limited generalizability to the broader NYC or United States population; enrollees in the WTCHR are a trauma-exposed population with a high prevalence of PTSD. Generalizability may be further limited because we excluded people with confusion or memory loss at wave 3, thereby lowering the proportions of confusion or memory loss at wave 4 as well as proportions of PTSD at wave 3; our study sample was healthier than the source population from which it was derived. Another limitation arises because we did not perform cognitive testing on enrollees, so we cannot easily compare our results to research that used this approach. A third limitation is that the questions from the WTCHR survey are very similar to those from the Behavioral Risk Factor Surveillance System [4,49], but they are not identical, so we cannot compare our numbers to those from the general population. Another limitation is that the validity of self-reported cognitive measures can be questionable, particularly for individuals who do have symptoms of impairment. However, those with mild cognitive impairment do not underreport their cognitive issues as much as those with dementia [50]. Also, our study sample is limited to middle-aged enrollees who are less likely to suffer from severe cognitive issues than older adults. Response bias and social desirability bias may lead to an underestimate of the outcome if individuals do not accurately report their confusion or memory loss as well. Finally, the probable PTSD group was much smaller than the not probable PTSD group (8% vs. 92% of total study sample, respectively), meaning that statistical power could have been limited for that group.

Strengths of this study include the fact that we were able to describe change in confusion or memory loss between wave 3 and wave 4, enabling us to approximate the outcome as mild cognitive decline. Also, the WTCHR cohort is a diverse cohort of approximately 71,000 people, giving us sufficient statistical power to detect relevant associations. Our results also support other research that has found that PTSD is an important risk factor for cognitive decline. Among our study sample, the incidence of confusion or memory loss among those with probable PTSD at wave 3 was 45%, while the incidence among those without probable PTSD was 20%.

5. Conclusions

There are elevated levels of PTSD among the WTCHR cohort [1,14]. Because PTSD is associated with cognitive impairment [6–12], we examined the degree to which confusion or memory loss was reported among our study sample. We were interested in how cognitive reserve levels might affect confusion or memory loss, as many of these factors are modifiable. Despite a high prevalence of PTSD among the source population, the majority of the cohort does not have PTSD; those individuals may still be at risk for cognitive decline. Our findings show that confusion and memory loss affect more than one in five enrollees in our study sample, and level of cognitive reserve affects likelihood of developing confusion or memory loss. Those with higher educational attainment, more social support, and greater levels of physical activity are less likely to report confusion or memory loss than those with less cognitive reserve overall. Three of the seven indicators used to create cognitive reserve levels in this study highlighted social support or social integration; their presence helps decrease likelihood of reporting symptoms of cognitive impairment. Results suggest that this is true for those with probable PTSD as well as those without probable PTSD, though the effects were stronger for those without probable PTSD. We believe that all members of the cohort could benefit from engaging in activities that promote cognitive reserve, resulting in lower likelihood of experiencing confusion or memory loss and improved overall health.

Author Contributions: Devising of research question and analytic plan: K.S., S.Y., H.A. Completion of data analysis: K.S. Manuscript drafting: K.S. Manuscript editing and finalizing: K.S., S.Y., H.A.

Funding: This publication was supported by Cooperative Agreement Numbers 2U50/OH009739 and 5U50/OH009739 from the National Institute for Occupational Safety and Health (NIOSH) of the Centers for Disease Control and Prevention (CDC); U50/ATU272750 from the Agency for Toxic Substances and Disease Registry (ATSDR, CDC), with support from the National Center for Environmental Health (CDC); and by the New York City Department of Health and Mental Hygiene (NYC DOHMH). Its contents are solely the responsibility of the authors and do not necessarily represent the official views of the NIOSH, CDC, or the Department of Health and Human Services.

Acknowledgments: The authors would like to acknowledge and thank Robert Brackbill for his assistance in formulating a research question and editing this manuscript. They also would like to thank Erin Takemoto for her help in checking and verifying the Results section.

Conflicts of Interest: The authors declare no conflict of interest.

References

1. Brackbill, R.M.; Hadler, J.L.; DiGrande, L.; Ekenga, C.C.; Farfel, M.R.; Friedman, S.; Perlman, S.E.; Stellman, S.D.; Walker, D.J.; Wu, D.; et al. Asthma and posttraumatic stress symptoms 5 to 6 years following exposure to the World Trade Center terrorist attack. *JAMA* **2009**, *302*, 502–516. [CrossRef]
2. Li, J.; Brackbill, R.M.; Jordan, H.T.; Cone, J.E.; Farfel, M.R.; Stellman, S.D. Effect of asthma and PTSD on persistence and onset of gastroesophageal reflux symptoms among adults exposed to the 11 September, 2001, terrorist attacks. *Am. J. Ind. Med.* **2016**, *59*, 805–814. [CrossRef] [PubMed]
3. Solan, S.; Wallenstein, S.; Shapiro, M.; Teitelbaum, S.L.; Stevenson, L.; Kochman, A.; Kaplan, J.; Dellenbaugh, C.; Kahn, A.; Biro, F.N.; et al. Cancer incidence in world trade center rescue and recovery workers, 2001–2008. *Environ. Health Perspect.* **2013**, *121*, 699–704. [CrossRef] [PubMed]
4. Taylor, C.A.; Bouldin, E.D.; McGuire, L.C. Subjective Cognitive Decline Among Adults Aged >/=45 Years—United States, 2015–2016. *Morb. Mortal. Wkly. Rep.* **2018**, *67*, 753–757. [CrossRef] [PubMed]
5. Langa, K.M.; Larson, E.B.; Karlawish, J.H.; Cutler, D.M.; Kabeto, M.U.; Kim, S.Y.; Rosen, A.B. Trends in the prevalence and mortality of cognitive impairment in the United States: Is there evidence of a compression of cognitive morbidity? *Alzheimers Dement. J. Alzheimers Assoc.* **2008**, *4*, 134–144. [CrossRef] [PubMed]
6. Ainamani, H.E.; Elbert, T.; Olema, D.K.; Hecker, T. PTSD symptom severity relates to cognitive and psycho-social dysfunctioning—A study with Congolese refugees in Uganda. *Eur. J. Psychotraumatol.* **2017**, *8*, 1283086. [CrossRef] [PubMed]
7. Clausen, A.N.; Francisco, A.J.; Thelen, J.; Bruce, J.; Martin, L.E.; McDowd, J.; Simmons, W.K.; Aupperle, R.L. PTSD and cognitive symptoms relate to inhibition-related prefrontal activation and functional connectivity. *Depress. Anxiety* **2017**, *34*, 427–436. [CrossRef] [PubMed]
8. Sumner, J.A.; Hagan, K.; Grodstein, F.; Roberts, A.L.; Harel, B.; Koenen, K.C. Posttraumatic stress disorder symptoms and cognitive function in a large cohort of middle-aged women. *Depress. Anxiety* **2017**, *34*, 356–366. [CrossRef] [PubMed]

9. Vasterling, J.J.; Brailey, K.; Constans, J.I.; Sutker, P.B. Attention and memory dysfunction in posttraumatic stress disorder. *Neuropsychology* **1998**, *12*, 125–133. [CrossRef] [PubMed]

10. Yaffe, K.; Vittinghoff, E.; Lindquist, K.; Barnes, D.; Covinsky, K.E.; Neylan, T.; Kluse, M.; Marmar, C. Posttraumatic stress disorder and risk of dementia among US veterans. *Arch. Gen. Psychiatry* **2010**, *67*, 608–613. [CrossRef]

11. Clouston, S.; Pietrzak, R.H.; Kotov, R.; Richards, M.; Spiro, A., 3rd; Scott, S.; Deri, Y.; Mukherjee, S.; Stewart, C.; Bromet, E.; et al. Traumatic exposures, posttraumatic stress disorder, and cognitive functioning in World Trade Center responders. *Alzheimers Dement. (N. Y.)* **2017**, *3*, 593–602. [CrossRef] [PubMed]

12. Brandes, D.; Ben-Schachar, G.; Gilboa, A.; Bonne, O.; Freedman, S.; Shalev, A.Y. PTSD symptoms and cognitive performance in recent trauma survivors. *Psychiatry Res.* **2002**, *110*, 231–238. [CrossRef]

13. Ranft, U.; Schikowski, T.; Sugiri, D.; Krutmann, J.; Kramer, U. Long-term exposure to traffic-related particulate matter impairs cognitive function in the elderly. *Environ. Res.* **2009**, *109*, 1004–1011. [CrossRef] [PubMed]

14. Clouston, S.A.; Kotov, R.; Pietrzak, R.H.; Luft, B.J.; Gonzalez, A.; Richards, M.; Ruggero, C.J.; Spiro, A., 3rd; Bromet, E.J. Cognitive impairment among World Trade Center responders: Long-term implications of re-experiencing the 9/11 terrorist attacks. *Alzheimers Dement. (Amst. Neth.)* **2016**, *4*, 67–75. [CrossRef]

15. Evans, I.E.M.; Martyr, A.; Collins, R.; Brayne, C.; Clare, L. Social Isolation and Cognitive Function in Later Life: A Systematic Review and Meta-Analysis. *J. Alzheimers Dis.* **2018**, 1–26. [CrossRef] [PubMed]

16. Evans, I.E.M.; Llewellyn, D.J.; Matthews, F.E.; Woods, R.T.; Brayne, C.; Clare, L. Social isolation, cognitive reserve, and cognition in healthy older people. *PLoS ONE* **2018**, *13*, e0201008. [CrossRef] [PubMed]

17. Ishiki, A.; Okinaga, S.; Tomita, N.; Kawahara, R.; Tsuji, I.; Nagatomi, R.; Taki, Y.; Takahashi, T.; Kuzuya, M.; Morimoto, S.; et al. Changes in Cognitive Functions in the Elderly Living in Temporary Housing after the Great East Japan Earthquake. *PLoS ONE* **2016**, *11*, e0147025. [CrossRef]

18. Lee, H.; Waite, L.J. Cognition in Context: The Role of Objective and Subjective Measures of Neighborhood and Household in Cognitive Functioning in Later Life. *Gerontologist* **2018**, *58*, 159–169. [CrossRef]

19. Yates, J.A.; Clare, L.; Woods, R.T. "You've got a friend in me": Can social networks mediate the relationship between mood and MCI? *BMC Geriatr.* **2017**, *17*, 144. [CrossRef] [PubMed]

20. Malek-Ahmadi, M.; Lu, S.; Chan, Y.; Perez, S.E.; Chen, K.; Mufson, E.J. Static and Dynamic Cognitive Reserve Proxy Measures: Interactions with Alzheimer's Disease Neuropathology and Cognition. *J. Alzheimers Dis. Parkinsonism* **2017**, *7*, 390.

21. Dodich, A.; Carli, G.; Cerami, C.; Iannaccone, S.; Magnani, G.; Perani, D. Social and cognitive control skills in long-life occupation activities modulate the brain reserve in the behavioural variant of frontotemporal dementia. *Cortex J. Devot. Study Nerv. Syst. Behav.* **2018**, *99*, 311–318. [CrossRef] [PubMed]

22. Harrison, S.L.; Sajjad, A.; Bramer, W.M.; Ikram, M.A.; Tiemeier, H.; Stephan, B.C. Exploring strategies to operationalize cognitive reserve: A systematic review of reviews. *J. Clin. Exp. Neuropsychol.* **2015**, *37*, 253–264. [CrossRef] [PubMed]

23. Opdebeeck, C.; Martyr, A.; Clare, L. Cognitive reserve and cognitive function in healthy older people: A meta-analysis. *Neuropsychol. Dev. Cogn. Sect. B Aging Neuropsychol. Cogn.* **2016**, *23*, 40–60. [CrossRef] [PubMed]

24. Robitaille, A.; van den Hout, A.; Machado, R.J.M.; Bennett, D.A.; Cukic, I.; Deary, I.J.; Hofer, S.M.; Hoogendijk, E.O.; Huisman, M.; Johansson, B.; et al. Transitions across cognitive states and death among older adults in relation to education: A multistate survival model using data from six longitudinal studies. *Alzheimers Dement. J. Alzheimers Assoc.* **2018**, *14*, 462–472. [CrossRef] [PubMed]

25. Reuser, M.; Willekens, F.J.; Bonneux, L. Higher education delays and shortens cognitive impairment: A multistate life table analysis of the US Health and Retirement Study. *Eur. J. Epidemiol.* **2011**, *26*, 395–403. [CrossRef]

26. Bento-Torres, N.V.; Bento-Torres, J.; Tomas, A.M.; Costa, V.O.; Correa, P.G.; Costa, C.N.; Jardim, N.Y.; Picanco-Diniz, C.W. Influence of schooling and age on cognitive performance in healthy older adults. *Braz. J. Med. Biol. Res. Rev. Bras. Pesqui. Med. Biol.* **2017**, *50*, e5892. [CrossRef] [PubMed]

27. Frankenmolen, N.L.; Fasotti, L.; Kessels, R.P.C.; Oosterman, J.M. The influence of cognitive reserve and age on the use of memory strategies. *Exp. Aging Res.* **2018**, *44*, 117–134. [CrossRef] [PubMed]

28. Lee, J.; Park, H.; Chey, J. Education as a Protective Factor Moderating the Effect of Depression on Memory Impairment in Elderly Women. *Psychiatry Investig.* **2018**, *15*, 70–77. [CrossRef] [PubMed]

29. Fratiglioni, L.; Wang, H.X. Brain reserve hypothesis in dementia. *J. Alzheimers Dis.* **2007**, *12*, 11–22. [CrossRef] [PubMed]

30. Stern, Y. Cognitive reserve and Alzheimer disease. *Alzheimers Dis. Assoc. Disord.* **2006**, *20*, 112–117. [CrossRef]

31. Stern, Y.; Tang, M.X.; Denaro, J.; Mayeux, R. Increased risk of mortality in Alzheimer's disease patients with more advanced educational and occupational attainment. *Ann. Neurol.* **1995**, *37*, 590–595. [CrossRef] [PubMed]

32. Blanchard, E.B.; Jones-Alexander, J.; Buckley, T.C.; Forneris, C.A. Psychometric properties of the PTSD Checklist (PCL). *Behav. Res. Ther.* **1996**, *34*, 669–673. [CrossRef]

33. Lanza, S.T.; Collins, L.M.; Lemmon, D.R.; Schafer, J.L. PROC LCA: A SAS Procedure for Latent Class Analysis. *Struct. Equ. Model. Multidiscip. J.* **2007**, *14*, 671–694. [CrossRef]

34. Lanza, S.T.; Dziak, J.J.; Huang, L.; Wagner, A.; Collins, L.M. *Proc LCA & Proc LTA Users' Guide (Version 1.3.2)*; The Methodology Center, Penn State: University Park, TX, USA, 2015; Available online: methodology.psu.edu (accessed on 22 October 2018).

35. Berglund, P.A. Latent Class Analysis Using Proc LCA: Paper 5500-2016. 2016. Available online: https://support.sas.com/resources/papers/proceedings16/5500-2016.pdf (accessed on 22 October 2018).

36. McNutt, L.A.; Wu, C.; Xue, X.; Hafner, J.P. Estimating the relative risk in cohort studies and clinical trials of common outcomes. *Am. J. Epidemiol.* **2003**, *157*, 940–943. [CrossRef] [PubMed]

37. Sekiguchi, A.; Kotozaki, Y.; Sugiura, M.; Nouchi, R.; Takeuchi, H.; Hanawa, S.; Nakagawa, S.; Miyauchi, C.M.; Araki, T.; Sakuma, A.; et al. Long-term effects of postearthquake distress on brain microstructural changes. *BioMed Res. Int.* **2014**, *2014*, 180468. [CrossRef] [PubMed]

38. Nyberg, L.; Sandblom, J.; Jones, S.; Neely, A.S.; Petersson, K.M.; Ingvar, M.; Backman, L. Neural correlates of training-related memory improvement in adulthood and aging. *Proc. Natl. Acad. Sci. USA* **2003**, *100*, 13728–13733. [CrossRef] [PubMed]

39. Speer, M.E.; Soldan, A. Cognitive reserve modulates ERPs associated with verbal working memory in healthy younger and older adults. *Neurobiol. Aging* **2015**, *36*, 1424–1434. [CrossRef] [PubMed]

40. Steffener, J.; Reuben, A.; Rakitin, B.C.; Stern, Y. Supporting performance in the face of age-related neural changes: Testing mechanistic roles of cognitive reserve. *Brain Imaging Behav.* **2011**, *5*, 212–221. [CrossRef]

41. Lopez-Higes, R.; Martin-Aragoneses, M.T.; Rubio-Valdehita, S.; Delgado-Losada, M.L.; Montejo, P.; Montenegro, M.; Prados, J.M.; de Frutos-Lucas, J.; Lopez-Sanz, D. Efficacy of Cognitive Training in Older Adults with and without Subjective Cognitive Decline Is Associated with Inhibition Efficiency and Working Memory Span, Not with Cognitive Reserve. *Front. Aging Neurosci.* **2018**, *10*, 23. [CrossRef] [PubMed]

42. Muir, S.W.; Gopaul, K.; Montero Odasso, M.M. The role of cognitive impairment in fall risk among older adults: A systematic review and meta-analysis. *Age Ageing* **2012**, *41*, 299–308. [CrossRef]

43. De Bruijn, R.F.; Akoudad, S.; Cremers, L.G.; Hofman, A.; Niessen, W.J.; van der Lugt, A.; Koudstaal, P.J.; Vernooij, M.W.; Ikram, M.A. Determinants, MRI correlates, and prognosis of mild cognitive impairment: The Rotterdam Study. *J. Alzheimers Dis.* **2014**, *42* (Suppl. 3), S239–S249. [CrossRef]

44. Ganguli, M. Depression, cognitive impairment and dementia: Why should clinicians care about the web of causation? *Indian J. Psychiatry* **2009**, *51* (Suppl. 1), S29–S34.

45. Caselli, R.J.; Chen, K.; Locke, D.E.; Lee, W.; Roontiva, A.; Bandy, D.; Fleisher, A.S.; Reiman, E.M. Subjective cognitive decline: Self and informant comparisons. *Alzheimers Dement. J. Alzheimers Assoc.* **2014**, *10*, 93–98. [CrossRef] [PubMed]

46. Schaefer, J.D.; Scult, M.A.; Caspi, A.; Arseneault, L.; Belsky, D.W.; Hariri, A.R.; Harrington, H.; Houts, R.; Ramrakha, S.; Poulton, R.; et al. Is low cognitive functioning a predictor or consequence of major depressive disorder? A test in two longitudinal birth cohorts. *Dev. Psychopathol.* **2017**, 1–15. [CrossRef] [PubMed]

47. Gatto, N.M.; Henderson, V.W.; Hodis, H.N.; St John, J.A.; Lurmann, F.; Chen, J.C.; Mack, W.J. Components of air pollution and cognitive function in middle-aged and older adults in Los Angeles. *Neurotoxicology* **2014**, *40*, 1–7. [CrossRef] [PubMed]

48. Lioy, P.J.; Weisel, C.P.; Millette, J.R.; Eisenreich, S.; Vallero, D.; Offenberg, J.; Buckley, B.; Turpin, B.; Zhong, M.; Cohen, M.D.; et al. Characterization of the dust/smoke aerosol that settled east of the World Trade Center (WTC) in lower Manhattan after the collapse of the WTC 11 September 2001. *Environ. Health Perspect.* **2002**, *110*, 703–714. [CrossRef] [PubMed]

49. Centers for Disease Control and Prevention (CDC). Self-reported increased confusion or memory loss and associated functional difficulties among adults aged >/= 60 years—21 States, 2011. *Morb. Mortal. Wkly. Rep.* **2013**, *62*, 347–350.

50. Farias, S.T.; Mungas, D.; Jagust, W. Degree of discrepancy between self and other-reported everyday functioning by cognitive status: Dementia, mild cognitive impairment, and healthy elders. *Int. J. Geriatr. Psychiatry* **2005**, *20*, 827–834. [CrossRef] [PubMed]

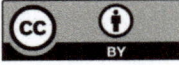

International Journal of
*Environmental Research
and Public Health*

MDPI

Article

Bronchodilator Response Predicts Longitudinal Improvement in Small Airway Function in World Trade Center Dust Exposed Community Members

Deepak Pradhan [1], Ning Xu [2], Joan Reibman [1], Roberta M. Goldring [1,3], Yongzhao Shao [2], Mengling Liu [2] and Kenneth I. Berger [1,3,*]

[1] Department of Medicine, Division of Pulmonary, Critical Care and Sleep Medicine, New York University School of Medicine, New York, NY 10016, USA; deepak.pradhan@nyumc.org (D.P.); joan.reibman@nyumc.org (J.R.); roberta.goldring@nyumc.org (R.M.G.)
[2] Department of Population Health, New York University School of Medicine, New York, NY 10016, USA; Nina.xu@bucknell.edu (N.X.); yongzhao.shao@nyumc.org (Y.S.); mengling.liu@nyumc.org (M.L.)
[3] André Cournand Pulmonary Physiology Laboratory, Bellevue Hospital, New York, NY 10016, USA
* Correspondence: kenneth.berger@nyumc.org; Tel.: +1-212-263-6407

Received: 27 February 2019; Accepted: 17 April 2019; Published: 20 April 2019

Abstract: The evolution of lung function, including assessment of small airways, was assessed in individuals enrolled in the World Trade Center Environmental Health Center (WTC-EHC). We hypothesized that a bronchodilator response at initial evaluation shown by spirometry or in small airways, as measured by forced oscillation technique (FOT), would be associated with improvement in large and small airway function over time. Standardized longitudinal assessment included pre and post bronchodilator (BD) spirometry (forced vital capacity, FVC; forced expiratory volume in 1 second, FEV_1) and FOT (resistance at 5 Hz, R_5; resistance at 5 minus 20 Hz, R_{5-20}). Longitudinal changes were assessed using linear mixed-effects modelling with adjustment for potential confounders (median follow-up 2.86 years; 95% measurements within 4.9 years). Data demonstrated: (1) parallel improvement in airflow and volume measured by spirometry and small airway function (R_5 and R_{5-20}) measured by FOT; (2) the magnitude of longitudinal improvement was tightly linked to the initial BD response; and (3) longitudinal values for small airway function on FOT were similar to residual abnormality observed post BD at initial visit. These findings suggest presence of reversible and irreversible components of small airway injury that are identifiable at initial presentation. These results have implications for treatment of isolated small airway abnormalities that can be identified by non-invasive effort independent FOT particularly in symptomatic individuals with normal spirometry indices. This study underscores the need to study small airway function to understand physiologic changes over time following environmental and occupational lung injury.

Keywords: airway physiology; dust; environmental health; forced oscillation; respiratory function; small airway disease

---

1. Introduction

The WTC Environmental Health Center (WTC-EHC) is a program for treatment of community members with medical and mental health symptoms as a result of exposure to the disaster that occurred in New York on 9/11, 2001. Lower respiratory symptoms (LRS) have been reported in WTC dust exposed community members and responders [1–10]. There are multiple reports of changes in spirometry associated with LRS, and importantly, small airway abnormalities have been associated with LRS even in the presence of normal spirometry [4–6,8,11–13]. Longitudinal improvement in LRS and spirometry is reported in many, although symptoms have often persisted [3,5,14,15]. Of note, structural changes within the airways and/or parenchyma have been demonstrated in community members, suggesting a potentially irreversible component of lung injury [16]. These findings suggest an admixture of reversible and irreversible components of lung injury in response to WTC dust exposure.

We hypothesized that a bronchodilator response at initial evaluation shown by spirometry or in small airways, as measured by forced oscillation technique (FOT), would be associated with improvement in large and small airway function over time. FOT was selected as a noninvasive test based on demonstrated ability to capture small airway dysfunction in WTC dust exposed populations even when airflow remains normal when assessed by spirometry [4,5,11,17,18]. Reduction of airflow on spirometry may not occur in the setting of isolated small airway disease due to the large aggregate cross-sectional area of the distal airways [19–21]. FOT overcomes this limitation by providing measures of non-uniformity of airflow distribution that reflect regional functional abnormalities in the small airways [22–24].

Based on the above considerations, longitudinal data for lung function using spirometry and FOT to capture small airway function were analyzed in community members enrolled in the WTC EHC. The study was designed to determine: (1) whether FOT measures of small airway function improved over time, and (2) whether the bronchodilator response at initial evaluation was associated with a reversible component of lung injury shown by longitudinal improvement in lung function.

2. Materials and Methods

2.1. Patients

Adult patients were self-referred to the WTC EHC with medical and/or mental health symptoms related to September 11, 2001 exposures as previously described [2]. Patients were included in this analysis if they had valid spirometry and FOT, which included bronchodilator testing at their initial evaluation and at least one subsequent spirometry and FOT evaluation. The Institutional Review Board of New York University School of Medicine approved the research database (NCT00404898), and only data from patients who provided informed consent were used for analysis.

2.2. Procedures

At initial visit to the WTC EHC patients completed a multi-dimensional interviewer-administered questionnaire that included questions relating to demographic characteristics, WTC-related dust exposures, presence and severity of respiratory symptoms, and history of tobacco use [2]. Patients were treated for asthma-like symptoms according to guidelines for asthma management [25], and evaluated with further additional studies if findings were inconsistent with asthma.

2.3. Spirometry and FOT Measurements

At initial visit all patients were referred for objective assessment of lung function using spirometry and FOT which was performed within a single location (André Cournand Pulmonary Physiology Laboratory, Bellevue Hospital). Spirometry and FOT were routinely performed on all patients before and 15 min after bronchodilator (BD) administration (2.5 mg albuterol sulfate delivered via nebulizer over 5 min) according to standard ATS/ERS guidelines [26,27]. FOT is a noninvasive test that measures the relationship between pressure and airflow fluctuations applied externally to the respiratory system during tidal breathing to determine the respiratory system resistance. Measurements included resistance assessed at an oscillating frequency of 5 Hz (R_5) and frequency dependence of resistance calculated as the difference between resistance at 5 and 20 Hz (R_{5-20}). R_{5-20} provides a measure of non-uniformity of airflow distribution that correlates with frequency dependence of compliance measured by invasive esophageal manometry, an established test of small airway function [22–24,28,29].

Predicted values for spirometry measures were derived from NHANES III [30]. and abnormal spirometry was defined by forced expiratory volume in 1 second (FEV_1), forced vital capacity (FVC), or FEV_1/FVC measurements below the lower limit of normal (LLN) [31]. A positive BD response

(+BD) on spirometry was defined according to ATS/ERS guidelines as a ≥12% and ≥200 cc increase in FEV_1 and/or FVC after bronchodilator [26]. FOT was performed under tidal breathing (Jaeger IOS®, Vyaire Medical, Yorba Linda, CA, USA). Measurements included respiratory resistance at 5 Hz (R_5) and the difference in resistance from 5 to 20 Hz (R_{5-20}) as an index of frequency dependence of resistance (FDR). Upper limits of normal (ULN) for R_5 and R_{5-20} (0.396 kPa/L/s and 0.075 kPa/L/s, respectively) were based on measures in asymptomatic non-smoking subjects with normal spirometry in our laboratory ($n = 80$) and the values are in the range of published estimates of normative data [18,32]. A positive BD response for IOS measurements was defined as a decrease in R_5 of ≥0.135 kPa/L/s, based on the 95th percentile for BD response in healthy adults in normative data on forced oscillation [32].

2.4. Definitions

WTC dust cloud exposure was defined by patient report of having been caught in a dust cloud created by a building collapse on 9/11. Patients were further classified as local residents, local workers or clean-up workers based on their description of location and activities. New-onset lower respiratory symptoms were defined by the presence of at least one symptom of wheezing, chest tightness, or dyspnea with onset after 11 September 2001. Symptomatic patients at initial presentation to the WTC EHC were defined based on a symptom frequency ≥2 times per week in the four preceding weeks. Patients were classified as a smoker if they had >5 pack year lifetime history of tobacco use.

2.5. Statistical Methods

Continuous variables were summarized using median and interquartile range (IQR) and compared across groups using nonparametric Kruskal-Wallis test. Categorical variables were summarized by counts and proportions and compared using Chi-squared test. A linear mixed-effects model was used to investigate longitudinal changes in lung function using each repeated spirometry and FOT measurement. In each model a fixed linear effect of the follow-up time (defined as duration since initial visit) on a measure of respiratory function was estimated with adjustment for potential confounders. Among the considered confounders, gender, race/ethnicity, income, WTC exposure category, dust cloud exposure did not substantively change the results and thus only age, BMI, and smoking history were included in the final models. Random intercept and slope were assumed to explain within-subject correlation among repeated measurements and among-subject heterogeneity.

Separate models were fit with pre-BD FVC, FVC% of predicted, FEV_1, FEV_1% of predicted, and FEV_1/FVC as dependent variables. To analyze longitudinal changes in FOT parameters, similar models were fit with pre-BD R_5 and R_{5-20} as the dependent variables. A p value < 0.05 was used to indicate statistical significance. Analyses were conducted using R (version 3.0.2, R Foundation for Statistical Computing, Vienna, Austria) and SPSS® (version 20.0, IBM® Corp, Armonk, NY, USA).

3. Results

3.1. Patient Demographics and Characteristics

A total of 1146 adult patients were enrolled in the WTC EHC between 29 October 2002 and 20 February 2013 who fit inclusion criteria. Patients were subsequently excluded from analysis if their studies were repeated within 180 days ($n = 133$), if post BD data were not available ($n = 119$), or if longitudinal data for either spirometry or FOT were not available ($n = 153$). The final analytic cohort consisted of 741 adult patients who met criteria for longitudinal study. Patient characteristics are shown in Table 1. The cohort had a median age of 51 at enrollment, with an equal distribution of males and females. Many patients were overweight with a median BMI of 28.1 (IQR 24.7–32.4) kg/m^2. The cohort was racially and ethnicity diverse, with the largest single group identifying themselves as Hispanic (36%). Less than a quarter (24%) of patients had a smoking history, with few (13%) reporting current tobacco use. The cohort included predominantly local workers (51%), with fewer local residents (20%)

and clean-up workers (17.0%). Over half (52%) were caught in the dust cloud caused by the collapse of the World Trade Center towers on 9/11. The group was highly symptomatic with 93% reporting LRS that began after 9/11 and persisted at the time of enrollment in the WTC EHC.

Table 1. Patient characteristics at initial visit ($n = 741$).

Characteristic	Value
Age, median (IQR)	51 (44–59)
Gender; (M/F, %)	50/50
BMI (kg/m^2), median (IQR)	28 (25–32)
Race/Ethnicity	
Hispanic	268 (36)
White	241 (33)
Black	155 (21)
Asian	52 (7)
Unspecified	25 (3)
Income/year $\leq$ $15,000	286 (39)
Smoking history	
>5 pack-year	177 (24)
Current smoker	96 (13)
WTC exposure category	
Local worker	378 (51)
Clean up worker	128 (17)
Resident	149 (20)
Rescue/recovery	25 (3)
Unspecified	61 (8)
Caught in WTC dust cloud	382 (52)
Lower respiratory symptoms	691 (93)

Data are presented at n (%) unless otherwise noted. IQR: interquartile range; BMI: body mass index; WTC: World Trade Center.

3.2. Lung Function at Initial Visit

The results of lung function evaluation at the initial visit are shown in Table 2. Median values for spirometry were within the normal range for pre-BD FVC, FEV$_1$, and FEV$_1$/FVC (median 92% predicted, 88% predicted, and 77% respectively). The percentage of individuals with values below the LLN for FVC, FEV$_1$, and FEV$_1$/FVC were 22, 28, and 20%, respectively. Only 58 patients (8%) met ATS/ERS criteria for a positive BD response on spirometry. Since 93% of the subjects developed respiratory symptoms after the WTC attack, data prior to the disaster were generally not available.

Table 2. Lung function at initial visit ($n = 741$).

	Pre-BD	Post-BD
Spirometry		
FVC (%predicted)	92 (81–103)	92 (81–103)
FEV$_1$ (%predicted)	88 (76–99)	92 (80–103)
FEV$_1$/FVC	77 (71–81)	79 (74–84)
FOT		
R$_5$ (kPa/L/s)	0.489 (0.375–0.615)	0.428 (0.328–0.527)
R$_{5-20}$ (kPa/L/s)	0.098 (0.055–0.168)	0.074 (0.041–0.128)

Data are presented at median (IQR). BD: bronchodilatory FOT: forced oscillation technique.

In contrast to spirometry measurements, the majority of patients had abnormal oscillometry measurements, with an elevated median pre-BD R$_5$ and R$_{5-20}$ (0.489 and 0.098 cm H$_2$O/L/sec, respectively), consistent with presence of airway dysfunction not evident on spirometry. The median decrease in these parameters after BD for the total cohort was 14% for R_5 and 23% for R_{5-20}. A positive BD response on oscillometry was noted 163 patients (22% of the cohort).

3.3. Longitudinal Spirometry Measurements

Patients were followed for a median of 2.86 years (IQR 1.8–3.7 years), with 95% of the repeated measurements occurring within 4.9 years. Table 3 shows the results from linear mixed-effects modeling adjusted for age, smoking, BMI, baseline pre-BD FEV_1 %predicted, and baseline pre-BD FVC %predicted. Spirometry measurements in the cohort improved over time for FVC and FEV_1 (36 ± 6 mL and 22 ± 4 mL/year respectively, $p < 0.001$); these changes in absolute values corresponded to an improvement in % of predicted FVC = 0.80 ± 0.17% per year and % of predicted FEV_1 = 0.60 ± 0.17% per year ($p < 0.001$ for both analyses). Subgroup analysis demonstrated that individuals with abnormal spirometry at initial visit had a significantly greater improvement in both FVC and FEV_1 over time than those with normal spirometry at initial visit ($p < 0.003$ for both variables, data not shown).

Table 3. Longitudinal change in spirometry parameters.

	Whole Cohort	Abnormal Spirometry		
	($n = 741$)	Total ($n = 270$)	(−) BD Response ($n = 212$)	(+) BD Response ($n = 58$)
ΔFVC (mL/year)	36 ± 6 *	43 ± 10 *	28 ± 9 **	122 ± 28 *
ΔFEV$_1$ (mL /year)	22 ± 4 *	29 ± 7 *	16 ± 7 **	91 ± 7 *

$* p < 0.001; ** p < 0.05.$

We evaluated whether patients with a positive BD response on spirometry at baseline had greater improvement in spirometry parameters over time compared with those who had a negative BD response. To conduct this analysis, data analyzed were limited to the 270 individuals with abnormal spirometry testing at baseline. Demographic characteristics did not differ between the group with (−) or (+) BD response at baseline. Initial values for FEV_1 and FEV_1/FVC were lower in patients with a (+) BD response compared with those with a (−) BD response (FEV_1 67% predicted [IQR 54–75] vs 74% predicted [IQR 67–82], $p < 0.001$; FEV_1/FVC 64% [IQR 59–71] vs 72% [IQR 67–81], $p < 0.001$). Whereas both groups showed improvement in FVC and FEV_1 over time, the improvement was greater in the individuals with a (+) BD response at baseline compared with those with a (−) BD response (ΔFVC = 122 ± 28 vs. 28 ± 9 mL/year; ΔFEV$_1$ 91 ± 7 vs. 16 ± 7 mL/year). Neither group demonstrated longitudinal change in FEV1/FVC. Although robust improvement in spirometry values were noted in the patients with (+) BD response, 70.7% demonstrated longitudinal values for FVC and/or FEV_1 that remained in the abnormal range.

3.4. Longitudinal FOT Measurements

Table 4 shows results for longitudinal assessment of lung function using oscillometry. In contrast to spirometry, the group as a whole failed to demonstrate change in either R_5 or R_{5-20}. Subgroup analysis of individuals who had abnormal oscillometry at initial evaluation demonstrated decline in resistance when assessed as R_5 (slope = −0.007 kPa/L/sec per year, $p < 0.05$).

Table 4. Longitudinal change in oscillometry parameters.

	Whole Cohort	Abnormal Oscillometry		
	($n = 741$)	Total ($n = 527$)	(−) BD Response ($n = 364$)	(+) BD Response ($n = 163$)
ΔR$_5$ (kPa/L/s/year)	−0.001 ± 0.002	−0.006 ± 0.003 *	0.002 ± 0.003 *	−0.027 ± 0.006 **
ΔR$_{5-20}$ (kPa/L/s/year)	0.001 ± 0.001	−0.001 ± 0.001	0.002 ± 0.001	−0.012 ± 0.004 *

$* p < 0.001; ** p < 0.05.$

The predictive value of a (+) BD response on FOT at baseline was evaluated in the cohort of 527 individuals with abnormal oscillometry testing at baseline. Demographic characteristics did not differ between the group with (−) or (+) BD response at baseline. Although oscillometry was abnormal in all of these patients, more abnormal pre BD values for R_5 and R_{5-20} were detected at the initial visit in individuals with a (+) BD response compared with those with a (−) BD response (R_5: 0.685 [IQR 0.573–0.816] vs 0.509 [IQR 0.441–0.597] kPa/L/s; R_{5-20}: 0.210 [IQR 0.123–0.302] vs 0.109 [IQR 0.068–0.165 kPa/L/s]. Table 4 and Figure 1 illustrate that while oscillometry variables remained stable in the group with (−) BD response at baseline, the group with (+) BD response at baseline showed significant longitudinal improvement over time ($\Delta R_5 = -0.027 \pm 0.006$ kPa/L/s/year, $p < 0.001$; $\Delta R_{5-20} = 0.012 \pm 0.004$ kPa/L/s/year, $p = 0.002$). Additional analysis demonstrated that the post-BD FOT values in these patients remained stable over time indicating that the residual abnormality noted post bronchodilator at baseline remained unchanged over time despite standard medical therapy.

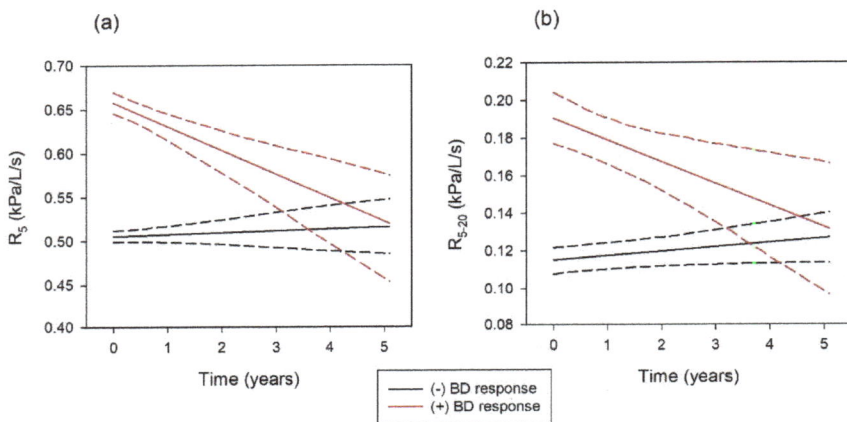

Figure 1. Panel (a) Longitudinal values and confidence interval for R_5 derived from mixed-effects modelling for the (−) BD and (+) BD groups. Panel (b) Longitudinal values and confidence interval for R_{5-20} derived from mixed-effects modelling for the (−) BD and (+) BD groups.

4. Discussion

The present study addressed the evolution of lung function including assessment of small airways in a cohort of community members enrolled in the WTC EHC with new onset lower respiratory symptoms following exposure to WTC dust. Improvement in respiratory function was demonstrated by parallel improvement in airflow and volume measured by spirometry as well as resistance (R_5) and FDR (R_{5-20}) measured by oscillometry. Moreover, the magnitude of improvement that occurred with therapy over time was tightly linked to a BD response at the initial visit. Lastly, the longitudinal values for small airway function observed on oscillometry were similar to the residual abnormality observed post BD at initial visit. These findings suggest the presence of reversible and irreversible components of small airway injury that are identifiable at initial presentation.

Data collected in numerous populations exposed to the WTC disaster demonstrate that in many the predominant site of injury is to the small airways. The most common abnormality noted on spirometry in exposed firefighters, workers at the WTC site, and community members was parallel reduction in both FVC and FEV_1 (i.e., without change in FEV_1/FVC) [1,2,4,6,8]. Small airway injury was implicated in these populations based on evidence for air trapping on plethysmography and/or computed tomography [1,6,33,34]. In accord with these findings, recent data show that exposure to inhaled ambient particulate matter at sizes below 2.5 μm and occupational toxins are also associated with small airway dysfunction as evidenced by parallel reduction in FVC and FEV_1 [35–40]. Furthermore, studies in WTC exposed populations using oscillometry demonstrate presence of FDR in accord with non-uniform distribution of airflow within small airways [4,11,41,42]. The presence of FDR is tightly correlated with presence of frequency dependence of compliance detected by esophageal manometry, an established marker of small airway dysfunction [11,28,29,43,44]. The clinical relevance of FDR in WTC dust exposed patients has been highlighted by association with magnitude of dust exposure, presence of wheeze and presence of systemic inflammation as assessed by serum C-reactive protein levels [4,17,18].

Longitudinal data from the present study indicate improvement in small airway function assessed by both spirometry and oscillometry. Spirometry assessments demonstrated parallel improvement of FVC and FEV_1 without change in FEV_1/FVC. This pattern is in accord with prior descriptions of a "volume response" following bronchodilator inhalation in patients with asthma and COPD, which has been attributed to improvement in small airway function with relief of air trapping [45–49]. In the present study, FOT was added to routine assessment of lung function by spirometry to directly assess the role and evolution of small airway function in WTC dust exposed individuals. Longitudinal assessment using FOT demonstrated improvement in FDR, in accord with improved small airway function over time. Of note, this improvement in small airway function was evident only in those individuals who had abnormal respiratory function at baseline with a reversible component, as evident by testing post administration of bronchodilator.

Prior studies in WTC dust exposed populations have indicated presence of both reversible and irreversible airways injury over time. Registry based longitudinal studies have indicated that resolution of lower respiratory symptoms over time is associated with improvement in measures of small airway function and conversely, persistence of LRS is associated with persistent small airway dysfunction [3,5]. In contrast, persistence of severe LRS has been documented despite a high level of respiratory medication use, including inhaled corticosteroid and long acting β-agonist [3]. Similarly, high rates of poorly or very poorly controlled asthma has been documented in numerous cohorts of individuals that were exposed to WTC dust [50–54]. We have previously demonstrated presence of sustained inflammation in WTC dust exposed community members based on peripheral eosinophilia and increased C-reactive protein levels, findings that were associated with persistent abnormality in small airway function [17,55]. Objective evidence for inhalation of particles to the distal lung and structural airway abnormalities has been demonstrated using analysis of induced sputum and by histologic assessment of lung tissue which showed peribronchiolar fibrosis and emphysematous changes [16,56,57]. Taken together these findings are consistent with a chronic disease syndrome due to disease in the small airways. Lack of complete improvement in small airway function may be due to chronic inflammation that is either not fully corrected by the current medical therapy and/or is located beyond the delivery range of conventional inhaled corticosteroid therapy. Alternatively, given the structural changes in the distal lung noted on histology, the residual small airway dysfunction observed over time could reflect irreversible structural damage that occurred prior to initial evaluation, presumably at time of injury.

There are some factors to consider when interpreting the data in the present study. First, there is significant heterogeneity within this population regarding amount and duration of WTC dust exposures, as well as other potential environmental exposures. However, data remained significant after adjustment for exposure categories, dust cloud exposure and smoking. Second, although medical therapy was prescribed by a standardized clinical algorithm, adherence to therapy was not documented. Of note, medications and provider visits were provided free-of-charge, theoretically minimizing financial and access to care issues as barriers to adherence. Despite these limitations, improvements in spirometry and FOT measures of small airway function were documented and were associated with presence of acute reversibility at baseline. Nevertheless, a contribution from non-adherence to medical therapy to the residual abnormality in both spirometry and FOT cannot be excluded. Third, modeling was performed with a linear time trend for changes in spirometry. These improvements would eventually be counterbalanced by normal age-related decline in spirometry, but analysis over a longer follow-up duration would be needed. In contrast, there are no data demonstrating age-related change in oscillometry in adult populations. Fourth, there is potential for bias as all patients were self-referred to the EHC with potential for follow-up bias as only 83% of patients with valid spirometry and oscillometry measurements at initial visit had subsequent valid spirometry and oscillometry measurements. Finally, this study was not designed to examine the association of longitudinal change in lung function with change in lower respiratory symptoms over time.

An additional limitation of this study relates to lack of interpretation of FOT data with respect to lung volume; change in values for resistance over time would occur if functional residual capacity (FRC) varied at each study visit. Although FRC was not measured in this study, the most likely explanation for variability over time would related to changing body weight. However, significant changes in body weight has not been evident in patients that have returned for routine monitoring within our WTC EHC population.

5. Conclusions

Inhalation of WTC dust was associated with small airway abnormalities in a cohort of exposed community members which showed incomplete improvement over time. Positive bronchodilator response in the small airways at presentation identified individuals with significant ability for improvement in lung function over time; however, residual abnormality noted post-BD at baseline identified an irreversible component of small airway injury. These results have implications for the treatment of isolated small airway abnormalities that can be readily identified by non-invasive effort independent FOT particularly in individuals who are symptomatic with normal spirometry indices. Finally, this study also underscores the need to study small airway function to understand physiologic changes over time for this and other environmental and occupational lung injuries.

Author Contributions: Conceptualization, D.P., J.R., R.M.G., Y.S., M.L. and K.I.B.; Methodology, D.P., J.R., R.M.G., and K.I.B.; Data analysis, N.X., Y.S. and M.L.; Writing—Original draft preparation, D.P.; Writing—Review and editing, J.R., R.M.G., Y.S., M.L. and K.I.B.; funding acquisition, J.R. and K.I.B.

Funding: This research was funded by National Institute for Occupational Safety and Health, grant number 1E11OH009630, Centers for Disease Control, contract numbers 200-2011-39413, 200-2017-93327, and 200-2017-93427.

Conflicts of Interest: The authors declare no conflict of interest. The funders had no role in the design of the study; in the collection, analyses, or interpretation of data; in the writing of the manuscript, or in the decision to publish the results.

References

1. Reibman, J.; Lin, S.; Hwang, S.A.; Gulati, M.; Bowers, J.A.; Rogers, L.; Berger, K.I.; Hoerning, A.; Gomez, M.; Fitzgerald, E.F. The World Trade Center residents' respiratory health study: New-onset respiratory symptoms and pulmonary function. *Environ. Health Perspect.* **2005**, *113*, 406–411. [CrossRef] [PubMed]

2. Reibman, J.; Liu, M.; Cheng, Q.; Liautaud, S.; Rogers, L.; Lau, S.; Berger, K.I.; Goldring, R.M.; Marmor, M.; Fernandez-Beros, M.E.; et al. Characteristics of a Residential and Working Community With Diverse Exposure to World Trade Center Dust, Gas, and Fumes. *J. Occup. Environ. Med.* **2009**, *51*, 234–541. [CrossRef] [PubMed]

3. Caplan-Shaw, C.; Kazeros, A.; Pradhan, D.; Berger, K.; Goldring, R.; Zhao, S.; Liu, M.; Shao, Y.; Fernandez-Beros, M.E.; Marmor, M.; et al. Improvement in severe lower respiratory symptoms and small airway function in World Trade Center dust exposed community members. *Am. J. Ind. Med.* **2016**, *59*, 777–787. [CrossRef] [PubMed]

4. Friedman, S.M.; Maslow, C.B.; Reibman, J.; Pillai, P.S.; Goldring, R.M.; Farfel, M.R.; Stellman, S.D.; Berger, K.I. Case-control study of lung function in World Trade Center Health Registry area residents and workers. *Am. J. Respir. Crit. Care Med.* **2011**, *184*, 582–589. [CrossRef]

5. Jordan, H.T.; Friedman, S.M.; Reibman, J.; Goldring, R.M.; Miller Archie, S.A.; Ortega, F.; Alper, H.; Shao, Y.; Maslow, C.B.; Cone, J.E.; et al. Risk factors for persistence of lower respiratory symptoms among community members exposed to the 2001 World Trade Center terrorist attacks. *Occup. Environ. Med.* **2017**, *74*, 449–455. [CrossRef] [PubMed]

6.   Prezant, D.J.; Weiden, M.; Banauch, G.I.; McGuinness, G.; Rom, W.N.; Aldrich, T.K.; Kelly, K.J. Cough and bronchial responsiveness in firefighters at the World Trade Center site. *N. Engl. J. Med.* **2002**, *347*, 806–815. [CrossRef]

7.   Webber, M.P.; Gustave, J.; Lee, R.; Niles, J.K.; Kelly, K.; Cohen, H.W.; Prezant, D.J. Trends in respiratory symptoms of firefighters exposed to the world trade center disaster: 2001–2005. *Environ. Health Perspect.* **2009**, *117*, 975–980. [CrossRef] [PubMed]

8.   Herbert, R.; Moline, J.; Skloot, G.; Metzger, K.; Baron, S.; Luft, B.; Markowitz, S.; Udasin, I.; Harrison, D.; Stein, D.; et al. The world Trade Center Disaster and the Health of Workers: Five-Year Assessment of a Unique Medical Screening Program. *Environ. Health Perspect.* **2006**, *114*, 1853–1858. [CrossRef] [PubMed]

9.   Maslow, C.B.; Friedman, S.M.; Pillai, P.S.; Reibman, J.; Berger, K.I.; Goldring, R.; Stellman, S.D.; Farfel, M. Chronic and acute exposures to the world trade center disaster and lower respiratory symptoms: Area residents and workers. *Am. J. Public Health* **2012**, *102*, 1186–1194. [CrossRef]

10.   Niles, J.K.; Webber, M.P.; Cohen, H.W.; Hall, C.B.; Zeig-Owens, R.; Ye, F.; Glaser, M.S.; Weakley, J.; Weiden, M.D.; Aldrich, T.K.; et al. The respiratory pyramid: From symptoms to disease in World Trade Center exposed firefighters. *Am. J. Ind. Med.* **2013**, *56*, 870–880. [CrossRef] [PubMed]

11.   Oppenheimer, B.V.; Goldring, R.M.; Herberg, M.E.; Hofer, I.S.; Reyfman, P.A.; Liautaud, S.; Rom, W.N.; Reibman, J.; Berger, K.I. Distal airway function in symptomatic subjects with normal spirometry following World Trade Center dust exposure. *Chest* **2007**, *132*, 1275–1282. [CrossRef] [PubMed]

12.   Weiden, M.D.; Kwon, S.; Caraher, E.; Berger, K.I.; Reibman, J.; Rom, W.N.; Prezant, D.J.; Nolan, A. Biomarkers of World Trade Center Particulate Matter Exposure: Physiology of Distal Airway and Blood Biomarkers that Predict FEV(1) Decline. *Semin. Respir. Crit. Care Me.* **2015**, *36*, 323–333. [CrossRef] [PubMed]

13.   de la Hoz, R.E.; Liu, X.; Doucette, J.T.; Reeves, A.P.; Bienenfeld, L.A.; Wisnivesky, J.P.; Celedon, J.C.; Lynch, D.A.; Sar Jose Estepar, R. Increased Airway Wall Thickness is Associated with Adverse Longitudinal First-Second Forced Expiratory Volume Trajectories of Former World Trade Center workers. *Lung* **2018**, *196*, 481–489. [CrossRef] [PubMed]

14.   Liu, M.; Qian, M.; Cheng, Q.; Berger, K.I.; Shao, Y.; Turetz, M.; Kazeros, A.; Parsia, S.; Goldring, R.M.; Caplan-Shaw, C.; et al. Longitudinal spirometry among patients in a treatment program for community members with World Trade Center-related illness. *J. Occup. Environ. Med.* **2012**, *54*, 1208–1213. [CrossRef] [PubMed]

15.   Zeig-Owens, R. Singh, A.; Aldrich, T.K.; Hall, C.B.; Schwartz, T.; Webber, M.P.; Cohen, H.W.; Kelly, K.J.; Nolan, A.; Prezant, D.J.; et al. Blood Leukocyte Concentrations, FEV1 Decline, and Airflow Limitation. A 15-Year Longitudinal Study of World Trade Center-exposed Firefighters. *Ann. Am. Thorac. Soc.* **2018**, *15*, 173–183. [CrossRef] [PubMed]

16.   Caplan-Shaw, C.E.; Yee, H.; Rogers, L.; Abraham, J.L.; Parsia, S.S.; Naidich, D.P.; Borczuk, A.; Moreira, A.; Shiau, M.C.; Ko, J.P.; et al. Lung pathologic findings in a local residential and working community exposed to World Trade Center dust, gas, and fumes. *J. Occup. Environ. Med.* **2011**, *53*, 981–991. [CrossRef]

17.   Kazeros, A.; Zhang, E.; Cheng, X.; Shao, Y.; Liu, M.; Qian, M.; Caplan-Shaw, C.; Berger, K.I.; Goldring, R.M.; Ghumman, M.; et al. Systemic Inflammation Associated With World Trade Center Dust Exposures and Airway Abnormalities in the Local Community. *J. Occup. Environ. Med.* **2015**, *57*, 610–616. [CrossRef] [PubMed]

18.   Berger, K.I.; Turetz, M.; Liu, M.; Shao, Y.; Kazeros, A.; Parsia, S.; Caplan-Shaw, C.; Friedman, S.M.; Maslow, C.B.; Marmor, M.; et al. Oscillometry complements spirometry in evaluation of subjects following toxic inhalation. *ERJ Open Res.* **2015**, *1*. [CrossRef]

19.   Mead, J. The lung's "quiet zone". *N. Engl. J. Med.* **1970**, *282*, 1318–1319. [CrossRef]

20.   Macklem, P.T. The physiology of small airways. *Am. J. Respir. Crit. Care Med.* **1998**, *157*, S181–S183. [CrossRef]

21.   Pedley, T.J.; Schroter, R.C.; Sudlow, M.F. The prediction of pressure drop and variation of resistance within the human bronchial airways. *Respir. Physiol.* **1970**, *9*, 387–405. [CrossRef]

22.   Fredberg, J.J.; Mead, J. Impedance of intrathoracic airway models during low-frequency periodic flow. *J. Appl. Physiol.* **1979**, *47*, 347–351. [CrossRef] [PubMed]

23.   Bates, J.H.; Lutchen, K.R. The interface between measurement and modeling of peripheral lung mechanics. *Respir. Physiol. Neurobiol.* **2005**, *148*, 153–164. [CrossRef]

24. Goldman, M.D.; Saadeh, C.; Ross, D. Clinical applications of forced oscillation to assess peripheral airway function. *Respir. Physiol. Neurobiol.* **2005**, *148*, 179–194. [CrossRef]

25. Bateman, E.D.; Hurley, S.S.; Barnes, P.J.; Bousquet, J.; Drazen, J.M.; FitzGerald, J.M.; Gibson, P.; Ohta, K.; O'Byrne, P.; Pedersen, S.E.; et al. Global strategy for asthma management and prevention: GINA executive summary. *Eur. Respir. J.* **2018**, *51*, 143–178. [CrossRef] [PubMed]

26. Miller, M.R.; Hankinson, J.; Brusasco, V.; Burgos, F.; Casaburi, R.; Coates, A.; Crapo, R.; Enright, P.; van der Grinten, C.P.; Gustafsson, P.; et al. Standardisation of spirometry. *Eur. Respir. J.* **2005**, *26*, 319–338. [CrossRef] [PubMed]

27. Oostveen, E.; MacLeod, D.; Lorino, H.; Farre, R.; Hantos, Z.; Desager, K.; Marchal, F. The forced oscillation technique in clinical practice: Methodology, recommendations and future developments. *Eur. Respir. J.* **2003**, *22*, 1026–1041. [CrossRef] [PubMed]

28. Oppenheimer, B.W.; Goldring, R.M.; Berger, K.I. Distal airway function assessed by oscillometry at varying respiratory rate: Comparison with dynamic compliance. *COPD* **2009**, *6*, 162–170. [CrossRef]

29. Kjeldgaard, J.M.; Hyde, R.W.; Speers, D.M.; Reichert, W.W. Frequency dependence of total respiratory resistance in early airway disease. *Am. Rev. Respir. Dis.* **1976**, *114*, 501–508. [PubMed]

30. Hankinson, J.L.; Odencrantz, J.R.; Fedan, K.B. Spirometric reference values from a sample of the general U.S. population. *Am. J. Respir. Crit. Care Med.* **1999**, *159*, 179–187. [CrossRef]

31. Pellegrino, R.; Viegi, G.; Brusasco, V.; Crapo, R.O.; Burgos, F.; Casaburi, R.; Coates, A.; van der Grinten, C.P.; Gustafsson, P.; Hankinson, J.; et al. Interpretative strategies for lung function tests. *Eur. Respir. J.* **2005**, *26*, 948–968. [CrossRef] [PubMed]

32. Oostveen, E.; Boda, K.; van der Grinten, C.P.; James, A.L.; Young, S.; Nieland, H.; Hantos, Z. Respiratory impedance in healthy subjects: Baseline values and bronchodilator response. *Eur. Respir. J.* **2013**, *42*, 1513–1523. [CrossRef]

33. Mendelson, D.S.; Roggeveen, M.; Levin, S.M.; Herbert, R.; de la Hoz, R.E. Air trapping detected on end-expiratory high-resolution computed tomography in symptomatic World Trade Center rescue and recovery workers. *J. Occup. Environ. Med.* **2007**, *49*, 840–845. [CrossRef]

34. Weiden, M.D.; Ferrier, N.; Nolan, A.; Rom, W.N.; Comfort, A.; Gustave, J.; Zeig-Owens, R.; Zheng, S.; Goldring, R.M.; Berger, K.I.; et al. Obstructive airways disease with air trapping among firefighters exposed to World Trade Center dust. *Chest* **2010**, *137*, 566–574. [CrossRef] [PubMed]

35. Churg, A.; Brauer, M.; del Carmen, A.; Fortoul, T.I.; Wright, J.L.; Churg, A.; Brauer, M.; Fortoul, T.I.; Wright, J.L. Chronic exposure to high levels of particulate air pollution and small airway remodeling. *Environ. Health Perspect.* **2003**, *111*, 714–718. [CrossRef]

36. Guerry-Force, M.L.; Muller, N.L.; Wright, J.L.; Wiggs, B.; Coppin, C.; Pare, P.D.; Hogg, J.C. A comparison of bronchiolitis obliterans with organizing pneumonia, usual interstitial pneumonia, and small airways disease. *Am. Rev. Respir. Dis.* **1987**, *135*, 705–712.

37. Chia, K.S.; Ng, T.P.; Jeyaratnam, J. Small airways function of silica-exposed workers. *Am. J. Ind. Med.* **1992**, *22*, 155–162. [CrossRef]

38. Mann, J.M.; Sha, K.K.; Kline, G.; Breuer, F.U.; Miller, A. World Trade Center dyspnea: Bronchiolitis obliterans with functional improvement: A case report. *Am. J. Ind. Med.* **2005**, *48*, 225–229. [CrossRef]

39. Rice, M.B.; Rifas-Shiman, S.L.; Litonjua, A.A.; Oken, E.; Gillman, M.W.; Kloog, I.; Luttmann-Gibson, H.; Zanobetti, A.; Coull, B.A.; Schwartz, J.; et al. Lifetime Exposure to Ambient Pollution and Lung Function in Children. *Am. J. Respir. Crit. Care Med.* **2016**, *193*, 881–888. [CrossRef]

40. Rice, M.B.; Ljungman, P.L.; Wilker, E.H.; Dorans, K.S.; Gold, D.R.; Schwartz, J.; Koutrakis, P.; Washko, G.R.; O'Connor, G.T.; Mittleman, M.A. Long-term exposure to traffic emissions and fine particulate matter and lung function decline in the Framingham heart study. *Am. J. Respir. Crit. Care Med.* **2015**, *191*, 656–664. [CrossRef] [PubMed]

41. Skloot, G.; Goldman, M.; Fischler, D.; Goldman, C.; Schechter, C.; Levin, S.; Teirstein, A. Respiratory symptoms and physiologic assessment of ironworkers at the World Trade Center disaster site. *Chest* **2004**, *125*, 1248–1255. [CrossRef] [PubMed]

42. Berger, K.I.; Reibman, J.; Oppenheimer, B.W.; Vlahos, I.; Harrison, D.; Goldring, R.M. Lessons from the world trade center disaster: Airway disease presenting as restrictive dysfunction. *Chest* **2013**, *144*, 249–257. [CrossRef]

43. van den Elshout, F.J.; van Herwaarden, C.L.; Folgering, H.T. Oscillatory respiratory impedance and lung tissue compliance. *Respir. Med.* **1994**, *88*, 343–347. [CrossRef]

44. Otis, A.B.; McKerrow, C.B.; Bartlett, R.A.; Mead, J.; McIlroy, M.B.; Selverstone, N.J.; Radford, E.P. Mechanical factors in distribution of pulmonary ventilation. *J. Appl. Physiol.* **1956**, *8*, 427–443. [CrossRef] [PubMed]

45. Woolcock, A.J.; Read, J. Lung volumes in exacerbations of asthma. *Am. J. Med.* **1966**, *41*, 259–273. [CrossRef]

46. Ayres, S.M.; Griesbach, S.J.; Reimold, F.; Evans, R.G. Bronchial component in chronic obstructive lung disease. *Am. J. Med.* **1974**, *57*, 183–191. [CrossRef]

47. Ramsdell, J.W.; Tisi, G.M. Determination of bronchodilation in the clinical pulmonary function laboratory. Role of changes in static lung volumes. *Chest* **1979**, *76*, 622–628. [CrossRef] [PubMed]

48. Pellegrino, R.; Rodarte, J.R.; Brusasco, V. Assessing the reversibility of airway obstruction. *Chest* **1998**, *114*, 1607–1612. [CrossRef]

49. Newton, M.F.; O'Donnell, D.E.; Forkert, L. Response of lung volumes to inhaled salbutamol in a large population of patients with severe hyperinflation. *Chest* **2002**, *121*, 1042–1050. [CrossRef]

50. Brackbill, R.M.; Hadler, J.L.; DiGrande, L.; Ekenga, C.C.; Farfel, M.R.; Friedman, S.; Perlman, S.E.; Stellman, S.D.; Walker, D.J.; Wu, D.; et al. Asthma and posttraumatic stress symptoms 5 to 6 years following exposure to the World Trade Center terrorist attack. *JAMA* **2009**, *302*, 502–516. [CrossRef]

51. Jordan, H.T.; Stellman, S.D.; Reibman, J.; Farfel, M.R.; Brackbill, R.M.; Friedman, S.M.; Li, J.; Cone, J.E. Factors associated with poor control of 9/11-related asthma 10-11 years after the 2001 World Trade Center terrorist attacks. *J. Asthma* **2015**, *52*, 630–637. [CrossRef]

52. Webber, M.P.; Glaser, M.S.; Weakley, J.; Soo, J.; Ye, F.; Zeig-Owens, R.; Weiden, M.D.; Nolan, A.; Aldrich, T.K.; Kelly, K.; et al. Physician-diagnosed respiratory conditions and mental health symptoms 7-9 years following the World Trade Center disaster. *Am. J. Ind. Med.* **2011**, *54*, 661–671. [CrossRef] [PubMed]

53. Wisnivesky, J.P.; Teitelbaum, S.L.; Todd, A.C.; Boffetta, P.; Crane, M.; Crowley, L.; de la Hoz, R.E.; Dellenbaugh, C.; Harrison, D.; Herbert, R.; et al. Persistence of multiple illnesses in World Trade Center rescue and recovery workers: A cohort study. *Lancet* **2011**, *378*, 888–897. [CrossRef]

54. Kim, H.; Herbert, R.; Landrigan, P.; Markowitz, S.B.; Moline, J.M.; Savitz, D.A.; Todd, A.C.; Udasin, I.G.; Wisnivesky, J.P. Increased rates of asthma among World Trade Center disaster responders. *Am. J. Ind. Med.* **2012**, *55*, 44–53. [CrossRef] [PubMed]

55. Kazeros, A.; Maa, M.T.; Patrawalla, P.; Liu, M.; Shao, Y.; Qian, M.; Turetz, M.; Parsia, S.; Caplan-Shaw, C.; Berger, K.I.; et al. Elevated peripheral eosinophils are associated with new-onset and persistent wheeze and airflow obstruction in world trade center-exposed individuals. *J. Asthma* **2013**, *50*, 25–32. [CrossRef] [PubMed]

56. Rom, W.N.; Weiden, M.; Garcia, R.; Yie, T.A.; Vathesatogkit, P.; Tse, D.B.; McGuinness, G.; Roggli, V.; Prezant, D. Acute eosinophilic pneumonia in a New York City firefighter exposed to World Trade Center dust. *Am. J. Respir. Crit. Care Med.* **2002**, *166*, 797–800. [CrossRef] [PubMed]

57. Fireman, E.M.; Lerman, Y.; Ganor, E.; Greif, J.; Fireman-Shoresh, S.; Lioy, P.J.; Banauch, G.I.; Weiden, M.; Kelly, K.J.; Prezant, D.J. Induced sputum assessment in New York City firefighters exposed to World Trade Center dust. *Environ. Health Perspect.* **2004**, *112*, 1564–1569. [CrossRef]

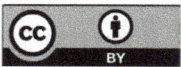

International Journal of
Environmental Research and Public Health

MDPI

Article

Time to Onset of Paresthesia Among Community Members Exposed to the World Trade Center Disaster

Sujata Thawani [1], Bin Wang [2,3], Yongzhao Shao [2,3], Joan Reibman [3,4] and Michael Marmor [1,2,*]

1 Department of Neurology, New York University School of Medicine, New York, NY 10017, USA; sujata.thawani@nyulangone.org
2 Department of Population Health, New York University School of Medicine, New York, NY 10016, USA; bin.wang@nyulangone.org (B.W.); yongzhao.shao@nyulangone.org (Y.S.)
3 Department of Environmental Medicine, New York University School of Medicine, New York, NY 10016, USA; joan.reibman@bellevue.nychhc.org
4 Department of Medicine, New York University School of Medicine, New York, NY 10016, USA
* Correspondence: michael.marmor@nyulangone.org; Tel.: +1-212-501-3374; Fax: +1-646-501-3681

Received: 12 March 2019; Accepted: 12 April 2019; Published: 22 April 2019

Abstract: We examined whether time to onset of paresthesia was associated with indicators of severity of World Trade Center (WTC) exposure. We analyzed data from 3411 patients from the Bellevue Hospital—WTC Environmental Health Center. Paresthesia was defined as present if the symptom occurred in the lower extremities with frequency "often" or "almost continuous." We plotted hazard functions and used the log-rank test to compare time to onset of paresthesia between different exposure groups. We also used Cox regression analysis to examine risk factors for time-to-paresthesia after 9/11/2001 and calculate hazard ratios adjusted for potential confounders. We found significantly elevated hazard ratios for paresthesia for (a) working in a job that required cleaning of WTC dust in the workplace; and (b) being heavily exposed to WTC dust on September 11, 2001, after adjusting for age, race/ethnicity, depression, anxiety, post-traumatic stress disorder, and body mass index. These observational data are consistent with the hypothesis that exposure to WTC dust or some other aspect of cleaning WTC dust in the workplace, is associated with neuropathy and paresthesia. Further neurological evaluations of this and other WTC-exposed populations is warranted.

Keywords: paresthesia; neuropathic symptoms; Cox regression; hazard function; World Trade Center exposure

---

1. Introduction

The World Trade Center (WTC) Environmental Health Center (EHC) serves community members exposed to the World Trade Center disaster of September 11, 2001. These individuals include local workers and residents, as well as other affected community members with potential exposure to WTC contaminants who developed physical or mental health symptoms after the event. The most common presenting complaints are aerodigestive symptoms [1,2]. However, within a few years after 9/11, patients seeking care at the Bellevue Hospital WTC EHC also reported paresthesias or sensations of tingling, prickling, or numbness in the extremities. Formal questions about paresthesias thus were added to the medical evaluation questionnaires around January 1, 2008 to evaluate for the potential for peripheral neuropathy associated with WTC toxic exposures.

Neuropathic symptoms were associated with sarin exposure that occurred during the terrorist attacks in Japan in 1994 and 1995 [3]. Of 155 individuals who required medical evaluation, 40 subjects required hospital admission due to severe exposure. These subjects had more frequent salivation, rhinorrhea, and diarrhea. 40% (16/40) of these subjects reported distal lower extremity dysesthesias and were noted to have reduced distal vibration on clinical exam. These signs and symptoms resolved at 3 months follow-up in the majority of cases.

Components of the WTC toxins provide biologic plausibility for the development of neuropathic disease. Heavy metals and environmental toxin exposures have been associated with distal symmetric polyneuropathy [4]. Examination of sciatic nerves from rats exposed to WTC dust also demonstrated reductions in conduction velocities of nerve action potentials when compared to controls [5]. WTC dust contained known neurotoxins including lead and complex hydrocarbons [6–9]. Workers involved in clean-up activities may also have been exposed to organic solvents. Distal sensory motor neuropathy is associated with lead poisoning, with a motor predominant neuropathy primarily seen following acute exposure [10]. Industrial exposure to n-hexane, an organic solvent, has been associated with paresthesia and distal symmetric, primarily axonal, large fiber polyneuropathy [11,12].

An earlier analysis of patients from the WTC EHC found that many reported paresthesias at enrollment 7–15 years after 9/11 [13]. These symptoms were associated with the severity of exposure to WTC dust on 9/11 and cleaning of workplaces after adjusting for known risk factors for paresthesia, including preexisting paresthesias, anxiety, and diagnoses of diabetes and cancer [3,12]. Paresthesias also were associated with respiratory symptoms and reduced lung function, which may have been surrogate measures of WTC exposure [4,14]. Paresthesia symptoms were associated with later (2013–2015) enrollment in the WTC EHC, suggesting a long latency period between exposure and development of symptoms in some patients. Neuropathic symptoms also were reported in a series of 16 first responders exposed to the WTC disaster [15]. 56% (9/16) of these patients had neuropathy that could not be explained by diabetes, B12 deficiency, or Lyme disease suggesting WTC exposure as a possible etiology. The present analyses aim to describe further paresthesia associated with WTC exposure by exploring time to paresthesia after the September 11, 2001 disaster and associations of time to paresthesia with measures of severity of WTC exposure.

2. Materials and Methods

2.1. Study Population

As previously described, we enrolled subjects for the present analysis from the Bellevue Hospital WTC Environmental Health Center (WTC EHC) [2]. Enrollment into the WTC EHC was open to individuals who were exposed to the disaster who reported medical or mental health symptoms certified as potentially due to exposure to the WTC event [2]. Paresthesias were not prerequisite symptoms for inclusion in the program. Patients of the WTC EHC primarily included individuals who worked in local businesses, lived in buildings near the WTC towers, or were traveling through the area of Manhattan south of Canal Street on the day of the disaster. A small proportion of the WTC EHC patient population were first-responders who were enrolled during the initiation of the program. Subsequently, separate programs were developed for first responders and community members [2]. Blood glucose was measured by the Bellevue Hospital Clinical Laboratory. Body mass index (BMI), post-traumatic stress disorder (PTSD), depression and anxiety were measured as previously described [16]. We limited the present analyses to subjects who responded to questions added around January 1, 2008 regarding paresthesia.

The New York University School of Medicine Institutional Review Board approved the research database used for these analyses. The present analyses used only data from patients who provided informed consent to allow the use of their data in research analyses.

2.2. Paresthesia

We investigated the incidence of paresthesia of the lower extremities. We defined paresthesia to be a positive response to the question, "In the past year, did you experience a prickling or tingling feeling, with or without an asleep feeling, in your feet or legs?" Moreover, we further limited persons with paresthesia to those who responded that they experienced this feeling "often" or "almost continuous". Persons who said they experienced this feeling "occasionally" or "never" were classified as not having paresthesia.

2.3. Time to Onset of Paresthesia

We inferred dates of onset of paresthesia after 9/11/2001 by two methods: Among subjects with a baseline visit only, we used subjects' self-reports of the number of months post-September 11, 2001 when they recalled first experiencing paresthesia of the lower extremities. For subjects who reported not having had paresthesia at their baseline enrollment interview but who then reported paresthesia at their first return visit, we estimated the date of onset of paresthesia as the midpoint between the dates of the baseline interview and the first return visit. We right-censored dates of onset of paresthesia of subjects in the following situations: (a) patients were considered as censored at initial baseline visit time for those who reported no paresthesia at the baseline visit and did not come back for a return visit; (b) patients who did not report paresthesia at both the baseline visit and return are considered as censored at return.

2.4. Statistical Analyses

Descriptive statistics were used to summarize the characteristics of the study population. Categorical variables (or categorized continuous variables) were summarized using counts and percentages. Initial analyses compared persons with follow-up visits to those without follow-up visits. We used the chi-squared test to compare categorical variables of subjects with and without follow-up. We used population hazard functions for paresthesia-free survival and the log-rank test to evaluate differences in time to onset of paresthesia among subjects with versus those without a job related to cleaning WTC dust. For multivariable analyses, we used Cox proportional hazards regression analysis to calculate hazard ratios associated with various risk factors after adjusting for potential confounders. We performed Cox regression analyses both including and excluding those subjects who reported "occasional" paresthesia without ever reporting "often" or "almost continuous" paresthesia. All statistical analyses were performed using SAS version 9.4 (SAS Institute, Cary, NC, USA).

3. Results

4165 subjects enrolled in the WTC EHC after January 1, 2008 when questions about paresthesia were first routinely included in the WTC EHC enrollment questionnaire. We excluded from our analyses, 11 subjects who were born after September 11, 2001, 132 subjects who reported paresthesia before September 11, 2001, and 458 subjects who reported diabetes, leaving 3564 individuals (Figure 1). After dropping subjects with diabetes, histories of cancer chemotherapy, paresthesia prior to 9/11 and those in utero on September 11, 2001, there remained for analysis data from 3411 individuals (Figure 1).

The median date of enrollment was January 19, 2010 (interquartile range [IQR] = September 19, 2007–May 1, 2014). Of the 3564, 38.5% (1373/3564) returned for follow-up at a median of 35 months (IQR = 23–47 months) after enrollment. The proportions returning for return visits were associated with age, year of enrollment, and race/ethnicity (all $p < 0.0001$) (Table 1).

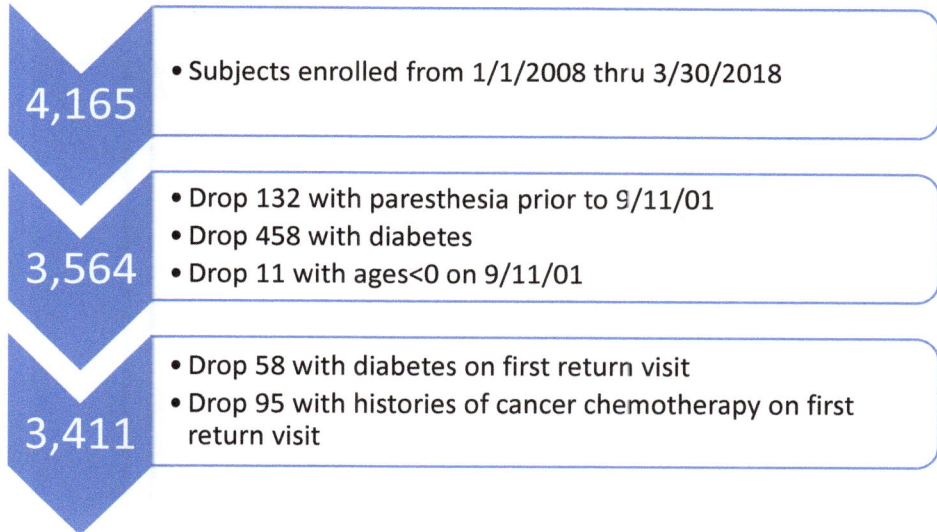

Figure 1. Flowchart of patients included in analyses of time to onset of paresthesia among patients of the Bellevue Hospital WTC (World Trade Center) EHC (Environmental Health Center).

Table 1. Baseline characteristics associated with returning percentage for a return visit (n = 3564).

Variable	Value	N at Baseline	N (%) with Return	N (%) without Return	p-Value
Gender					0.4
	Female	1811	711 (39.3)	1100 (60.7)	
	Male	1753	662 (37.8)	1091 (62.2)	
Age on 911					<0.0001
	<35	967	302 (31.2)	665 (68.8)	
	35–44	1155	452 (39.1)	703 (60.9)	
	45–54	1022	435 (42.6)	587 (57.4)	
	55–64	356	156 (43.8)	200 (56.2)	
	≥65	64	28 (43.8)	36 (56.2)	
Year of enrollment					<0.0001
	2008–2010	1432	746 (52.1)	686 (47.9)	
	2011–2013	817	381 (46.6)	436 (53.4)	
	2014–2015	538	197 (36.6)	341 (63.4)	
	2016–2018	777	49 (6.3)	728 (93.7)	
Race/Ethnicity					<0.0001
	Hispanic	799	382 (47.8)	417 (52.2)	
	Non-Hispanic Caucasian	1713	566 (33.0)	1147 (67.0)	
	Non-Hispanic African-American	705	294 (41.7)	411 (58.3)	
	Asian	263	93 (35.4)	170 (64.6)	
	Other or Native American	47	16 (34.0)	31 (66.0)	
	Missing race/ethnicity	37			

Among the 3411 subjects included in the present analyses, 50.7% were female, 48% were Caucasian, and 78% were non-Hispanic (Table 2). The median age was 53 (IQR = 44–61) years. At baseline, 605 (17.7%) reported feeling "often" or "almost continuous" symptoms of paresthesia of the lower extremities and these 605 were regarded as having had paresthesia at the number of months post-September 11, 2001 that each subject recalled having first noticed the symptom. The remaining 2806 (82.3%) were classified as not having paresthesia at baseline in our analysis. These 2806 subjects included 1004 (35.7%) who answered "occasionally" at either the baseline or return visit.

Table 2. Characteristics of subjects at the baseline visit (*n* = 3411).

Variable	Value	N (Column %)
Gender		
	Male	1681 (49.3)
	Female	1730 (50.7)
Age at enrollment (years)		
	<25	138 (4.0)
	25–34	231 (6.8)
	35–44	552 (16.2)
	45–54	1006 (29.5)
	55–64	1001 (29.3)
	≥65	483 (14.2)
Median age at enrollment (IQR) 53(44–61)		
Year of enrollment	2008–2010	1372 (40.2)
	2011–2013	776 (22.8)
	2014–2015	499 (14.6)
	2016–2018	764 (22.4)
Race and ethnicity		
	Hispanic	765 (22.4)
	Non-Hispanic Caucasian	1635 (47.9)
	Non-Hispanic African- American	675 (19.8)
	Asian	258 (7.6)
	Other or Native American	44 (1.3)
	Missing	34 (1.0)
Subjects reported paresthesia	Yes	605 (17.7)
	No	2806 (82.3)

3.1. Time to Onset of Paresthesia: Nonparametric Analysis

To examine potential change in the hazard rate (or incidence rate) of paresthesia, we used nonparametric estimates of the Kaplan–Meier survival functions and the cumulative hazard functions for times-to-paresthesia after 9/11 in our study population. As is well known, the Kaplan–Meier survival functions are nonparametric estimates of the survival probabilities and the cumulative hazard function (Figure 2) is just the negative logarithm of the estimated survival functions. The nonparametric analysis is based on the 605 paresthesia cases reported at initial visit and the 159 new cases from M1. The above nonparametric cumulative hazard function of paresthesia-free survival suggests a long-term and continuing risk of paresthesia 17 years or more after the WTC disaster. More specifically, the slope for the cumulative hazard function in Figure 2 suggests a near-constant incidence rate of paresthesia in this population over the study period.

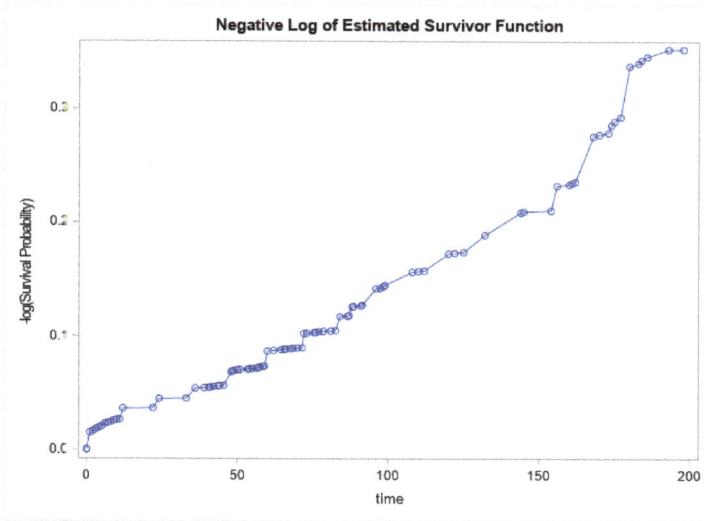

Figure 2. Nonparametric hazard function of paresthesia-free survival (*n* = 3411).

3.2. Time to Onset of Paresthesia: Multivariate Cox Regression

Multivariable Cox proportional hazards regression analysis indicated a significantly elevated hazard ratio (HR = 1.369, *p* = 0.003) for paresthesia associated with having worked in a job that required cleaning of WTC dust after adjusting for age, race-ethnicity, depression, anxiety, post-traumatic stress disorder, and elevated body mass index (Table 3). These associations remained if we analyzed data only from the baseline questionnaire without considering data from the return visit. Blood glucose concentrations were not significant and thus did not enter into the model.

Table 3. Multivariable Cox proportional hazards regression using both Baseline and Return Visit data (*n* = 3411).

Variable		Hazard Ratio	95% Confidence Interval		*p*-Value
Gender	F vs. M	1.14	0.99	1.33	0.08
Age on 911 (years)	Per unit increase	1.01	1.01	1.02	<0.0001
Race-Ethnicity (vs. Non-Hispanic Caucasian)	Hispanic	1.24	1.03	1.50	0.03
	Non-Hispanic African-American	1.12	0.92	1.37	0.2
	Asian	0.85	0.61	1.18	0.3
	Other or Native-American	1.83	1.07	3.13	0.03
Cleaning Job	Yes vs. No	1.37	1.11	1.69	0.003
Covered in Dust	Much vs. Little	1.09	0.94	1.27	0.2
Body mass index (kg/m^2)	Per unit increase	1.02	1.01	1.03	0.001
Anxiety (vs. <1.75)	≥1.75	1.37	1.10	1.71	0.006
	Missing	1.45	0.28	7.58	0.7
Post-Traumatic Stress Disorder (vs. PCL*- < 44)	PCL ≥ 44	1.29	1.04	1.59	0.02
	Missing	0.98	0.19	5.14	0.9
Depression (vs. <1.75)	≥1.75	1.41	1.13	1.76	0.002
	Missing	1.45	0.28	7.58	0.7

* PCL is Post-Traumatic Stress Disorder Check List.

Nonparametric hazard functions (Figure 3) comparing the 422 subjects who worked in a job that required cleaning of WTC dust (red curve) to the 2915 subjects who did not have such jobs (blue curve) showed a significant difference between the two groups (*p* < 0.0001, log-rank test).

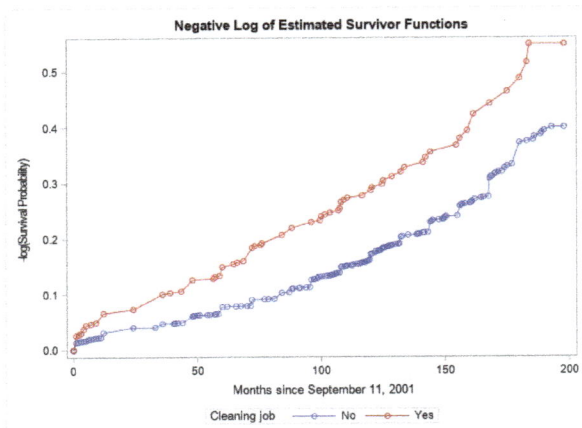

Figure 3. Nonparametric hazard functions of paresthesia-free survival stratified by cleaning job.

The nonparametric hazard curves in Figure 3 indicate significantly higher risk in time to onset of paresthesia among persons who worked in jobs that required cleaning of WTC dust in the workplace after adjusting for potential confounders.

The Cox model shown in Table 3 categorized as paresthesia-free those subjects who reported paresthesia with frequencies of "none" or "occasional". This might have weakened the observed statistical associations because some persons with "occasional" paresthesia might indeed have had the same condition as subjects with paresthesia of frequency "often" or "almost continuous". We therefore analyzed the data excluding 1004 subjects with one or two reports of paresthesia of frequency "occasional" but who never reported paresthesia of frequency "often" or "almost continuous". Cox regression analysis of the reduced data set (Table 4) showed significant associations of time to paresthesia with being employed in a job that required cleaning of WTC dust and with being heavily covered with dust on the day of the WTC disaster, September 11, 2001. The hazard ratio for working in a job that required cleaning of WTC dust increased from 1.35 (95% confidence interval CI = 1.11–1.69) in the model that included all subjects to 1.52 (95% CI = 1.24–1.87) in the model that excluded subjects with "occasional" paresthesia.

Table 4. Multivariable Cox proportional hazards regression using Baseline and Return Visit data, excluding subjects with "occasional" paresthesia (*n* = 2407).

Variable		Hazard Ratio	95% Confidence Interval		*p*-Value
Gender	F vs. M	1.22	1.05	1.41	0.01
Age on 911 (years)	Per unit increase	1.01	1.01	1.02	<0.0001
Race-Ethnicity (vs. Non-Hispanic Caucasian)	Hispanic	0.85	0.61	1.18	0.3
	Non-Hispanic African-American	1.32	1.09	1.59	0.004
	Asian	1.29	1.06	1.57	0.0106
	Other or Native-American	1.75	1.02	2.99	0.04
Cleaning Job	Yes vs. No	1.52	1.24	1.87	<0.0001
Covered in Dust	Much vs. Little	1.19	1.03	1.38	0.02
Body mass index (kg/m²)	Per unit increase	1.02	1.01	1.03	0.0007
Anxiety (vs. <1.75)	≥1.75	1.51	1.21	1.89	0.0002
	Missing	1.10	0.25	4.82	0.9
Post-Traumatic Stress Disorder (vs. PCL < 44)	PCL ≥ 44	1.35	1.09	1.67	0.006
	Missing	1.42	0.32	6.27	0.6
Depression (vs. <1.75)	≥1.75	1.49	1.19	1.85	0.0004
	Missing	1.10	0.25	4.82	0.9

4. Discussion

Among WTC survivors from the general community, we found significantly shorter time to onset of paresthesia among persons who worked in jobs that required cleaning of WTC dust in the workplace, or who were heavily covered with dust on the day of the disaster, after adjusting for potential confounders. Paresthesia was a common problem in this population, with 17.7% of subjects reporting symptoms of paresthesia at initial visit, even after excluding from the case definition those who reported paresthesias only of the upper extremities, and restricting the case definition to those who experienced the symptom with a frequency of "often" or "almost continuous". The slope of the estimated cumulative hazard function was approximately constant, indicating a long latency period before onset of paresthesia among many subjects and a flat incidence rate in the WTC affected populations many years after 9/11.

Results of a previous analysis of risk factors for paresthesia among WTC EHC patients that did not take into account times to events were similar to those of one of the present models in finding significant associations of paresthesias with both working in jobs that required cleaning of WTC dust in the workplace and heavy exposure to WTC dust on September 11, 2001 after adjusting for potential confounders [13]. Of these two risk factors, only work in a job that required cleaning of WTC dust was significant in our initial Cox regression model that counted subjects with "occasional" paresthesia as paresthesia-free. The finding that being heavily covered with dust also was significant in the model that excluded subjects with "occasional" paresthesia suggests that exposures of some of the "occasional" paresthesia subjects were similar to those of subjects with "often" or "almost continuous" paresthesia. Categorization of subjects with "occasional" paresthesia as paresthesia-free during the study period appears to have reduced the statistical power of the analysis that included these subjects.

The present findings cannot establish a causal relationship between WTC exposure and paresthesia. The findings are consistent, however, with the hypothesis that exposure to the WTC event during cleaning of dust in the workplace increased the subsequent risk of paresthesia and that the hazard continued to be relatively constant over extended times through approximately 17 years.

Our hazard function plots of survival times paresthesia-free suggest a long-term and continuing risk 17 years or more after the WTC disaster of paresthesia. Few instances of exposure to a time-limited event, including environmental disasters with neurotoxic consequences, have been reported and most exposures to neurotoxins result in symptoms within weeks or months [3,17,18]. In some instances, it is difficult to untangle whether a latency period precedes symptom expression of neuropathy or if a certain level of dose must be accumulated. Chemotherapy-associated neuropathy, for example, is more likely to develop in patients who have received larger doses over longer periods [19]. Occupational exposure to n-hexanes and low boiling point hydrocarbons have been associated with the development of a sub-acute neuropathy [20,21]. Removal of exposure of the occupational neurotoxins and cancer chemotherapy has been reported to improve neuropathic symptoms and in some cases also reverse the neuropathy or improve it [19,22]. The increased occurrence of symptoms over time might be due to other causes, including the onset of diabetes. Our available serum values did not suggest poor glycemic control in this population. While most patients fasted before blood donation, we did not record whose samples were provided after fasting and which were not.

One conceptual model for our finding is that WTC exposure resulted in inhalation or ingestion of neurotoxins on airborne particulate matter and that these particulates became embedded in lung or other tissues, with slow leaching of the neurotoxins from these particles into the bloodstream over years, eventually leading to adequate bioaccumulation to cause expression of neurologic symptoms. Slow leaching of lead from retained bullet fragments has been associated with elevated blood lead levels [23]. Perhaps the delayed onset of symptoms in WTC subjects may be mediated by a delay in cumulative dose since the event, or may be due to a combination of industrial and environmental toxins related to the WTC disaster.

Symptoms of paresthesia resolved or decreased in a subset of subjects between the enrollment and first return visits. This finding may be due to removal of the toxic exposure and subsequent reduction in symptoms. Another possibility may be due to medication for neuropathic symptoms with improvement in symptoms. Another consideration is that subjects started treatment for known etiologies of neuropathy that may have alleviated neuropathic symptoms.

Hispanic ethnicity, older age, active mental health issues, and BMI also were associated with significantly elevated hazard ratios of paresthesia. Diabetes and pre-diabetes are the most common etiologies of neuropathy, specifically distal symmetric polyneuropathy of the lower extremities [24,25]. Although elevated BMI is associated with a greater risk of diabetes and pre-diabetes, serum glucose concentrations were not associated with time to paresthesia, suggesting that neither diabetes nor pre-diabetes were responsible for the reported paresthesias.

Mood disorders are associated with different variants of neuropathy from diabetic, inflammatory, and chemotherapy-associated neuropathy [26–28]. The prevalence of depression is also greater in diabetics who have neuropathy [29,30]. The significant association of time to paresthesia with WTC exposure variables after controlling for covariates including measures of depression, anxiety, post-traumatic stress disorder and BMI, suggests a role of WTC-associated exposure.

There are limitations to our study. We used a standard question for paresthesias that may not be specific for neuropathy and our question was not supplemented with complete neurological examinations, serum studies to search for etiologies of neuropathy, or additional investigations such as electromyography and nerve conduction study, or skin biopsy for evaluation of small fiber polyneuropathy. The questionnaire data also did not specifically address unilateral lower limb from bilateral limb paresthesia. Paresthesias due to other etiologies that would be considered independent of WTC exposure, such as unilateral lumbar radiculopathy, may have been included in our case definition. However, to improve the accuracy of our case definition, we only counted as cases those subjects who reported frequent symptoms. Counting subjects who reported paresthesia with frequency of "occasional" as paresthesia-free, however, likely weakened the statistical associations we observed compared with the model we created that excluded such subjects. We lacked a control group without exposure to the WTC disaster. Only 36% of subjects had follow-up visits. Whereas some subjects had two or more return visits during this period, the numbers were too small to warrant inclusion in this analysis and the subset of patients returning for earlier, follow-up visits might have been over-weighted with those with more severe symptoms. In addition, dates of onset of paresthesia were inferred from self-reports among subjects without return visits, and were calculated from the mid-points between visits for those with incident paresthesia at recall. Another limitation of the current study is that a portion of the reported paresthesia cases might be symptoms that are transient in nature. The patterns of symptom persistence and/or recurrence of paresthesia are worthy of further studies using more comprehensive follow up data.

Paresthesia is a common symptom of neuropathy, but the estimated prevalence of neuropathy in the general population is only 2.4%–7% [31,32]. The higher prevalence of paresthesia in the present study sample strongly suggests that something about exposure to the WTC event or employment in jobs requiring cleaning of WTC dust increased the risk of neuropathy and paresthesia.

5. Conclusions

Reports of paresthesia symptoms are common in the WTC EHC population. We also found significantly higher risk in time to onset of paresthesia for (a) working in a job that required cleaning of WTC dust in the workplace; and (b) being heavily exposed to WTC dust on September 11, 2001, after adjusting for potential confounders. This study suggests that WTC exposure is associated with the development of paresthesias and underscores the importance of further evaluating this population clinically to search for a possible mechanism.

Author Contributions: Conceptualization, J.R. and M.M.; Formal analysis, S.T., B.W., Y.S. and M.M.; Funding acquisition, M.M.; Methodology, S.T., J.R. and M.M.; Writing—original draft, S.T., B.W., Y.S. and M.M.; Writing—review & editing, S.T., B.W., Y.S., J.R. and M.M.

Funding: This research was funded by cooperative agreement U01 OH010395 from the National Institute for Occupational Health and Safety, Centers for Disease Control and Prevention to NYU School of Medicine; and NIOSH contracts 200-2017-93327 (Data Center) and 200-2017-93427 (Clinical Center of Excellence) to NYC Health + Hospitals, Bellevue Hospital Center; and Center Grant 5P30ES000260 from the National Institute of Environmental Health Sciences to NYU School of Medicine.

Conflicts of Interest: The authors declare no conflict of interest.

References

1. Reibman, J.; Levy-Carrick, N.; Miles, T.; Flynn, K.; Hughes, C.; Crane, M.; Lucchini, R.G. Destruction of the World Trade Center Towers. Lessons Learned from an Environmental Health Disaster. *Ann. Am. Thoracic Soc.* **2016**, *13*, 577–583. [CrossRef] [PubMed]

2. Reibman, J.; Liu M.; Cheng, Q.; Liautaud, S.; Rogers, L.; Lau, S.; Berger, K.I.; Goldring, R.M.; Marmor, M.; Fernandez-Beros, M.E.; et al. Characteristics of a residential and working community with diverse exposure to World Trade Center dust, gas, and fumes. *J. Occup. Environ. Med.* **2009**, *51*, 534–541. [CrossRef] [PubMed]

3. Yanagisawa, N.; Morita, H.; Nakajima, T. Sarin experiences in Japan: Acute toxicity and long-term effects. *J. Neurol. Sci.* **2006**, *249*, 76–85. [CrossRef] [PubMed]

4. Callaghan, B.C.; Price, R.S.; Feldman, E.L. Distal Symmetric Polyneuropathy: A Review. *JAMA* **2015**, *314*, 2172–2181. [CrossRef] [PubMed]

5. Stecker, M.; Segelnick, J.; Wilkenfeld, M. Analysis of short-term effects of World Trade Center dust on rat sciatic nerve. *J. Occup. Environ. Med.* **2014**, *56*, 1024–1028. [CrossRef] [PubMed]

6. Lippmann, M.; Cohen, M.D.; Chen, L.C. Health effects of World Trade Center (WTC) Dust: An unprecedented disaster's inadequate risk management. *Crit. Rev. Toxicol.* **2015**, *45*, 492–530. [CrossRef]

7. Lioy, P.J.; Weisel, C.P.; Millette, J.R.; Eisenreich, S.; Vallero, D.; Offenberg, J.; Buckley, B.; Turpin, B.; Zhong, M.; Cohen, M.D.; et al. Characterization of the dust/smoke aerosol that settled east of the World Trade Center (WTC) in lower Manhattan after the collapse of the WTC 11 September 2001. *Environ. Health Perspect.* **2002**, *110*, 703–714. [CrossRef] [PubMed]

8. Soffritti, M.; Falcioni, L.; Bua, L.; Tibaldi, E.; Manservigi, M.; Belpoggi, F. Potential carcinogenic effects of World Trade Center dust after intratracheal instillation to Sprague-Dawley rats: First observation. *Am. J. Ind. Med.* **2013**, *56*, 155–162. [CrossRef] [PubMed]

9. Yiin, L.M.; Millette, J.R.; Vette, A.; Ilacqua, V.; Quan, C.; Gorczynski, J.; Kendall, M.; Chen, L.C.; Weisel, C.P.; Buckley, B.; et al Comparisons of the dust/smoke particulate that settled inside the surrounding buildings and outside on the streets of southern New York City after the collapse of the World Trade Center, September 11, 2001. *J. Air Waste Manag. Assoc.* **2004**, *54*, 515–528. [CrossRef] [PubMed]

10. Thomson, R.M.; Parry, G.J. Neuropathies associated with excessive exposure to lead. *Muscle Nerve* **2006**, *33*, 732–741. [CrossRef] [PubMed]

11. Herskowitz, A.; Ishii, N.; Schaumburg, H. N-hexane neuropathy. A syndrome occurring as a result of industrial exposure. *N. Engl. J. Med.* **1971**, *285*, 82–85. [CrossRef] [PubMed]

12. Tenenbein, M.; deGroot, W.; Rajani, K.R. Peripheral neuropathy following intentional inhalation of naphtha fumes. *Can. Med. Assoc. J.* **1984**, *131*, 1077–1079.

13. Marmor, M.; Shao, Y.; Bhatt, D.H.; Stecker, M.M.; Berger, K.I.; Goldring, R.M.; Rosen, R.L.; Caplan-Shaw, C.; Kazeros, A.; Pradhan, D.; et al. Paresthesias Among Community Members Exposed to the World Trade Center Disaster. *J. Occup. Environ. Med.* **2017**, *59*, 389–396. [CrossRef]

14. Macefield, G.; Burke, D. Paraesthesiae and tetany induced by voluntary hyperventilation. Increased excitability of human cutaneous and motor axons. *Brain* **1991**, *114 Pt 1B*, 527–540. [CrossRef]

15. Stecker, M.M.; Yu, H.; Barlev, R.; Marmor, M.; Wilkenfeld, M. Neurologic Evaluations of Patients Exposed to the World Trade Center Disaster. *J. Occup. Environ. Med.* **2016**, *58*, 1150–1154. [CrossRef]

16. Rosen, R.L.; Levy-Carrick, N.; Reibman, J.; Xu, N.; Shao, Y.; Liu, M.; Ferri, L.; Kazeros, A.; Caplan-Shaw, C.E.; Pradhan, D.R.; et al. Elevated C-reactive protein and posttraumatic stress pathology among survivors of the 9/11 World Trade Center attacks. *J. Psychiatr. Res.* **2017**, *89*, 14–21. [CrossRef]

17. De Cauwer, H.; Somville, F. Neurological disease in the aftermath of terrorism: A review. *Acta. Neurol. Belg.* **2018**, *118*, 193–199. [CrossRef]

18. Barth, S.K.; Kang, H.K.; Bullman, T.A.; Wallin, M.T. Neurological mortality among U.S. veterans of the Persian Gulf War: 13-year follow-up. *Am. J. Ind. Med.* **2009**, *52*, 663–670. [CrossRef] [PubMed]

19. Herskovitz, S.S.H. Neuropathy caused by drugs. In *Peripheral Neuropathy*, 4th ed.; Dyck, P.J., Thomas, P.K., Eds.; Elsevier Inc.: Philadelphia, PA, USA, 2005.

20. Cianchetti, C.; Abbritti, G.; Perticoni, G.; Siracusa, A.; Curradi, F. Toxic polyneuropathy of shoe-industry workers. A study of 122 cases. *J. Neurol. Neurosurg. Psychiatry* **1976**, *39*, 1151–1161. [CrossRef] [PubMed]

21. Wang, C.; Chen, S.; Wang, Z. Electrophysiological follow-up of patients with chronic peripheral neuropathy induced by occupational intoxication with n-hexane. *Cell Biochem. Biophys.* **2014**, *70*, 579–585. [CrossRef] [PubMed]

22. Berger, A.R.; Schaumburg, H.H. Human toxic neuropathy caused by industrial agents. In *Peripheral Neuropathy*, 4th ed.; Dyck, P.J., Thomas, P.K., Eds.; Elsevier Inc.: Philadelphia, PA, USA, 2005.

23. Weiss, D.; Tomasallo, C.D.; Meiman, J.G.; Alarcon, W.; Graber, N.M.; Bisgard, K.M.; Anderson, H.A. Elevated Blood Lead Levels Associated with Retained Bullet Fragments—United States, 2003–2012. *MMWR Morb. Mortal. Wkly. Rep.* **2017**, *66*, 130–133. [CrossRef]

24. Johannsen, L.; Smith, T.; Havsager, A.M.; Madsen, C.; Kjeldsen, M.J.; Dalsgaard, N.J.; Gaist, D.; Schroder, H.D.; Sindrup, S.H. Evaluation of patients with symptoms suggestive of chronic polyneuropathy. *J. Clin. Neuromuscul. Dis.* **2001**, *3*, 47–52. [CrossRef]

25. Lubec, D.; Mullbacher, W.; Finsterer, J.; Mamoli, B. Diagnostic work-up in peripheral neuropathy: An analysis of 171 cases. *Postgrad. Med. J.* **1999**, *75*, 723–727. [CrossRef]

26. Mengel, D.; Fraune, L.; Sommer, N.; Stettner, M.; Reese, J.P.; Dams, J.; Glynn, R.J.; Balzer-Geldsetzer, M.; Dodel, R.; Tackenberg, B. Costs of illness in chronic inflammatory demyelinating polyneuropathy in Germany. *Muscle Nerve* **2018**, *58*, 681–687. [CrossRef]

27. Rajabally, Y.A.; Seri, S.; Cavanna, A.E. Neuropsychiatric manifestations in inflammatory neuropathies: A systematic review. *Muscle Nerve* **2016**, *54*, 1–8. [CrossRef]

28. Kerckhove, N.; Collin, A.; Conde, S.; Chaleteix, C.; Pezet, D.; Balayssac, D. Long-Term Effects, Pathophysiological Mechanisms, and Risk Factors of Chemotherapy-Induced Peripheral Neuropathies: A Comprehensive Literature Review. *Front Pharmacol.* **2017**, *8*, 86. [CrossRef]

29. Salinero-Fort, M.A.; Gomez-Campelo, P.; San Andres-Rebollo, F.J.; Cardenas-Valladolid, J.; Abanades-Herranz, J.C.; Carrillo de Santa Pau, E.; Chico-Moraleja, R.M.; Beamud-Victoria, D.; de Miguel-Yanes, J.M.; Jimenez-Garcia, R.; et al. Prevalence of depression in patients with type 2 diabetes mellitus in Spain (the DIADEMA Study): Results from the MADIABETES cohort. *BMJ Open* **2018**, *8*, e020768. [CrossRef]

30. Zafeiri, M.; Tsioutis, C.; Kleinaki, Z.; Manolopoulos, P.; Ioannidis, I.; Dimitriadis, G. Clinical Characteristics of Patients with co-Existent Diabetic Peripheral Neuropathy and Depression: A Systematic Review. *Exp. Clin. Endocrinol. Diabetes* **2018**. [CrossRef]

31. Bharucha, N.E.; Bharucha, A.E.; Bharucha, E.P. Prevalence of peripheral neuropathy in the Parsi community of Bombay. *Neurology* **1991**, *41*, 1315–1317. [CrossRef]

32. Savettieri, G.; Rocca, W.A.; Salemi, G.; Meneghini, F.; Grigoletto, F.; Morgante, L.; Reggio, A.; Costa, V.; Coraci, M.A.; Di Perri, R. Prevalence of diabetic neuropathy with somatic symptoms: A door-to-door survey in two Sicilian municipalities. Sicilian Neuro-Epidemiologic Study (SNES) Group. *Neurology* **1993**, *43*, 1115–1120. [CrossRef]

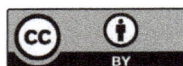

International Journal of
Environmental Research and Public Health

MDPI

Article

Metabolic Syndrome Biomarkers of World Trade Center Airway Hyperreactivity: A 16-Year Prospective Cohort Study

Sophia Kwon [1], George Crowley [1], Mena Mikhail [1], Rachel Lam [1], Emily Clementi [1], Rachel Zeig-Owens [2,3,4], Theresa M. Schwartz [2,3], Mengling Liu [5,6], David J. Prezant [2,3] and Anna Nolan [1,2,5,*]

[1] Department of Medicine, Division of Pulmonary, Critical Care and Sleep Medicine, New York University, School of Medicine, New York, NY 10016, USA; Sophia.kwon@nyumc.org (S.K.); George.crowley@nyumc.org (G.C.); mena.mikhail@nyumc.org (M.M.); Rachel.Lam@nyumc.org (R.L.); Emily.clementi@nyumc.org (E.C.)

[2] Bureau of Health Services and Office of Medical Affairs, Fire Department of New York, Brooklyn, NY 11201, USA; Rachel.zeig-owens@fdny.nyc.gov (R.Z.-O.); Theresa.Schwarz@fdny.nyc.gov (T.M.S.); David.Prezant@fdny.nyc.gov (D.J.P.)

[3] Pulmonary Medicine Division, Department of Medicine, Montefiore Medical Center and Albert Einstein College of Medicine, Bronx, NY 10461, USA

[4] Department of Epidemiology and Population Health, Albert Einstein College of Medicine, Bronx, NY 10461, USA

[5] Department of Environmental Medicine, New York University, School of Medicine, New York, NY 10016, USA; Mengling.liu@nyumc.org

[6] Division of Biostatistics, Departments of Population Health, New York University School of Medicine, New York, NY 10016, USA

[*] Correspondence: anna.nolan@med.nyu.edu; Tel.: +01-212-263-7283

Received: 19 March 2019; Accepted: 18 April 2019; Published: 26 April 2019

Abstract: Airway hyperreactivity (AHR) related to environmental exposure is a significant public health risk worldwide. Similarly, metabolic syndrome (MetSyn), a risk factor for obstructive airway disease (OAD) and systemic inflammation, is a significant contributor to global adverse health. This prospective cohort study followed $N = 7486$ World Trade Center (WTC)-exposed male firefighters from 11 September 2001 (9/11) until 1 August 2017 and investigated $N = 539$ with newly developed AHR for clinical biomarkers of MetSyn and compared them to the non-AHR group. Male firefighters with normal lung function and no AHR pre-9/11 who had blood drawn from 9 September 2001–24 July 2002 were assessed. World Trade Center-Airway Hyperreactivity (WTC-AHR) was defined as either a positive bronchodilator response (BDR) or methacholine challenge test (MCT). The electronic medical record (EMR) was queried for their MetSyn characteristics (lipid profile, body mass index (BMI), glucose), and routine clinical biomarkers (such as complete blood counts). We modeled the association of MetSyn characteristics at the first post-9/11 exam with AHR. Those with AHR were significantly more likely to be older, have higher BMIs, have high intensity exposure, and have MetSyn. Smoking history was not associated with WTC-AHR. Those present on the morning of 9/11 had 224% increased risk of developing AHR, and those who arrived in the afternoon of 9/11 had a 75.9% increased risk. Having ≥3 MetSyn parameters increased the risk of WTC-AHR by 65.4%. Co-existing MetSyn and high WTC exposure are predictive of future AHR and suggest that systemic inflammation may be a contributor.

Keywords: metabolic syndrome; airway hyperreactivity; World Trade Center

1. Introduction

Metabolic syndrome (MetSyn) is a clinical diagnosis made by fulfilment of at least three of the five following comorbidity criteria: Abdominal obesity, insulin resistance, hypertriglyceridemia, low high density lipoproteins (HDL), and hypertension [1,2]. MetSyn and particulate matter (PM) exposure are known independent risk factors in the development of many diseases including cardiovascular disease and cancer [3]. MetSyn, classically a risk factor for cardiovascular disease, is now being investigated as a risk factor for pulmonary disease [4].

Obesity, one component of MetSyn, has been typically linked to restrictive patterns of lung disease through mechanical stress and mass loading. However, many recent studies have focused on the systemic effects of MetSyn, through hormonal and immunoinflammatory mediators, and their association with pollution exposure and subsequent respiratory disease [5–11]. One study suggests that adipose tissue and adipokines such as C-reactive protein (CRP) and tumor necrosis factor-α (TNF-α) may contribute to a systemic low-grade inflammatory process leading to airway hyperreactivity (AHR) [12].

The association between MetSyn and the development of AHR has been seen in several studies [13]. Multiple cross-sectional studies have shown an increased prevalence of MetSyn or its constituents amongst those with diagnosed asthma or asthma-like symptoms [14–16]. A meta-analysis that included cohorts in the United States (US), Canada, and Europe reported that odds of incident asthma are increased by 50% in obese individuals, and that risk increased with body weight [17]. Two prospective studies investigated adults who were asthma-free at baseline and showed that obesity and insulin resistance were MetSyn risk factors that contributed to eventual asthma or asthma-like symptoms [17,18]. Murine studies showed that mice that developed insulin resistance from a high fat diet had increased airway resistance at baseline and after methacholine provocation, indicating a component of AHR [19].

AHR and PM exposure have also been strongly linked in numerous studies. In a cohort of asthmatic and non-asthmatic children exposed to freeway and non-freeway air pollution, there was a positive association between air pollution exposure and asthmatic children [20]. In a cohort study of 40 asthmatic children who attended school in close proximity to expressways, there was an increased risk of wheezing and shortness of breath [21]. In a cross-sectional study of adults over 50 years of age in low resource countries, 5.12% of cases were secondary to PM exposure, and the prevalence ratio of asthma after each 10 μg/m^3 increase of PM$_{2.5}$ was 1.05 [22]. The World Trade Center (WTC) complex destruction on 11 September 2001 (9/11) led to the release of over 11,000 tons of PM, and exposed over 300,000 local workers, residents, and rescue and recovery workers [23]. An early study monitoring pulmonary function in firefighters from the Fire Department of the City of New York (FDNY) with World Trade Center Particulate Matter (WTC-PM) exposure had AHR prevalence of 40%, and over half of the studied group had persistent AHR in a follow-up exam 10 years later [24,25]. These studies established a significant association between exposure level and AHR [26].

Our initial work focused on inflammatory biomarkers, such as GM-CSF and MDC, in WTC-PM-exposed firefighters [27]. We also investigated amylin, leptin, and lipids in a subset of exposed firefighters with WTC lung injury (WTC-LI) as defined by a loss of forced expiratory volume in 1 second (FEV$_1$) to less than the lower limit of normal (LLN), and recently validated our findings of MetSyn associated with WTC-LI in the larger exposed group [4,28]. We now investigate the impact of MetSyn on the development of WTC-associated AHR.

2. Materials and Methods

Study Design: Demographics, clinical information and serial spirometry obtained as part of the Fire Department of New York World Trade Center Health Program (FDNY WTC-HP) was extracted from the FDNY electronic medical record [29]. All WTC-exposed FDNY rescue/recovery workers (baseline cohort; N = 12,781) were included if they were firefighters, had research consent, FEV$_1$ ≥ lower limits of normal, no AHR on available lung function testing pre-9/11, fasting blood drawn prior to WTC site closure on 24 July 2002, and available clinical endpoints, yielding a source cohort of $N = 7486$ (Figure 1) [30]. Exposure to WTC-PM, defined per the FDNY WTC-HP, was based on first arrival at the WTC site and considered the highest if arrived in the morning of 9/11 during the collapse of the WTC, intermediate arriving the afternoon of 9/11, and lower intensity if arriving on or after 9/12 [31]. All subjects consented to analysis of their information for research at the time of enrolment. All data was collected in compliance with the Code of Federal Regulations, Title 21, Part 11 and the Montefiore Medical Center/Albert Einstein College of Medicine (#07-09-320) and New York University (#16-01412) Institutional Review Boards have approved this study. All participants gave informed written consent.

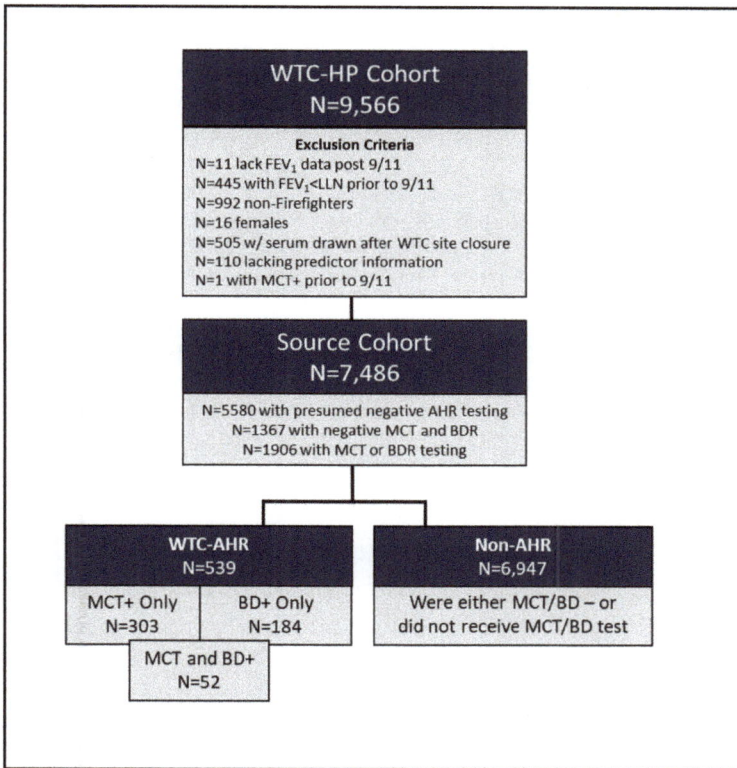

Figure 1. Study Design. Fire Department of New York (FDNY) rescue workers exposed to World Trade Center (WTC) particulates and enrolled in the WTC Health Program.

AHR Definition. The cohort was followed longitudinally until 1 August 2017 and $N = 1906$ had either a pulmonary function test (PFT) with assessment of bronchodilator response (BDR) or methacholine challenge test (MCT) administered. World Trade Center Airway Hyperreactivity (WTC-AHR) was defined at the earliest positive BDR or MCT after WTC exposure. In general, a bronchoprovocation test such as an MCT may be utilized to assess hyperreactivity, whereas a bronchodilator test may indicate reversibility consistent with asthma. MCTs were positive when the cumulative methacholine dose that reduced the FEV_1 by 20%, (PC_{20}) was equivalent or was less than 16 mg/mL [32]. BD was positive when post-bronchodilator FEV_1 change exceeded 12% and at least 200 mL [33]. Those without AHR ($N = 6947$) were defined as those who either had a negative study or were presumed negative if they did not have subspecialty testing.

MetSyn Phenotypic Definition. Diagnosis of MetSyn was based on National Cholesterol Education Program Adult Treatment Panel III (NCEP ATP III) guidelines and optimized for our cohort by having at least 3 of 5 following criteria: Systolic blood pressure (SBP) ≥130 mmHg or diastolic blood pressure (DBP) ≥85 mmHg; HDL <40 mg/dL; triglycerides ≥150 mg/dL; insulin resistance, as glucose ≥100 mg/dL; or body mass index (BMI) ≥30 kg/m^2. BMI ≥30 kg/m^2 was used as surrogate for central adiposity as per Word Health Organization (WHO) guidelines [34]. Smoking information and exposure intensity were self-reported and collected from questionnaires administered during medical monitoring exams. Clinical parameters including DBP, glucose, and lipid panel were measured at WTC-HP entry. All of the above criteria were from data points obtained pre-9/11 and prior to any measurements of post-9/11 AHR.

Additional Clinical Biomarkers. We investigated the correlation between AHR and other clinical biomarkers. Absolute counts of differentiated white blood cells (WBC) such as neutrophils and eosinophils present at the first post-9/11 evaluation. A cutoff of at least 500 eosinophils was utilized, consistent with definition of clinical hyper-eosinophilia. Cholesterol/HDL ratio ≥3.5, a predictor of ischemic heart disease risk, and its association with AHR was also investigated [35–37].

Statistical Analysis. SPSS-23 (IBM) was used for primary data handling and statistics. Continuous variables are expressed as mean (standard deviation (SD)), and compared by two-sample t-test. Categorical data was summarized as count and proportions, and compared using Pearson-χ^2. Smoking data was categorized into a dichotomous variable of ever or never a smoker, as previously described [38–42]. The primary endpoint of all analyses was development of WTC-AHR based on a positive BDR or MCT any time after 9/11. Survival interval was determined by time from 9/11 to positive AHR test or until 1 August 2017, the administrative censoring date of the study closure, if they did not have AHR. Association of endpoints and MetSyn, smoking, BMI, and exposure level were analyzed using the Cox proportional hazards regression and are represented as hazard ratio (HR) and 95% confidence interval (CI). We assigned a cut point of ≥500 eosinophils/μL as a marker of clinically significant eosinophilia for Cox modeling. All models were adjusted for age at 9/11, exposure intensity, and smoking status, and considered significant if $p < 0.05$. Omnibus testing was used to assess the quality of the comparisons. Time-to-event curves were determined by the Kaplan–Meier method and compared with the log-rank test. There were no dropouts in this study.

3. Results

3.1. WTC-AHR Cohort

Of the $N = 1906$ individuals with subspecialty pulmonary testing, $N = 891$ had a MCT while $N = 1168$ had BDR testing, and 153 individuals had both tests (Figure 1). Of the $N = 539$ participants that had WTC-AHR, 303 were positive on MCT only, 184 had a positive BDR only and 52 were positive on both tests, yielding a total of $N = 355$ who were MCT positive and $N = 236$ who were BDR positive (Figure 1). Demographic and clinical measures were compared between those with and without AHR (Tables 1 and 2). Years of service information was only available on $N = 5029/6947$ non-AHR and $N = 418/539$ AHR. There was no difference between a positive MCT and a positive BDR in age, BMI, smoking status, or clinical measures except for total cholesterol. A positive MCT had a slightly higher cholesterol of mean (SD) of 217.4 (40.1) compared to positive BDR 210.2 (36.0), $p = 0.03$. AHR and non-AHR were not significantly different in race or smoking status; those with AHR were significantly older by a mean of 1 year, had an average of three fewer years of service compared to non-AHR, and had a higher percentage present in the morning of 9/11 (Table 1).

Spirometry was compared in those with AHR and non-AHR at both the most recent pre-9/11 and first post-9/11 examination showed significantly lower FEV$_1$% predicted, Forced Vital Capacity (FVC) % predicted, and FEV$_1$/FVC ratios in AHR, but the differences were clinically insignificant and were not indicative of OAD (Table 1).

Table 1. Demographic and pulmonary function test data of group.

Measure		MCT+ N = 355	BD+ N = 236	Non-AHR N = 6947	WTC-AHR N = 539	p
Age on 9/11		40.3 (6.3)	40.9 (6.8)	39.5 (7.5)	40.5 (6.5)	0.004
Years of service *		19.3 (7.3)	20.1 (7.2)	22.8 (6.5)	19.7 (7.3)	<0.001
Ever smokers		122 (34%)	89 (38%)	2531 (36%)	191 (35%)	0.643
Race	Caucasian	342 (96%)	220 (93%)	6529 (94%)	512 (95%)	
	African American	3 (1%)	6 (3%)	183 (3%)	9 (2%)	0.560
	Hispanic	9 (3%)	10 (4%)	215 (3%)	17 (3%)	
	Asian/other	1 (.3%)	0 (0%)	20 (0.3%)	1 (0.2%)	
Exposure group	Morning of 9/11	79 (22%)	59 (25%)	1124 (16%)	123 (23%)	
	Afternoon of 9/11	211 (59%)	134 (57%)	3749 (54%)	317 (59%)	<0.001
	On or after 9/12	65 (18%)	43 (18%)	2074 (30%)	99 (18%)	
Pre-9/11	FEV_1% pred.	101.5 (11.6)	101.5 (13.5)	106.3 (13.0)	101.7 (12.4)	<0.001
	FVC% pred.	97.7 (10.9)	98.4 (12.7)	99.6 (12.1)	98.2 (11.7)	0.017
	Ratio	82.9 (5.7)	82.4 (5.4)	85.3 (4.9)	82.7 (5.6)	<0.001
WTC-HP entry	FEV% pred.	91.8 (13.4)	90.7 (14.8)	98.1 (13.1)	91.6 (13.9)	<0.001
	FVC% pred.	89.6 (12.0)	89.3 (21.1)	92.4 (11.8)	89.6 (12.2)	<0.001
	Ratio	82.0 (6.0)	81.2 (6.6)	84.6 (4.9)	81.7 (6.3)	<0.001

Values are in mean (SD) or N (%) as indicated. *p* calculated by *t*-test or Chi-square as appropriate, comparing airway hyperreactivity (AHR) and non-AHR. * Data available on N = 5029/6947 non-AHR, N = 418/539 AHR.

Table 2. Clinical measures of inflammation and metabolic syndrome.

Measure	MCT+ N = 355	BD+ N = 236	Non-AHR N = 6947	WTC-AHR N = 539	p
Systolic BP, mmHg	118.0 (12.5)	118.3 (12.6)	117.1 (12.5)	118.0 (12.7)	0.092
Diastolic BP, mmHg	73.4 (8.0)	74.3 (8.3)	73.4 (8.4)	73.6 (8.2)	0.598
BMI at WTC-HP entry, kg/m^2	29.2 (3.2)	28.9 (3.0)	28.6 (3.3)	29.1 (3.2)	0.001
White blood cells × 10^9 cells/L *	6.5 (1.9)	6.5 (1.8)	6.3 (1.6)	6.5 (1.9)	0.021
Neutrophils (ANC)	3809.8 (1654.5)	3697.7 (1400.1)	3664.6 (1290.1)	3758.1 (1524.8)	0.113
Lymphocytes (ALC)	1818.9 (534.4)	1861.8 (590.2)	1830.9 (540.3)	1843.4 (561.2)	0.608
Eosinophils (AEC)	227.8 (149.9)	227.2 (160.3)	187.1 (130.9)	229.3 (156.6)	<0.001
Monocytes (AMC)	579.4 (194.3)	605.7 (216.2)	581.3 (193.2)	591.1 (204.8)	0.263
Glucose	92.9 (18.8)	91.7 (10.4)	91.6 (13.9)	92.5 (16.4)	0.177
Triglyceride	195.7 (139.1)	190.7 (126.0)	185.1 (136.6)	197.4 (137.9)	0.046
HDL	48.0 (12.6)	47.1 (12.1)	48.1 (11.7)	47.6 (12.4)	0.351
LDL	133.1 (34.5)	128.3 (32.4)	128.3 (33.5)	131.6 (33.7)	0.028
Cholesterol	217.4 (40.1)	210.2 (36.0)	210.8 (38.7)	216.3 (38.5)	0.009
Cholesterol/HDL ratio	4.8 (1.5)	4.7 (1.3)	4.6 (1.4)	4.8 (1.4)	0.007
MetSyn definition	82 (23%)	54 (23%)	1329 (19%)	123 (23%)	<0.001
SBP ≥ 130 and/or DBP ≥ 85 mmHg	78 (22%)	56 (24%)	1384 (20%)	119 (22%)	0.229
HDL < 40 mg/dL	94 (27%)	72 (31%)	1667 (24%)	151 (28%)	0.036
Triglycerides ≥ 150 mg/dL	194 (55%)	123 (52%)	3428 (49%)	294 (55%)	0.020
Glucose ≥ 100 mg/dL	72 (20%)	45 (19%)	1269 (18%)	106 (20%)	0.419
BMI ≥ 30 kg/m^2	130 (30%)	78 (33%)	2040 (29%)	193 (36%)	0.002

Values are in mean (SD) or N (%) as indicated; *p* calculated by t-test or Chi-square as appropriate, comparing AHR and non-AHR; * Data available on N = 6896/6947 non-AHR, N = 532/537 AHR, differentials expressed as absolute counts, cells/µL.

Participants with a positive MCT had a PC_{20} mean (SD) of 5.6 (4.7) mg/mL. Participants with a positive BDR had a mean (SD) gain of FEV_1 % predicted of 18.6% (9.9%), and 661.0 (274.0) mL. Participants with AHR also had a slightly higher average BMI (29.1 vs. 28.6 kg/m^2; *p* = 0.001), triglycerides (*p* = 0.046), low-density lipoprotein (*p* = 0.028), and cholesterol (*p* = 0.009) compared to non-AHR (Table 2). A higher proportion of subjects with AHR also had MetSyn; subgroup analyses by Maentel–Haenszel odds ratio estimates shows that triglyceride ≥150 mg/dL (OR 21.6, 95% CI of 17.5–26.76, *p* < 0.001), obesity defined as BMI ≥30kg/m^2 (OR 13.07, 95% CI 11.41–14.97, *p* < 0.001), and

HDL <40 had OR of 12.25 (10.75–13.97), $p < 0.001$, were the most likely to meet the definition of MetSyn. SBP/DBP ≥130/85 had OR of 6.85 (6.03–7.79), $p < 0.001$, and glucose ≥ 100 OR 5.96 (5.24–6.78), $p < 0.001$.

Complete blood count and differentials were also compared on available samples between 532/537 AHR and 6896/6947 non-AHR (Table 2). AHR displayed higher WBC count and absolute eosinophil counts (AEC) compared to non-AHR. Of the $N = 196$ subjects with AEC > 500 cells/μL, $N = 26$ had AHR whereas $N = 154$ had at least one MetSyn risk factor.

3.2. Model Development

Cox proportional hazard models were used to estimate univariate hazard ratio of individual clinical biomarkers on developing WTC-AHR, with the adjustment of age, smoking, and WTC-exposure intensity (Table 3). AEC ≥500 cells/μL increased the risk of development of AHR by 94% (CI 1.31–2.88). The clinically utilized ratio of cholesterol/HDL ratio ≥3.5 was similarly correlated with a 33% increased risk of development of AHR. Similar to what was originally identified by t-test, dyslipidemia and obesity were significant risk factors for development of AHR, whereas hypertension or insulin resistance were not significant. This also mirrors the subgroup analyses where the most significant contributors to MetSyn definition were from dyslipidemia and obesity.

Table 3. Cox proportional hazards of univariate metabolic risk factors of AHR.

Measure		Hazards (95% CI)
Cholesterol/HDL ratio ≥ 3.5		1.332 (1.057–1.679)
BMI ≥ 30 kg/m^2		1.329 (1.114–1.585)
Glucose ≥ 100 mg/dL		1.062 (0.857–1.315)
Lipids mg/dL	HDL < 40	1.237 (1.025–1.492)
	Triglycerides ≥ 150	1.204 (1.016–1.427)
Blood pressure mmHg	Systolic ≥ 130	1.079 (0.872–1.335)
	Diastolic ≥ 85	0.970 (0.718–1.309)
Number of MetSyn risk factors	1	1.441 (1.124–1.847)
	2	1.690 (1.310–2.151)
	3+	1.654 (1.268–2.158)
Exposure intensity	Morning of 9/11	2.240 (1.719–2.919)
	Afternoon of 9/11	1.759 (1.403–2.205)
	After 9/12	Reference
Ever smoker		1.759 (1.403–2.205)
Age (per year)		1..017 (1.005–1.029)

All models were adjusted for age, smoking, and exposure intensity. Exposure, age, and smoking RR refer to RR in final model of combined MetSyn risk factors.

The final MetSyn model, adjusted for age, smoking, and exposure intensity, assessed the total number of MetSyn risk factors predicting AHR. Having at least two or three MetSyn risk factors had 69% and 65% increased risk of developing AHR, respectively (Table 3). Having high exposure, being present in the morning of 9/11, increased odds of developing AHR by 2.24 times, whereas being present in the afternoon increased odds by 1.76 times. Age also had an associated risk of development of AHR by 1.7% for every increasing year. Smoking was not significantly associated with AHR (Table 3).

Survival curves were plotted and time to divergence calculations from having no MetSyn risk factors showed that having one MetSyn risk factor diverged three years post-9/11, compared to having two risk factors, and divergence occurred within the first year post-9/11 (Figure 2). Kaplan–Meier curves were also assessed for subgroups of each MetSyn factors. BMI ≥30 kg/m^2, triglycerides ≥150 mg/dL, HDL <40 mg/dL, and having the highest exposure to WTC-PM by being present at the site on the morning of 9/11 carried significantly higher risk of developing of AHR (Figure 3A–D).

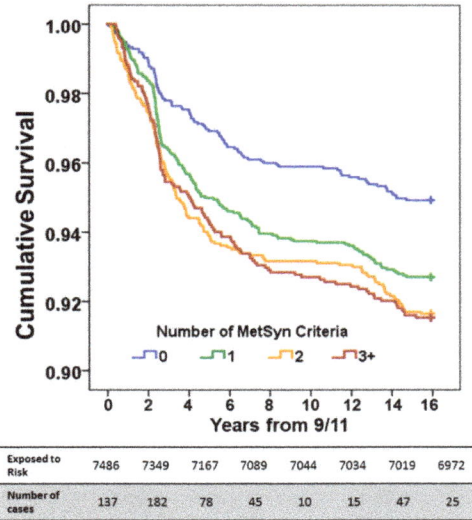

Figure 2. Cumulative AHR survival curves by total number of MetSyn biomarkers. Cumulative disease-free survival is expressed on the *y*-axis and time in years from their WTC exposure is on the *x*-axis. Life table expresses the number of individuals at risk in 2-year intervals.

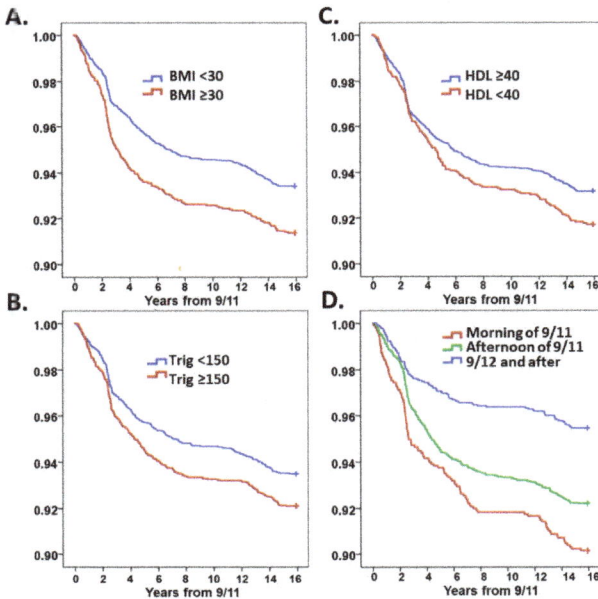

Figure 3. Kaplan–Meier survival curves stratified by (**A**). BMI $\geq$30 kg/m^2 ($p = 0.001$ by log rank), (**B**). Triglycerides $\geq$150 mg/dL ($p = 0.019$), (**C**). HDL <40 mg/dL ($p = 0.038$), and (**D**). Exposure intensity ($p < 0.001$). Cumulative disease-free survival is expressed on the *y*-axis and time in years from their WTC exposure is on the *x*-axis. Log rank was not significant for SBP, DBP, and glucose, and were not included in this graph.

We examined the reproducibility of the model in the cohort of $N = 1906$ who had MCT/BD testing. Even in this restricted cohort we found that having two or three MetSyn risk factors also yielded an increased risk of developing AHR by 54.4% and 39.6% ($p = 0.001$ and 0.014) respectively. Having one MetSyn risk factor had 25% increased risk but was not statistically significant ($p = 0.08$), and exposure was not a significant risk factor in the smaller cohort.

4. Discussion

The WTC-exposed FDNY rescue/recovery workers represent the largest longitudinally assessed first responder cohort with pre and post lung function assessments following a high PM exposure. They continue to have their health adversely impacted even after 18 years [26–28,43–54]. Our previous work focused on the contribution of MetSyn in the development of WTC-LI [4,28]. We now show that metabolically active biomarkers and markers of inflammation (such as eosinophils) predict AHR in the WTC-exposed firefighter cohort [55–57].

This study represents the only longitudinal study to our knowledge investigating the temporal relationship of MetSyn, PM exposure, and AHR. We demonstrate that MetSyn is an independent risk factor for the development of AHR, as all study participants were categorized as having or not having MetSyn prior to the development of AHR. A prior cross-sectional study investigating MetSyn, PM exposure, and cardiovascular risk found no significant associations with inflammatory markers of CRP or WBC [3].

Our earlier model showed that dyslipidemia and heart rate independently increased the odds of developing WTC-LI [4,28]. While WTC-LI and AHR both fall under the umbrella of OAD, there is little overlap in these populations. When examining a subgroup analysis of the WTC-LI cases, only $N = 203/1204$ (16.8%) also have AHR. This strongly suggests that MetSyn is implicated in multiple pathways in the development of OAD. Although MetSyn risk factors and cholesterol/HDL ratios are classically predictors of cardiovascular disease, their implications in affecting future lung disease are novel. Moreover, these represent reversible risk factors that may be potential therapeutic targets to alter the outcome of other obstructive lung disease.

Our current investigation shows the associations of MetSyn biomarkers with the development of WTC-AHR. We also show obesity having similar ability to predict AHR, an unexpected finding given the vast literature of restrictive patterns in obesity. However, this fits in the growing body of literature showing that obesity has hormonal pathways that influence the pulmonary environment. Another unexpected finding, but similar to our prior investigation of MetSyn predictor of WTC-LI, was that glucose was not a significant predictor of WTC-AHR [28]. Specifically, in our current study with cut-points of 100 and 126 mg/dL, there was no significantly increased risk of lung injury in our cohort. Studies in non-exposed individuals have shown an association between insulin resistance and OAD [58].

A strength of this study is the rigorously characterized prospective cohort, with a clearly defined time of exposure (9/11), pre and post exposure lung function measurements, blood drawn soon after exposure, and MetSyn categorization done prior to AHR measurements. Another strength of this study is that the development of AHR was post-exposure in that FDNY firefighters are excluded at hire and during annual medical monitoring if they have signs or symptoms of airways obstruction or AHR [59]. A key strength of this study is in the study design that allowed us to explore multiple aspects of WTC-AHR. Since the decision to administer BDR or MCT tests to determine disease is often a clinician's judgement, it was reassuring to have found little difference between the two groups, those with only a positive BDR and those with only a positive MCT. This suggests that our findings are plausible and potentially reproducible in other cohorts. Examining the model for reproducibility in the smaller cohort of $N = 1906$ also bolsters our findings that MetSyn is an independent risk factor for development of future AHR.

Using the clinical markers of MetSyn as predictors of AHR is advantageous in several ways. These biomarkers are easily attainable, cost effective, and can be replicated in many cohorts. Dyslipidemia, insulin resistance, obesity, and hypertension are also all potentially reversible causes of end-organ disease. Extending statin therapy, for example, and increasing glycemic control can be the target of future studies focused on their mitigating effects in progressive lung disease. Furthermore, our group is currently studying dietary effects on pulmonary function and biomarker profile of the FDNY exposed cohort. MetSyn also has global reach and can be investigated in other cohorts with similar pollutant or PM exposure.

Eosinophilia, while a significant risk factor of AHR, did not augment the predictive model investigating MetSyn. Subgroup analysis shows that although only 13% of the hyper-eosinophilia group had overlap with the AHR population, 78.5% ($N = 154/196$) had at least one MetSyn risk factor. This was somewhat surprising because the literature reflects that obesity-related lung dysfunction is often a neutrophil-mediated process [60]. This may indicate the need for further studies in eosinophilia-mediated pathways in MetSyn.

There are several limitations to this study. We focus on a male-only cohort. Interestingly, MetSyn and asthma have been shown to have stronger associations in female-only cohorts [18,61]. An additional limitation is that we classified participants as not having AHR if they had negative tests or even if they had no testing of AHR. The presumption of negative AHR in the absence of direct measurement, while a limitation, biased our results towards the null. We also used a broad definition of AHR by requiring either a positive BDR or a positive MCT. This combined definition could have biased our results away from the null and towards a positive finding but we believe this combined definition is the most clinically relevant, and also accounts for those that may have only had one type of test due to clinical contraindications [32].

We also caution on over-interpretation of the results of individual components of MetSyn. We use a one-time fasting blood level at the earliest time point after exposure to 9/11 to make predictions of future lung injury. Future studies can focus on repeated measures of MetSyn, dyslipidemia, fasting blood glucose, and AHR to control for other possible confounders and aid in understanding the associations of individual components of MetSyn and AHR and their temporal relationships. The lack of medication history could also cause under-identification of those with MetSyn risk factors. Having this information could improve the sensitivity of those at risk of AHR and specificity of the model. Alternatively, it can help to determine if attenuation of MetSyn risk factors through pharmacologic methods impacted pulmonary health.

5. Conclusions

In summary, MetSyn biomarkers are predictors of future WTC-AHR in a large cohort of WTC-exposed FDNY firefighters followed over 16 years. These metabolically active biomarkers are associated with dyslipidemia, insulin resistance, and cardiovascular disease, and suggest that MetSyn may contribute to systemic inflammation that leads to future development of AHR. Our data supports the hypothesis and contributes to the growing body of literature investigating the complex associations between potentially reversible MetSyn risk factors and lung injury. We are strongly encouraged by our results indicating that pathways involved in metabolism have broad impacts on the immune and hormonal environment in the lung.

Author Contributions: A.N. and S.K. participated in study conception and design; A.N. was the primary investigator; S.K., T.M.S., R.Z.-O., A.N. and D.J.P. were responsible for data collection; A.N. and S.K. were responsible for data validation; A.N. and S.K. participated in data analysis; S.K., M.L. and A.N. undertook the statistical analysis. All authors participated in data interpretation, writing and revision of the report, and approval of the final version.

Funding: This research was funded by NHLBI R01HL119326, CDC/NIOSH U01-OH11300, Clinical Center of Excellence 200-2017-93426, Data Center 200-2017-93326.

Acknowledgments: We are thankful to the FDNY rescue workers for their selfless dedication.

Conflicts of Interest: The authors declare no conflict of interest.

Abbreviations

AHR	Airway hyperreactivity
ATP III	Adult treatment panel III
BDR	Bronchodilator response
BMI	Body mass index
CRP	C-reactive protein
CI	Confidence interval
DBP	Diastolic blood pressure
EMR	Electronic medical record
FDNY	Fire Department of City of New York
FEV_1	Forced expiratory volume over 1 second
FVC	Forced vital capacity
HDL	High density lipoprotein
HR	Hazards ratio
LDL	Low density lipoprotein
LLN	Lower limit of normal
MCT	Methacholine test
MetSyn	Metabolic syndrome
NCEP	National Cholesterol Education Program
OAD	Obstructive Airways Disease
PC_{20}	Methacholine dose required to reduce FEV_1 by 20%.
PFT	Pulmonary function test
PM	Particulate matter
SBP	Systolic blood pressure
SD	Standard deviation
TNF	Tumor necrosis factor
US	United States
WBC	White blood cell
WHO	World Health Organization
WTC	World Trade Center
WTC-AHR	World Trade Center-airway hyperreactivity
WTC-HP	World Trade Center-health program
WTC-LI	WTC-lung injury

References

1. Grundy, S.M.; Cleeman, J.I.; Daniels, S.R.; Donato, K.A.; Eckel, R.H.; Franklin, B.A.; Gordon, D.J.; Krauss, R.M.; Savage, P.J.; Smith, S.C., Jr.; et al. Diagnosis and management of the metabolic syndrome: An American Heart Association/National Heart, Lung, and Blood Institute Scientific Statement. *Circulation* **2005**, *112*, 2735–2752. [CrossRef] [PubMed]
2. Aguilar, M.; Bhuket, T.; Torres, S.; Liu, B.; Wong, R.J. Prevalence of the metabolic syndrome in the United States, 2003–2012. *JAMA* **2015**, *313*, 1973–1974. [CrossRef] [PubMed]
3. Dabass, A.; Talbott, E.O.; Rager, J.R.; Marsh, G.M.; Venkat, A.; Holguin, F.; Sharma, R.K. Systemic inflammatory markers associated with cardiovascular disease and acute and chronic exposure to fine particulate matter air pollution (PM2.5) among US NHANES adults with metabolic syndrome. *Environ. Res.* **2018**, *161*, 485–491. [CrossRef] [PubMed]
4. Kwon, S.; Crowley, G.; Caraher, E.J.; Haider, S.H.; Lam, R.; Veerappan, A.; Yang, L.; Liu, M.; Zeig-Owens, R.; Schwartz, T.; et al. Validation of Predictive Metabolic Syndrome Biomarkers of World Trade Center Lung Injury: A 16-Year Longitudinal Study. *Chest* **2019**. [CrossRef] [PubMed]
5. Wallwork, R.S.; Colicino, E.; Zhong, J.; Kloog, I.; Coull, B.A.; Vokonas, P.; Schwartz, J.D.; Baccarelli, A.A. Ambient Fine Particulate Matter, Outdoor Temperature, and Risk of Metabolic Syndrome. *Am. J. Epidemiol.* **2017**, *185*, 30–39. [CrossRef] [PubMed]

6. Brook, R.D.; Sun, Z.; Brook, J.R.; Zhao, X.; Ruan, Y.; Yan, J.; Mukherjee, B.; Rao, X.; Duan, F.; Sun, L.; et al. Extreme Air Pollution Conditions Adversely Affect Blood Pressure and Insulin Resistance: The Air Pollution and Cardiometabolic Disease Study. *Hypertension* **2016**, *67*, 77–85. [CrossRef]

7. Leone, N.; Courbon, D.; Thomas, F.; Bean, K.; Jego, B.; Leynaert, B.; Guize, L.; Zureik, M. Lung function impairment and metabolic syndrome: The critical role of abdominal obesity. *Am. J. Respir. Crit. Care Med.* **2009**, *179*, 509–516. [CrossRef] [PubMed]

8. Fiordelisi, A.; Piscitelli, P.; Trimarco, B.; Coscioni, E.; Iaccarino, G.; Sorriento, D. The mechanisms of air pollution and particulate matter in cardiovascular diseases. *Heart Fail. Rev.* **2017**, *22*, 337–347. [CrossRef] [PubMed]

9. Zammit, C.; Liddicoat, H.; Moonsie, I.; Makker, H. Obesity and respiratory diseases. *Int. J. Gen. Med.* **2010**, *3*, 335–343. [CrossRef] [PubMed]

10. Baffi, C.W.; Wood, L.; Winnica, D.; Strollo, P.J., Jr.; Gladwin, M.T.; Que, L.G.; Holguin, F. Metabolic Syndrome and the Lung. *Chest* **2016**, *149*, 1525–1534. [CrossRef]

11. Peters, U.; Suratt, B.T.; Bates, J.H.T.; Dixon, A.E. Beyond BMI: Obesity and Lung Disease. *Chest* **2017**, *153*, 702–709. [CrossRef]

12. Garmendia, J.V.; Moreno, D.; Garcia, A.H.; De Sanctis, J.B. Metabolic syndrome and asthma. *Recent Pat. Endocr. Metab. Immune Drug Discov.* **2014**, *8*, 60–66. [CrossRef] [PubMed]

13. Chen, W.L.; Wang, C.C.; Wu, L.W.; Kao, T.W.; Chan, J.Y.; Chen, Y.J.; Yang, Y.H.; Chang, Y.W.; Peng, T.C. Relationship between lung function and metabolic syndrome. *PLoS ONE* **2014**, *9*, e108989. [CrossRef]

14. Lee, E.J.; In, K.H.; Ha, E.S.; Lee, K.J.; Hur, G.Y.; Kang, E.H.; Jung, K.H.; Lee, S.Y.; Kim, J.H.; Lee, S.Y.; et al. Asthma-like symptoms are increased in the metabolic syndrome. *J. Asthma* **2009**, *46*, 339–342. [CrossRef] [PubMed]

15. Adeyeye, O.O.; Ogbera, A.O.; Ogunleye, O.O.; Brodie-Mens, A.T.; Abolarinwa, F.F.; Bamisile, R.T.; Onadeko, B.O. Understanding asthma and the metabolic syndrome—A Nigerian report. *Int. Arch. Med.* **2012**, *5*, 20. [CrossRef] [PubMed]

16. Ko, S.H.; Jeong, J.; Baeg, M.K.; Han, K.D.; Kim, H.S.; Yoon, J.S.; Kim, H.H.; Kim, J.T.; Chun, Y.H. Lipid profiles in adolescents with and without asthma: Korea National Health and nutrition examination survey data. *Lipids Health Dis.* **2018**, *17*, 158. [CrossRef] [PubMed]

17. Thuesen, B.H.; Husemoen, L.L.; Hersoug, L.G.; Pisinger, C.; Linneberg, A. Insulin resistance as a predictor of incident asthma-like symptoms in adults. *Clin. Exp.* **2009**, *39*, 700–707. [CrossRef]

18. Brumpton, B.M.; Camargo, C.A., Jr.; Romundstad, P.R.; Langhammer, A.; Chen, Y.; Mai, X.M. Metabolic syndrome and incidence of asthma in adults: The HUNT study. *Eur. Respir. J.* **2013**, *42*, 1495–1502. [CrossRef]

19. Singh, V.P.; Aggarwal, R.; Singh, S.; Banik, A.; Ahmad, T.; Patnaik, B.R.; Nappanveettil, G.; Singh, K.P.; Aggarwal, M.L.; Ghosh, B.; et al. Metabolic Syndrome Is Associated with Increased Oxo-Nitrative Stress and Asthma-Like Changes in Lungs. *PLoS ONE* **2015**, *10*, e0129850. [CrossRef]

20. Urman, R.; Eckel, S.; Deng, H.; Berhane, K.; Avol, E.; Lurmann, F.; McConnell, R.; Gilliland, F. Risk Effects of near-Roadway Pollutants and Asthma Status on Bronchitic Symptoms in Children. *Environ. Epidemiol.* **2018**, *2*. [CrossRef]

21. Spira-Cohen, A.; Chen, L.C.; Kendall, M.; Lall, R.; Thurston, G.D. Personal exposures to traffic-related air pollution and acute respiratory health among Bronx schoolchildren with asthma. *Environ. Health Perspect.* **2011**, *119*, 559–565. [CrossRef]

22. Ai, S.; Qian, Z.M.; Guo, Y.; Yang, Y.; Rolling, C.A.; Liu, E.; Wu, F.; Lin, H. Long-term exposure to ambient fine particles associated with asthma: A cross-sectional study among older adults in six low- and middle-income countries. *Environ. Res.* **2019**, *168*, 141–145. [CrossRef] [PubMed]

23. Rom, W.N.; Reibman, J.; Rogers, L.; Weiden, M.D.; Oppenheimer, B.; Berger, K.; Goldring, R.; Harrison, D.; Prezant, D. Emerging exposures and respiratory health: World Trade Center dust. *Proc. Am. Thorac. Soc.* **2010**, *7*, 142–145. [CrossRef]

24. Berger, K.I.; Kalish, S.; Shao, Y.; Marmor, M.; Kazeros, A.; Oppenheimer, B.W.; Chan, Y.; Reibman, J.; Goldring, R.M. Isolated small airway reactivity during bronchoprovocation as a mechanism for respiratory symptoms in WTC dust-exposed community members. *Am. J. Ind. Med.* **2016**, *59*, 767–776. [CrossRef]

25. Aldrich, T.K.; Weakley, J.; Dhar, S.; Hall, C.B.; Crosse, T.; Banauch, G.I.; Weiden, M.D.; Izbicki, G.; Cohen, H.W.; Gupta, A.; et al. Bronchial Reactivity and Lung Function After World Trade Center Exposure. *Chest* **2016**, *150*, 1333–1340. [CrossRef] [PubMed]

26. Prezant, D.J.; Weiden, M.; Banauch, G.I.; McGuinness, G.; Rom, W.N.; Aldrich, T.K.; Kelly, K.J. Cough and bronchial responsiveness in firefighters at the World Trade Center site. *N. Engl. J. Med.* **2002**, *347*, 806–815. [CrossRef]

27. Edelman, P.; Osterloh, J.; Pirkle, J.; Caudill, S.P.; Grainger, J.; Jones, R.; Blount, B.; Calafat, A.; Turner, W.; Feldman, D.; et al. Biomonitoring of chemical exposure among New York City firefighters responding to the World Trade Center fire and collapse. *Environ. Health Perspect.* **2003**, *111*, 1906–1911. [CrossRef] [PubMed]

28. Weiden, M.D.; Naveed, B.; Kwon, S.; Cho, S.J.; Comfort, A.L.; Prezant, D.J.; Rom, W.N.; Nolan, A. Cardiovascular biomarkers predict susceptibility to lung injury in World Trade Center dust-exposed firefighters. *Eur. Respir. J.* **2013**, *41*, 1023–1030. [CrossRef] [PubMed]

29. Liu, X.; Yip, J.; Zeig-Owens, R.; Weakley, J.; Webber, M.P.; Schwartz, T.M.; Prezant, D.J.; Weiden, M.D.; Hall, C.B. The Effect of World Trade Center Exposure on the Timing of Diagnoses of Obstructive Airway Disease, Chronic Rhinosinusitis, and Gastroesophageal Reflux Disease. *Front. Public Health* **2017**, *5*, 2. [CrossRef]

30. Crapo, R.O.; Casaburi, R.; Coates, A.L.; Enright, P.L.; Hankinson, J.L.; Irvin, C.G.; MacIntyre, N.R.; McKay, R.T.; Wanger, J.S.; Anderson, S.D.; et al. Guidelines for methacholine and exercise challenge testing-1999. This official statement of the American Thoracic Society was adopted by the ATS Board of Directors, July 1999. *Am. J. Respir. Crit. Care Med.* **2000**, *161*, 309–329. [CrossRef] [PubMed]

31. Pellegrino, R.; Viegi, G.; Brusasco, V.; Crapo, R.O.; Burgos, F.; Casaburi, R.; Coates, A.; van der Grinten, C.P.; Gustafsson, P.; Hankinson, J.; et al. Interpretative strategies for lung function tests. *Eur. Respir. J.* **2005**, *26*, 948–968. [CrossRef]

32. Alberti, K.G.; Zimmet, P.Z. Definition, diagnosis and classification of diabetes mellitus and its complications. Part 1: Diagnosis and classification of diabetes mellitus provisional report of a WHO consultation. *Diabet. Med.* **1998**, *15*, 539–553. [CrossRef]

33. Ingelsson, E.; Schaefer, E.J.; Contois, J.H.; McNamara, J.R.; Sullivan, L.; Keyes, M.J.; Pencina, M.J.; Schoonmaker, C.; Wilson, P.W.; D'Agostino, R.B.; et al. Clinical utility of different lipid measures for prediction of coronary heart disease in men and women. *JAMA* **2007**, *298*, 776–785. [CrossRef]

34. Lemieux, I.; Lamarche, B.; Couillard, C.; Pascot, A.; Cantin, B.; Bergeron, J.; Dagenais, G.R.; Despres, J.P. Total cholesterol/HDL cholesterol ratio vs. LDL cholesterol/HDL cholesterol ratio as indices of ischemic heart disease risk in men: The Quebec Cardiovascular Study. *Arch. Intern. Med.* **2001**, *161*, 2685–2692. [CrossRef] [PubMed]

35. Keil, U.; Liese, A.D.; Hense, H.W.; Filipiak, B.; Doring, A.; Stieber, J.; Lowel, H. Classical risk factors and their impact on incident non-fatal and fatal myocardial infarction and all-cause mortality in southern Germany—Results from the MONICA Augsburg cohort study 1984–1992. *Eur. Heart J.* **1998**, *19*, 1197–1207. [CrossRef]

36. Weiden, M.D.; Ferrier, N.; Nolan, A.; Rom, W.N.; Comfort, A.; Gustave, J.; Zeig-Owens, R.; Zheng, S.; Goldring, R.M.; Berger, K.I.; et al. Obstructive airways disease with air trapping among firefighters exposed to World Trade Center dust. *Chest* **2010**, *137*, 566–574. [CrossRef] [PubMed]

37. Naveed, B.; Comfort, A.L.; Ferrier, N.; Kasturiarachchi, K.J.; Rom, W.N.; Prezant, D.J.; Weiden, M.D.; Nolan, A. Biomarkers of metabolic syndrome predict accelerated decline of lung function in NYC firefighters that were exposed to WTC particulates. *Am. J. Respir. Crit. Care Med.* **2011**, *183*, A4795. [CrossRef]

38. Kwon, S.; Naveed, B.; Comfort, A.L.; Ferrier, N.; Rom, W.N.; Prezant, D.J.; Nolan, A.; Weiden, M.D. Elevated MMP-3, MMP-12, and TIMP-3 in serum are biomarkers predictive of world trade center-lung injury in New York city firefighters. *Am. J. Respir. Crit. Care Med.* **2012**, *185*, A2019. [CrossRef]

39. Naveed, B.; Kwon, S.; Comfort, A.L.; Ferrier, N.; Rom, W.N.; Prezant, D.J.; Weiden, M.D.; Nolan, A. Cardiovascular serum biomarkers predict world trade center lung injury in NYC firefighters. *Am. J. Respir. Crit. Care Med.* **2012**, *185*, A4894.

40. Naveed, B.; Weiden, M.D.; Kwon, S.; Gracely, E.J.; Comfort, A.L.; Ferrier, N.; Kasturiarachchi, K.J.; Cohen, H.W.; Aldrich, T.K.; Rom, W.N.; et al. Metabolic syndrome biomarkers predict lung function impairment: A nested case-control study. *Am. J. Respir. Crit. Care Med.* **2012**, *185*, 392–399. [CrossRef]

41. Landgren, O.; Zeig-Owens, R.; Giricz, O.; Goldfarb, D.; Murata, K.; Thoren, K.; Ramanathan, L.; Hultcrantz, M.; Dogan, A.; Nwankwo, G.; et al. Multiple Myeloma and Its Precursor Disease Among Firefighters Exposed to the World Trade Center Disaster. *JAMA Oncol.* **2018**, *4*, 821–827. [CrossRef]

42. Haider, S.H.; Kwon, S.; Lam, R.; Lee, A.K.; Caraher, E.J.; Crowley, G.; Zhang, L.; Schwartz, T.M.; Zeig-Owens, R. Liu, M.; et al. Predictive Biomarkers of Gastroesophageal Reflux Disease and Barrett's Esophagus in World Trade Center Exposed Firefighters: A 15 Year Longitudinal Study. *Sci. Rep.* **2018**, *8*, 3106. [CrossRef]

43. Hena, K.M.; Yip, J.; Jaber, N.; Goldfarb, D.; Fullam, K.; Cleven, K.; Moir, W.; Zeig-Owens, R.; Webber, M.P.; Spevack, D.M.; et al. Clinical Course of Sarcoidosis in World Trade Center-Exposed Firefighters. *Chest* **2018**, *153*, 114–123. [CrossRef]

44. Cho, S.J.; Echevarria, G.C.; Kwon, S.; Naveed, B.; Schenck, E.J.; Tsukiji, J.; Rom, W.N.; Prezant, D.J.; Nolan, A.; Weiden, M.D. One airway: Biomarkers of protection from upper and lower airway injury after World Trade Center exposure. *Respir. Med.* **2014**, *108*, 162–170. [CrossRef]

45. Nolan, A.; Naveed, B.; Comfort, A.L.; Ferrier, N.; Hall, C.B.; Kwon, S.; Kasturiarachchi, K.J.; Cohen, H.W.; Zeig-Owens, R.; Glaser, M.S.; et al. Inflammatory biomarkers predict airflow obstruction after exposure to World Trade Center dust. *Chest* **2012**, *142*, 412–418. [CrossRef]

46. Lippman, M.; Cohen, M.D.; Chen, L.C. Health effects of World Trade Center (WTC) Dust: An unprecedented disaster with inadequate risk management. *Critical Reviews in Toxicology.* **2015**, *45*, 492–530. [CrossRef]

47. Crowley, G.; Kwon, S.; Haider, S.H.; Caraher, E.J.; Lam, R.; St-Jules, D.E.; Liu, M.; Prezant, D.J.; Nolan, A. Metabolomics of World Trade Center-Lung Injury: A machine learning approach. *BMJ Open Respir. Res.* **2018**, *5*, e000274 [CrossRef]

48. Lioy, P.J.; Weisel, C.P.; Millette, J.R.; Eisenreich, S.; Vallero, D.; Offenberg, J.; Buckley, B.; Turpin, B.; Zhong, M.; Cohen, M.D.; et al. Characterization of the dust/smoke aerosol that settled east of the World Trade Center (WTC) in lower Manhattan after the collapse of the WTC 11 September 2001. *Environ. Health Perspect* **2002**, *110*, 703–714. [CrossRef]

49. Levin, S.; Herbert, R.; Skloot, G.; Szeinuk, J.; Teirstein, A.; Fischler, D.; Milek, D.; Piligian, G.; Wilk-Rivard, E.; Moline, J. Health effects of World Trade Center site workers. *Am. J. Ind. Med.* **2002**, *42*, 545–547. [CrossRef]

50. Banauch, G.I.; Dhala, A.; Alleyne, D.; Alva, R.; Santhyadka, G.; Krasko, A.; Weiden, M.; Kelly, K.J.; Prezant, D.J. Bronchial hyperreactivity and other inhalation lung injuries in rescue/recovery workers after the World Trade Center collapse. *Crit. Care Med.* **2005**, *33*, S102–S106. [CrossRef]

51. Landrigan, P.J.; Lioy, P.J.; Thurston, G.; Berkowitz, G.; Chen, L.C.; Chillrud, S.N.; Gavett, S.H.; Georgopoulos, P.G.; Geyh, A.S.; Levin, S.; et al. Health and environmental consequences of the world trade center disaster. *Environ. Health Perspect.* **2004**, *112*, 731–739. [CrossRef]

52. Farfel, M.; DiGrande, L.; Brackbill, R.; Prann, A.; Cone, J.; Friedman, S.; Walker, D.J.; Pezeshki, G.; Thomas, P.; Galea, S.; et al. An overview of 9/11 experiences and respiratory and mental health conditions among World Trade Center Health Registry enrollees. *J. Urban Health* **2008**, *85*, 880–909. [CrossRef]

53. Aldrich, T.K.; Vossbrinck, M.; Zeig-Owens, R.; Hall, C.B.; Schwartz, T.M.; Moir, W.; Webber, M.P.; Cohen, H.W.; Nolan, A.; Weiden, M.D.; et al. Lung Function Trajectories in World Trade Center-Exposed New York City Firefighters Over 13 Years: The Roles of Smoking and Smoking Cessation. *Chest* **2016**, *149*, 1419–1427. [CrossRef] [PubMed]

54. Niles, J.K.; Webber, M.P.; Cohen, H.W.; Hall, C.B.; Zeig-Owens, R.; Ye, F.; Glaser, M.S.; Weakley, J.; Weiden, M.D.; Aldrich, T.K.; et al. The respiratory pyramid: From symptoms to disease in World Trade Center exposed firefighters. *Am. J. Ind. Med.* **2013**, *56*, 870–880. [CrossRef] [PubMed]

55. Zeig-Owens, R.; Singh, A.; Aldrich, T.K.; Hall, C.B.; Schwartz, T.; Webber, M.P.; Cohen, H.W.; Kelly, K.J.; Nolan, A.; Prezant, D.J.; et al. Blood Leukocyte Concentrations, FEV1 Decline, and Airflow Limitation. A 15-Year Longitudinal Study of World Trade Center-exposed Firefighters. *Ann. Am. Thorac. Soc.* **2018**, *15*, 173–183. [CrossRef] [PubMed]

56. Kerkhof, M.; Tran, T.N.; van den Berge, M.; Brusselle, G.G.; Gopalan, G.; Jones, R.C.M.; Kocks, J.W.H.; Menzies-Gow, A.; Nuevo, J.; Pavord, I.D.; et al. Association between blood eosinophil count and risk of readmission for patients with asthma: Historical cohort study. *PLoS ONE* **2018**, *13*, e0201143. [CrossRef] [PubMed]

57. Price, D.B.; Rigazio, A.; Campbell, J.D.; Bleecker, E.R.; Corrigan, C.J.; Thomas, M.; Wenzel, S.E.; Wilson, A.M.; Small, M.B.; Gopalan, G.; et al. Blood eosinophil count and prospective annual asthma disease burden: A UK cohort study. *Lancet Respir. Med.* **2015**, *3*, 849–858. [CrossRef]

58. Bolton, C.E.; Evans, M.; Ionescu, A.A.; Edwards, S.M.; Morris, R.H.; Dunseath, G.; Luzio, S.D.; Owens, D.R.; Shale, D.J. Insulin resistance and inflammation—A further systemic complication of COPD. *J. Chron. Obstruct. Pulm. Dis.* **2007**, *4*, 121–126. [CrossRef] [PubMed]

59. Caraher, E.J.; Kwon, S.; Haider, S.H.; Crowley, G.; Lee, A.; Ebrahim, M.; Zhang, L.; Chen, L.C.; Gordon, T.; Liu, M.; et al. Receptor for advanced glycation end-products and World Trade Center particulate induced lung function loss: A case-cohort study and murine model of acute particulate exposure. *PLoS ONE* **2017**, *12*, e0184331. [CrossRef]

60. Scott, H.A.; Gibson, P.G.; Garg, M.L.; Wood, L.G. Airway inflammation is augmented by obesity and fatty acids in asthma. *Eur. Respir. J.* **2011**, *38*, 594–602. [CrossRef]

61. Wadden, D.; Allwood Newhook, L.A.; Twells, L.; Farrell, J.; Gao, Z.W. Sex-Specific Association between Childhood BMI Trajectories and Asthma Phenotypes. *Int. J. Pediat.* **2018**, *2018*, 9057435. [CrossRef] [PubMed]

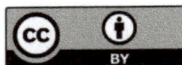

International Journal of
*Environmental Research
and Public Health*

MDPI

Article

A Quality Improvement Assessment of the Delivery of Mental Health Services among WTC Responders Treated in the Community

Mayer Bellehsen [1], Jacqueline Moline [2,*], Rehana Rasul [3], Kristin Bevilacqua [2],
Samantha Schneider [2], Jason Kornrich [4] and Rebecca M. Schwartz [5]

[1] Department of Psychiatry, Unified Behavioral Health Center and World Trade Center Health Program,
    Northwell Health, 132 East Main Street, Bay Shore, NY 11706, USA; mbellehsen@northwell.edu
[2] Department of Occupational Medicine, Epidemiology and Prevention, Northwell Health, 175 Community
    Drive, Great Neck, NY 11021, USA; kbevilacqu@northwell.edu (K.B.); sschneide5@northwell.edu (S.S.)
[3] Department of Biostatistics and Department of Occupational Medicine, Epidemiology and Prevention,
    Northwell Health, 175 Community Drive, Great Neck, NY 11021, USA; rrasul@northwell.edu
[4] World Trade Center Health Center, Northwell Health, 97-77 Queens Blvd, Rego Park, NY 11374, USA;
    jkornrich@northwell.edu
[5] Feinstein Institute for Medical Research, Department of Occupational Medicine, Epidemiology and
    Prevention and Northwell Health and Joint Center for Trauma, Disaster Health and Resilience at Mount
    Sinai, Stony Brook University, and Northwell Health, 175 Community Drive, Great Neck, NY 11021, USA;
    rschwartz3@northwell.edu
* Correspondence jmoline@northwell.edu; Tel.: +1-516-465-2639

Received: 28 February 2019; Accepted: 24 April 2019; Published: 30 April 2019

Abstract: The World Trade Center Health Program (WTCHP) provides mental health services through diverse service delivery mechanisms, however there are no current benchmarks to evaluate utilization or quality. This quality improvement (QI) initiative sought to examine the delivery and effectiveness of WTCHP mental health services for World Trade Center (WTC) responders who receive care through the Northwell Health Clinical Center of Excellence (CCE), and to characterize the delivery of evidence-based treatments (EBT) for mental health (MH) difficulties in this population. Methods include an analysis of QI data from the Northwell CCE, and annual WTCHP monitoring data for all responders certified for mental health treatment. Nearly 48.9% of enrolled responders with a WTC-certified diagnosis utilized treatment. The majority of treatment delivered was focused on WTC-related conditions. There was significant disagreement between provider-reported EBT use and independently-evaluated delivery of EBT (95.6% vs. 54.8%, $p \leq 0.001$). EBT delivery was associated with a small decrease in Posttraumatic Stress Disorder (PTSD) symptoms over time. Providers engaged in the process of data collection, but there were challenges with adherence to outcome monitoring and goal setting. Data from this report can inform continued QI efforts in the WTCHP, as well as the implementation and evaluation of EBT.

Keywords: disaster mental health; evidence-based treatment; mental health service utilization; quality improvement

1. Introduction

1.1. WTC Responders' Mental Health

Following the September 11, 2001 attacks on the World Trade Center (WTC), an estimated 90,000 World Trade Center responders (WTC responders) provided emergency services at Ground Zero, where they were exposed to unprecedented traumatic events [1] while providing rescue, recovery, demolition, debris removal, and related support services in the aftermath of the attack. Symptoms of PTSD, depression, panic disorder, and anxiety have been observed in WTC responders over 10 years after the events of 9/11 [2–14].

The rate of PTSD among WTC responders continues to be significantly higher than in the general population, and is the most prevalent mental health (MH) diagnosis for responders and clean-up workers at Ground Zero [2]. One study found that 9.7% of WTC responders interviewed 11–13 years after 9/11 met the criteria for current PTSD [7], compared to the estimated lifetime PTSD prevalence in the general United States population of 6.4% [15]. Furthermore, a study of over 10,000 WTC responders found that nearly 7% experienced a delayed onset of symptoms up to 8 years after 9/11, and the risk of stable or worsening PTSD among first responders is supported in the literature [16].

Limited research has been conducted on treatment for PTSD in a first responder population [17]. Three studies have examined the efficacy of specific treatment modalities among WTC responders, including combined prolonged exposure and paroxetine [18], cognitive behavioral treatment [19], and virtual reality exposure therapy [20]. These studies have been limited in several important ways including the use of diverse exposure assessment tools limiting comparability and small sample sizes [21]. The generalizability of these studies to clinical settings is somewhat limited, in that these studies examine treatment outcomes within a clinical trial, and can speak to treatment efficacy. However, they do not necessarily reflect MH utilization and treatment outcomes among WTC responders obtaining routine treatment for PTSD, thereby hindering conclusions regarding clinical effectiveness. In addition, the studies were university-based, and not reflective of care provided in the community. To our knowledge, no studies have focused on the evaluation of treatments for other mental health difficulties (besides PTSD), specifically among WTC responders, including depression and anxiety [21]. Little is also known as to the extent to which WTC responders are obtaining recommended evidence-based treatments (EBTs) for their mental health diagnoses, including PTSD, or the impact of treatment upon their symptoms.

1.2. Mental Health Service Provision for WTC Responders

The WTC Health Program (WTCHP) (previously known as the Medical Monitoring and Treatment Program) was established in 2002 to address the physical and mental health needs of WTC responders through annual medical monitoring, and then through the delivery of no-cost medical services [1]. WTC responders treated through the WTCHP (WTCHP responders) include traditional first responder professionals, such as police, paramedics and non-FDNY firefighters, as well as non-traditional responders like construction workers and vehicle maintenance workers. To date, an estimated 45,894 WTC responders have had at least one monitoring visit as part of the WTCHP. The structure of the program's service delivery efforts rests on partnerships between hospital systems and community practitioners to meet the needs of the population. Clinical Centers of Excellence (CCE) are responsible for monitoring the well-being of participants, and then authorizing physical and mental health treatment in the community. Mental health services coordinated by CCEs are delivered through a provider network that is comprised of health system-attached clinics and private practice-based clinicians enrolled by the CCE. A recent report [22] indicated that in 2017, about 5% of continuously-enrolled WTCHP responders utilized MH services (excluding pharmacy), and 99% of these services were delivered in an outpatient setting. However, utilization rates varied among sub-groups of members and by each individual CCE, and little is known about the quality and effectiveness of the treatment provided. This gap warrants attention, given the high prevalence of PTSD, depression, and anxiety in this population.

Mental health programs and systems of care that have focused on improving the quality of services and effectiveness of treatment have broadly targeted two areas for intervention: Supporting evidence-based practice implementation (EBPI), and measurement-based quality improvement (MBQI) [23,24]. Treatment recommendations for PTSD include first-line recommendation on the delivery of trauma-focused EBTs (TF-EBTs), such as Prolonged Exposure therapy and Cognitive

Processing Therapy [25,26]. Despite these recommendations, it is known that, in general, providers do not sufficiently use research to inform practice [27].

Prior to a heavy investment by the Veterans Administration (VA) to support implementation of EBTs for PTSD, one survey showed that as few as 10% of PTSD specialists and general MH providers utilized evidence-based treatments for PTSD [28]. Since the VA investment in implementation of TF-EBTs in 2006, progress has been made, yet penetration of these treatments is highly variable, and challenges remain [29,30].

1.3. Quality Improvement Initiative

The provision of no-cost MH services to a large cohort of responders and the longitudinal, standardized monitoring of a large cohort of WTC responders through the WTCHP presents a unique opportunity to better understand the delivery and effectiveness of mental health care services for this population. The current analysis aims to characterize the provision of mental health services to WTC responders within the Northwell Health Queens World Trade Center Health Program, also referred to as the Northwell Clinical Center of Excellence (CCE). Data for this analysis relies on a quality improvement project that was initiated in late 2017. It entails modification of treatment plan data collected in the course of administering the program to obtain information on the interventions being utilized, and to require greater movement towards measurement-based care. In addition, WTCHP annual monitoring and claims data can be used to verify the information and findings from the treatment plan data. The goal of the quality improvement project is to characterize the mental health services delivered to clients, to begin implementing an MBQI process, and to explore delivery of recommended EBT for PTSD and other WTC-certified mental health diagnoses to WTCHP responders being treated for mental health difficulties by community providers. Upon characterizing the population and understanding baseline data, program interventions can be designed to promote engagement in care, as well as enhanced services and outcomes for the population.

2. Materials and Methods

2.1. Data Sources

This is a quality improvement initiative, focused on a subset of community mental health providers who provide psychotherapy to World Trade Center Health Program (WTCHP) responders (i.e., WTC responders to 9/11, excluding FDNY firefighters) served by the Northwell Center of Excellence (CCE). The Northwell CCE Treatment Plan Database was started in December 2017 to monitor mental health treatment delivery and outcomes, and consider targets for quality improvement. Community mental health providers for the Northwell CCE include psychiatrists, psychologists, and clinical social workers spread across the community, some of whom are attached to a Northwell Health ambulatory program. Due to logistical challenges, such as administrative burden, and the fact that the ambulatory programs have their own processes for QI, efforts were initiated with just psychotherapists located in private practices in the community. Within this group, 100% of providers were able to provide treatment plan data. The project was submitted to the Northwell Health IRB for evaluation as research, and deemed as non-human subjects research, due to its quality improvement (QI) focus. Providers had already been completing treatment plans regarding the mental health treatment of WTCHP responders, but these were not developed or analyzed in a systematic manner. Members of this team modified the plans to ensure that they include items to assess modality of treatment, descriptions of treatment, including whether or not the provider believed that the treatment was evidence based, goals for treatment, scores on standardized measures of symptoms, expected duration of treatment, and explanation of the connection between treatment and 9/11 exposure. Providers were engaged prior to the modifications of the treatment plans, and then again after the plans were modified, to inform them of changes to the treatment plans, and to answer questions. The Northwell CCE team was also available for questions as they arose. Follow-up treatment plans are completed every four months, and the data is inputted into the database by a Northwell CCE staff member. For the current analysis, data from baseline (Review 1) and the first four month follow-up time point (Review 2) were used.

Data from annual monitoring visits collected for the WTCHP General Responder Cohort for all Northwell CCE responders certified for mental health treatment were also obtained and linked to the Treatment Plan Database, to provide annual survey and administrative claims data, which included demographics, mental health diagnoses, standardized scores of mental health symptoms, and mental healthcare utilization data.

2.2. Treatment Plan Data

Data reported from the Northwell CCE community provider network included provider-reported used of evidence-based treatments (EBT) (yes/no), goals requested in a specific (or simple), measureable, achievable, relevant, and time-framed (SMART) format, treatment modality (i.e., individual weekly, family, group, medication management) type of therapy used, whether treatment was WTC-focused, and the expected length of further treatment. Mental health symptom scores were also reported.

Primary variables of interest: To evaluate whether recommended EBT was delivered to the WTCHP responder, treatment plans were reviewed by two independent psychologists with backgrounds in EBT for mental health (MH) disorders, with particular expertise in working with responders. A standardized decision process was formulated to make this decision. This included alignment between diagnosis and indicated EBT, that the provider was utilizing as per the American Psychological Association (APA), Veterans Administration/Department Of Defense (VA/DOD), and National Institute for Health and Care Excellence treatment recommendations, where available [31–33]. Information from other sections of the treatment plan was also utilized. For example, reference to exposure-based goals (for Posttraumatic Stress Disorder (PTSD)) was indicative of some EBT use. Therapy was categorized by reviewers as: Cognitive Behavioral Therapy (CBT), Trauma-Focused Evidence-Based Therapies (e.g., Prolonged Exposure, Cognitive Processing Therapy etc.), non-trauma focused evidence-based therapies for PTSD (e.g., Interpersonal Psychotherapy, Stress Inoculation Therapy, etc.), eclectic/supportive therapy, mindfulness/relaxation therapy, psychodynamic therapy, and non-recommended therapies for PTSD (e.g., "Emotional Freedom Technique"). The determinations for which therapies are considered recommended for PTSD, were those based on the treatment guidelines noted above. Therapies which did not meet any criteria for a recommendation based on these guidelines may still have an evidence base, but it was categorized as non-recommended. The variable (i.e., independent reviewer assessment of recommended EBT delivery) was labeled *EBT Delivered* and categorized as: Yes, No, Elements of EBT-Delivered, and Cannot Interpret from Clinician's Report. For analysis, EBT-Delivered was dichotomized as Yes (Yes or Elements of EBT-Delivered), or No. Cases where EBT-Delivered could not be interpreted from the clinician's report ($n = 4$), were excluded for analysis for this variable.

Reviewers also independently evaluated provider-reported therapy, use of SMART goals, and whether or not treatment had a WTC focus. Providers were expected to list goals in SMART format, which is frequently used as a frame for goal setting across disciplines. This format facilitates the reporting of measurable progress for WTCHP responders, even in the absence of EBT and standardized symptom measurement. Providers were also asked to elaborate on whether or not their treatment had a WTC focus, which was then reviewed.

Lastly, providers were asked to include symptom severity scores by utilizing self-report instruments with clients, summing the items to calculate symptom scores, and then including the final score in their treatment plans. For PTSD symptom severity, providers used the Posttraumatic Stress Disorder Checklist-5 (PCL-5)—a 20 item measure of PTSD (range = 0–80) [34]. For depression symptom severity, providers used the Patient Health Questionnaire-9 (PHQ-9)—a nine item measure of depressive symptoms (range = 0–27) [35]. For anxiety symptom severity, providers utilized the General Anxiety Disorder-7 Item (GAD-7)—a seven item measure of anxiety symptoms [36].

2.3. WTCHP Annual Medical-Monitoring Data

Mental healthcare utilization was extracted from administrative claims out of the WTC annual monitoring data for all Northwell CCE responders certified for MH (*N* = 477). Utilization during 2018 was defined as having at least one claim for psychotherapeutic services, diagnostic evaluation, or medication management. Psychotherapy treatment modality (individual, family), length of treatment session (20–30 min, 45–60 min), and number of medication management appointments, were also tabulated. The number of sessions per WTCHP responder within each year was also determined.

The WTCHP Annual Medical-Monitoring data also provided demographics including age, sex (male/female), race, ethnicity, and education (<high school (HS), ≥HS). ICD-9 and ICD-10 codes were extracted to define WTC-related certified mental health diagnoses of PTSD, anxiety and depression. PTSD, anxiety and depression symptom scores were measured annually, using the PCL-S (specific to the WTC terrorist attacks on 9/11, PHQ-9, and GAD-7 scales, respectively. For each instrument separately, items were summed to create symptom severity scores for PTSD (range = 17–85) [37], depression (range = 0–27) [35], and anxiety (range = 0–21) [36]. In our sample, the reliability of these instruments was high (Cronbach's alpha: PCL-S = 0.949, GAD-7 = 0.914, PHQ-9 = 0.921).

2.4. Statistical Analysis

From the WTCHP Annual medical-monitoring data, mental healthcare utilization rates and number of sessions per WTCHP responder were described for 2018 overall, and for the responders treated by the Northwell CCE community provider network. In the Treatment Plan Database, WTCHP responder characteristics at first review were compared by EBT-Delivered, using the Mann-Whitney Rank Sum test for continuous variables, and Fisher's exact test for categorical variables. McNemar's test and the Kappa statistic were used to evaluate any agreement between provider-reported EBT and EBT-Delivered.

For WTCHP responders where MH symptom scores at both review 1 and 2 were available, the change in mental health symptom scores between the reviews were described using mean differences overall, and were stratified by EBT-Delivered. To assess the sensitivity of the Treatment Plan Database results, the change between MH symptom scores between the last two annual monitoring visits from the WTC-data monitoring data, was also analyzed. For this analysis, WTCHP responders from the Treatment Plan Database were linked to their annual monitoring visit data, and included if they had two annual visits from 2016 to 2018 (*N* = 86). Analyses were conducted using SAS software, version 9.4 (SAS Institute, Cary, NC, USA).

3. Results

Of the 477 WTCHP responders certified for MH, 48.9% utilized mental healthcare in 2018 (Table 1). WTCHP responders utilized: Diagnostic evaluation (14.9%), psychotherapeutic services (41.3%), and/or medication management (8.2%). Of WTCHP responders who utilized psychotherapeutic services (*n* = 197), all had individual sessions, and 92.4% of them lasted between 45–60 min. Only 3% also had a family session. About one third of WTCHP responders (35.5%) also had diagnostic evaluation or medication management. WTCHP responders had a median number of 17 (IQR = 5–34) individual therapy sessions in 2018. As expected, utilization rates were high among WTCHP responders captured through the Treatment Plan Database.

From the Northwell Treatment Plan Database, data were collected from 16 providers on 129 WTCHP responders at the first review, and of those, 103 had a second review. During the four month review period, providers conducted a median of 11 sessions (IQR = 2–37, range = 1–64), and saw a median of 5.6 (range = 1–29) WTCHP responders. WTCHP responders were 55.3 (SD = 9.6) years old on average, 32.8% female, and 40.2% white (Table 2). Most were diagnosed with PTSD (74.4%) and some had anxiety (24.8%) and depression (34.1%) diagnoses. The majority underwent weekly individual therapy

(72.1%), and the estimated length of further treatment was 12 months for 61.7% of WTCHP responders. Two WTCHP responders were indicated to have group therapy as well.

Providers reported that nearly 94% of services delivered were evidence-based treatments with the majority of providers reporting delivering CBT (74.4%), and mindfulness or relaxation therapy (19.4%). Notably, despite reporting delivery of EBTs, providers also reported delivering eclectic/supportive therapy (which are not categorized as EBTs) 23.3% of the time. Based on the independent QI review, treatment was determined to be largely WTC-focused (85.3%). However, some of the provider responses were characterized as "unclear" (14%).

Table 1. Mental healthcare utilization by service type from January 2018–December 2018.

Type	Northwell Health CCE Responders (N = 477)			Community Provider Network (N = 124 [a])		
	n	%	No. Sessions/WTCHPR Med (IQR)	n	% [b]	No. Sessions/WTCHPR Med (IQR)
Overall MH Utilization	233	48.9	13 (3–30)	118	95.2	27 (15–43)
Diagnostic Evaluation	71	14.9	1 (1–2)	7	5.7	2 (1–2)
Medication Management	39	8.2	4 (2–8)	19	15.3	6 (2–8)
Psychotherapeutic Services	197	41.3	17 (5–34)	117	94.4	27 (16–40)
Family	6	1.3	1 (1–2)	6	4.8	1 (1–2)
Individual	197	41.3	15 (5–34)	117	94.4	26 (13–40)
20–30 min TX	37	7.8	2 (1–4)	15	12.1	3 (1–4)
45–60 min TX	182	38.2	18.5 (6–35)	114	91.9	27 (15–40)

MH = mental health. TX = treatment. No. = number. WTCHPR = World Trade Center Health Program Responder. Med = median. IQR = Interquartile range. [a] Of the 129 WTCHP responders in the Treatment Database, those who were transferred out of the Northwell CCE were not included in the WTCHP Annual Monitoring data (n = 5). [b] Mental healthcare utilization was not 100% for WTCHP responders in the Treatment Database. This may be due to the lag time in processing claims in the annual monitoring data.

Almost all providers in the community provider network (96.0) reported using EBT. For those providers that indicated the use of EBT, treatment plans were reviewed by independent Northwell CCE reviewers to determine EBT-Delivered status. Sixteen WTCHP responders (12.4%) were assessed to have likely received EBT, and 52 (40.3%) were assessed to have likely received elements of EBT at baseline. There was also a significant disagreement between provider-reported EBT use and an independently-evaluated delivery of EBT (95.6% vs. 54.8%, McNemar's test $p < 0.001$, Kappa coefficient = 0.097 (95% CI = 0.015–0.179)). Demographics and WTC-certified diagnoses were similar across WTCHP responders, with EBT-Delivered compared to not (Table 2). Use of SMART goals (70.6% vs. 24.6%) and number of SMART goals ≥3 (89.71% vs. 59.7%), were more frequent with patients who had EBT delivery. Additionally, when EBT was not delivered, WTCHP responders had higher levels of missing documentation of goal progress (35.1% vs. 14.7%), and a longer length of further treatment (80.7% vs. 43.9%).

Among all WTCHP responders where MH symptom scores at both review 1 and 2 were available, PTSD anxiety, and depression symptom scores improved by 1.81, 0.46, and 0.03 points, respectively. When compared by EBT Delivered, similar changes were noted. PTSD symptom scores decreased 2.29 points in the four month period for those with EBT-Delivered. There was also a weaker mean decrease of 1.42 points among the group without EBP delivery. WTCHP responders with and without EBT-Delivered also had small decreases from review 1 to review 2 in mean anxiety and depression symptom scores (Table 3). The analysis of the WTC annual monitoring data also indicated small symptom changes over time by EBT provision (Table 3).

Table 2. Characteristics (%) compared by reviewer-assessed EBT delivery.

Variable	Category	Total (N = 129)		EBT = No (N = 57) [a]		EBT = Yes (N = 68) [a]		p Value
		n	%	n	%	n	%	
Demographics								
Age, mean (SD) [b]		55.3 (9.6)		55.1 (11.6)		55.1 (7.8)		0.984
Gender	Male	82	67.2	38	71.7	40	61.5	0.329
	Female	40	32.8	15	28.3	25	38.5	
Race [c]	White or Caucasian	49	40.2	22	41.5	26	40.0	0.244
	Black or African American	20	16.4	10	18.9	8	12.3	
	Other/Unknown	53	43.5	21	39.7	31	47.7	
Ethnicity [c]	Non-Hispanic	48	53.3	24	64.9	22	44.0	0.082
	Hispanic	42	46.7	13	35.1	28	56.0	
Education [c]	<HS	17	15.9	5	11.4	12	20.3	0.288
	≥HS	90	84.1	39	88.6	47	79.7	
Language [c]	English	95	78.5	47	88.7	45	70.3	**0.023**
	Spanish	26	21.5	6	11.3	19	29.7	
Certified MH Conditions								
Anxiety	No	97	75.2	47	82.5	47	69.1	0.099
	Yes	32	24.8	10	17.5	21	30.9	
Depression	No	85	65.9	35	61.4	49	72.1	0.252
	Yes	44	34.1	22	38.6	19	27.9	
PTSD	No	33	25.6	12	21.1	20	29.4	0.311
	Yes	96	74.4	45	79.0	48	70.6	
Treatment Related								
World Trade Center (WTC) Focus [c]	Yes	110	85.3	39	68.4	67	98.5	**<0.001**
	No	1	0.8	1	1.8	0	0.0	
	Unclear	18	14.0	17	29.8	1	1.5	
SMART Goals present [c]	SMART Goals Present	25	19.4	3	5.3	22	32.4	**<0.001**
	Some SMART Goals Present	37	28.7	11	19.3	26	38.2	
	Goals, Not SMART	42	32.6	32	56.1	9	13.2	
	Goals, partially SMART	22	17.1	9	15.8	11	16.2	
	No Goals	3	2.3	2	3.5	0	0.0	

Table 2. *Cont.*

Variable	Category	Total (N = 129)		EBT = No (N = 57) [a]		EBT = Yes (N = 68) [a]		p Value
		n	%	n	%	n	%	
Number of SMART Goals	<3	33	25.6	23	40.4	7	10.3	**<0.001**
	≥3	96	74.4	34	59.7	61	89.7	
Length of further treatment (months) [c]	≤8	48	37.8	11	19.3	37	56.1	**<0.001**
	≥12	79	62.2	46	80.7	29	43.9	
Documented Progress on ≥ 1 goal [c]	Yes	66	51.6	29	50.9	35	51.5	**0.001**
	No	31	24.2	20	35.1	10	14.7	
	Can't Interpret from clinician's report	19	14.8	8	14.0	11	16.2	
	Initial Goal	12	9.4	0	0.0	12	17.7	
Treatment type [c]	Weekly individual therapy	93	72.1	43	75.4	46	67.7	0.428
	<Weekly individual therapy	36	27.9	14	24.6	22	32.4	

EBT = reviewer assessed evidence-based treatment. SD = standard deviation. MH = mental health. HS = high school. PTSD = Post-traumatic stress disorder. SA = substance abuse. TX = treatment. Med = median. IQR = Interquartile range. [a] Four WTCHP responders are missing an EBP-Delivered classification, because reviewers could not determine it from the clinician's report. [b] *p* Value for continuous variables based on the Mann Whitney Rank Sum test. [c] *p* Value for categorical variables based on Fisher's exact test. Bold: *p* < 0.05.

Table 3. Mental health symptom scores at review 1 and review 2 compared by study variables.

MH Symptom Score	EBT	N	Period 1 Mean (SD)	Period 2 Mean (SD)	Mean Change
Using TX Plan Data with Four Month Follow Up					
PTSD symptom score (using PCL-5)	No	24	33.04 (17.21)	31.63 (17.12)	−1.42
	Yes	28	38.61 (16.09)	36.32 (15.76)	−2.29
Anxiety symptom score	No	27	9.56 (5.06)	9.44 (5.44)	−0.11
	Yes	25	12.44 (5.51)	11.56 (5.42)	−0.88
Depression symptom score	No	27	9.81 (5.21)	9.74 (5.1)	−0.07
	Yes	24	10.54 (5.45)	10.38 (5.25)	−0.17
Using Monitoring Data with One Year Follow Up					
PTSD symptom score (using PCL-S)	No	28	43.52 (15.25)	45.16 (16.01)	1.64
	Yes	33	53.06 (13.17)	55.41 (13.74)	2.35
Anxiety symptom score	No	17	8.53 (4.05)	8.18 (4.79)	−0.35
	Yes	24	9.71 (4.29)	10 (3.6)	0.29
Depression symptom score	No	27	9.08 (5.32)	8.34 (5.23)	−0.75
	Yes	30	10.26 (5.84)	10.24 (6.06)	−0.02

MH = mental health. EBT = reviewer-assessed evidence based treatment. Med = Median. IQR = Interquartile range. PTSD = Posttraumatic stress disorder. TX = treatment. PCL-5 = Posttraumatic Stress Disorder Checklist-5.

4. Discussion

This project has yielded numerous findings and considerations for future efforts. Consistent with a recent HRA report on service utilization, our team found that among WTCHP responders with a WTC-certified mental health diagnosis, nearly 49% utilized mental health care [22]. That report found the Northwell CCE had service utilization of 55%, but their analysis included the removal of responders that may have unenrolled in the program, or were deceased. This information was not available to us for this project, and it is likely that if this information were accounted for, the overall cohort would shrink, and the utilization rate would further rise. This level of service utilization meets the national average [22] for access indicated in the HRA report, and speaks to the value of using a community provider network to ensure access for WTCHP responders.

It was also meaningful that most providers (85%) were providing treatment that was deemed as targeted towards the WTC-attributed diagnosis. Consistent with the literature, the most prominent MH diagnosis for the overall cohort at the Northwell CCE was PTSD. Most providers indicated that they were working on goals that were related to the sequelae of 9/11, such as PTSD and its associated impact on interpersonal functioning. This is a difficult variable to assess, as treatment is not being directly observed, but these findings are promising for adherence to WTCHP objectives.

This QI project was also notable for the high rate of participation by providers in the process. The providers were familiar with completing some information for treatment plans as part of past program expectations, but this project included a more robust overhaul of the treatment plan process. There were challenges with framing goals in a SMART format, and with ensuring the collection of all outcome data, but most providers completed numerous data elements for the treatment plans, despite the extra reporting requirements. For example, almost no providers submitted treatment plans without goals, and the majority of providers documented progress on at least one goal. Even among providers who had missing outcome measures, many of these providers completed some data points. Importantly, the providers whose treatment plans were evaluated, were also engaged in the development of the plans. Quality improvement is seen as a bottom up process, and stakeholder engagement is therefore critical to implementing systems change, which likely contributed to this high participation [24].

The finding that there was an association among providers between delivering EBT services and a greater use of SMART goals was interesting. Without further exploration into this association, it is difficult to say why this occurred, but it may reflect some underlying shared attribute among those providers towards utilization of measurable objectives and provision of EBT services. Frequent utilization of measurement tools is consistent with expectations of EBTs, and may help explain this association. Informal conversations with providers who had difficulty around both the SMART goal format and reporting on outcome measures, indicated numerous challenges, such as confusion about what SMART formats entailed, and challenges obtaining measures from WTCHP responders. Future efforts of this QI project should include further education of providers on how to meet these types of objectives and engage with providers on problem solving challenges to obtain outcome measurements.

Interestingly, nearly all providers in this project claimed to be providing EBT to the majority of their clients. This is a higher number than expected, and was unforeseen for numerous reasons. As noted earlier, even when providers are trained in EBTs, and are provided institutional support to execute these treatments, penetration is challenging [29]. Furthermore, it has been often reported that there is a gap between clinical research and practice [27]. Additionally, while providers endorsed utilizing an EBT, a significant number of them endorsed utilizing eclectic/supportive therapies, and many indicated utilizing therapies for PTSD that are not recommended as EBTs for PTSD. It is therefore not surprising that upon independent review by Northwell CCE psychologists, there was significant disagreement with the provider report. Only about 12% of WTCHP responders were deemed to have likely been in receipt of a recommended EBT, and an additional 40% were considered to have likely received some elements of an EBT, such as cognitive restructuring or exposure therapy. Notably, even these numbers may be an over-representation of true EBT delivery, as treatment was not observed directly, and no treatment fidelity checks were in place.

Additionally, many of the clients were deemed by providers to require an additional 12 months of treatment, and the median number of sessions per WTCHP annual monitoring data for 2018 was 27 sessions. This would be inconsistent with expectations of many EBTs that typically range from 8 to 20 sessions. Accurate assessment of EBT delivery is a challenging endeavor that will continue to require attention if this is an area of priority for the WTCHP.

When recommended EBT or components of EBT were deemed to have been delivered, the WTCHP responders demonstrated small improvements in measures of PTSD symptoms. This was notable for PCL-5 scores that were attained using the Treatment Plan Database, however, these changes were below the 10 point change that is considered a clinically significant change [38]. Additionally, no significant changes in PTSD symptoms were observed with the data collected from the annual monitoring exam. While the time between measurements on the annual monitoring exam is about one year, as compared to the four months in the Treatment Plan Database, the overall negligible movement in the measurement of symptoms warrants further exploration. It may be that even in cases of clients deemed to be receiving recommended EBTs, they are not receiving them with great fidelity, which speaks to program effectiveness, as opposed to efficacy. If this is the case, greater investment on the part of WTCHP in supporting the dissemination of EBTs for this cohort may lead to an improved delivery of these treatments.

The findings from this report suggest that future QI projects within the Northwell CCE should explore mechanisms for increasing engagement in outcome monitoring and support of EBT interventions. Additionally, future research among the Northwell CCE clients, and in the larger WTCHP mental health cohort, is needed to explore patterns of change in outcomes for those engaged in treatment. While those in treatment may not be demonstrating substantial improvements in symptoms on self-report measures, those who are being seen for an extended duration may be obtaining maintenance treatment that could be preventing any exacerbation of symptoms. It may also be the case that treatment is not being delivered as effectively as desired, or that there are unique challenges to understand with this responder cohort, which explain the lack of demonstrable progress on these measures. For instance, this population may have a high degree of medical co-morbidity, as well as exposure to multiple and severe traumas, that may be hindering the treatment progress [7,13].

Several limitations should be noted. Firstly, this is a quality improvement project that included an analysis of our institution's administrative data, and should be interpreted as such. We did not formally adjust significance values for multiple comparisons. Secondly, not all providers overseen by the Northwell CCE were included at this step of the QI process, and may not be accessible without further administrative mandates, given that the providers who did not participate were also part of other systems of care with a high level of administrative burden. This made it difficult to obtain the necessary information without adding to the administrative burden of those providers. Accordingly, the data obtained could reflect a potential response bias. Thirdly, even among those who did complete treatment plan data, the information provided was the report of the provider, and not from direct observation. Specifically, outcome data were self-report measures that providers collected, scored, and then reported on, as opposed to data to which the team had direct access. Furthermore, EBT delivery was captured through an analysis of treatment plans, as opposed to fidelity checks of treatment which would have been prohibitive. These issues were compensated for by evaluating data from the annual monitoring report, where feasible. Finally, a high level of missing data was present for mental health outcomes, and we were not able to model changes in outcomes. Instead, unadjusted analyses were used to compare differences in symptom scores across time, and whether those changes were different by use of EBT Delivered. This hampered our ability to adjust for potential confounding variables as well. Therefore, the results from the analysis represent a signal to be explored further to determine if it reflects the larger treatment plan population, or the WTC responder population more broadly.

Many of the limitations listed above are to be expected in a QI project that does not allow for rigorous controls of treatment setting and delivery. Instead, this project reflects a real-world delivery setting for services, and offers meaningful first steps towards assuring quality of treatment in a WTCHP CCE, that could have implications for other CCEs and the larger MH treatment population. Untreated PTSD and other mental health conditions can have a debilitating impact on functioning, and come at a significant cost to society [39]. It is therefore important that the CCEs consider opportunities for improving services among their providers. These services are often delivered in very different contexts, such as in ambulatory programs of hospital systems, and in private practices of community providers. Systems of care and individuals can vary widely in the quality and consistency of the services delivered. This poses a challenge in assuring the quality of services for enrollees in the WTCHP both across and within CCEs.

The Substance Abuse and Mental Health Services Administration (SAMHSA) has directed significant attention towards supporting the adoption of evidence-based practices and collecting and utilizing data to inform policy and practice [40]. Progress has also been made towards a broad standardization of outcome measures, such as those undertaken in collaboration with the National Quality Forum [41] and the National Committee for Quality Assurance [42]. The WTC programs, given their unique funding structure, allow for greater flexibility and oversight to develop QI initiatives and encourage provision of EBTs by community providers, who provide the care, with the assurance that they will be paid for their clinical service.

Should the WTCHP move towards more standardized metrics for MH, and/or support for any implementation of evidence-based therapies, QI processes are an ideal mechanism for measurement and intervention [23,24]. Unfortunately, it is unclear as to what would constitute ideal targets for an improvement of program performance. As noted, mental health utilization in the Northwell CCE meets the national average target, but it is not clear as to what would be the ideal performance measures for outcome monitoring or EBT delivery. In addition, demands and priorities should be sensitive to the contexts in which they are implemented. It is important to bear in mind that even robust implementation programs have had significant challenges. Furthermore, EBT implementation and quality assurance processes have greater chances of success when the stakeholders' voices and the contexts of implementation are factored into the process of change [43,44]. Due to the various demands imposed on providers, and the diverse contexts within which the WTCHP operates, modifications should be selective in targeting particular outcomes that will have the greatest value to the WTC MH cohort. Given the high proportion of responders with PTSD, this will likely require consideration of interventions that enhance services and outcomes for that population.

5. Conclusions

This project has leveraged the usage of quality improvement mechanisms to characterize service delivery, evaluate both EBT provision and the implementation of outcome monitoring in a community provider network for the WTCHP. The initial findings include: Robust access to psychotherapeutic services, adherence to program objectives of treating WTC-related conditions, and an engagement of providers in the process. However, the findings also point towards areas for improvement in both EBT delivery and measurement based care, with implications for the well-being of members served. Priorities for program performance need to be set by the WTCHP, but information gleaned from this project in the Northwell CCE provide some areas for consideration. Providers could be engaged in more outcome-based measurement, and could be given more support for EBT training and delivery. Close coordination of these changes with relevant stakeholders (i.e., CCEs, providers, and clients) could ensure effective implementation of any desired objectives.

Author Contributions: Conceptualization, M.B., J.M., R.R. and R.M.S.; Methodology, M.B., R.R., and R.M.S.; Formal Analysis, R.R. and R.M.S.; Resources, J.M. and J.K.; Writing—Original Draft Preparation, M.B., R.R., K.B., S.S. and R.M.S.; Writing—Review & Editing, M.S., J.M., R.R., K.B., S.S. and R.M.S.; Supervision, M.S., J.M. and R.M.S.; Project Administration, M.B., J.M. and R.M.S.

Funding: This research received no external funding.

Conflicts of Interest: The authors declare no conflict of interest.

References

1. Herbert, R.; Moline, J.; Skloot, G.; Metzger, K.; Baron, S.; Luft, B.; Markowitz, S.; Udasin, I.; Harrison, D.; Stein, D.; et al. The World Trade Center disaster and the health of workers: Five-year assessment of a unique medical screening program. *Environ. Health Perspect.* **2006**, *114*, 1853–1858. [CrossRef]

2. Stellman, J.M.; Smith, R.P.; Katz, C.L.; Sharma, V.; Charney, D.S.; Herbert, R.; Moline, J.; Luft, B.J.; Markowitz, S.; Udasin, I.; et al. Enduring Mental Health Morbidity and Social Function Impairment in World Trade Center Rescue, Recovery, and Cleanup Workers: The Psychological Dimension of an Environmental Health Disaster. *Environ. Health Perspect.* **2008**, *116*, 1248–1253. [CrossRef] [PubMed]

3. Brackbill, R.M.; Hadler, J.L.; DiGrande, L.; Ekenga, C.C.; Farfel, M.R.; Friedman, S.; Perlman, S.E.; Stellman, S.D.; Walker, D.J.; Wu, D.; et al. Asthma and Posttraumatic Stress Symptoms 5 to 6 Years Following Exposure to the World Trade Center Terrorist Attack. *JAMA* **2009**, *302*, 502–516. [CrossRef] [PubMed]

4. Perrin, M.A.; DiGrande, L.; Wheeler, K.; Thorpe, L.; Farfel, M.; Brackbill, R. Differences in PTSD Prevalence and Associated Risk Factors Among World Trade Center Disaster Rescue and Recovery Workers. *AJP* **2007**, *164*, 1385–1394. [CrossRef] [PubMed]

5. Pietrzak, R.H.; Van Ness, P.H.; Fried, T.R.; Galea, S.; Norris, F.H. Trajectories of posttraumatic stress symptomatology in older persons affected by a large-magnitude disaster. *J. Psychiatr. Res.* **2013**, *47*, 520–526. [CrossRef]

6. Gross, R.; Neria, Y.; Tao, X.G.; Massa, J.; Ashwell, L.; Davis, K.; Geyh, A. Posttraumatic stress disorder and other psychological sequelae among world trade center clean up and recovery workers. *Ann. N. Y. Acad. Sci.* **2006**, *1071*, 495–499. [CrossRef] [PubMed]

7. Bromet, E.J.; Hobbs, M.J.; Clouston, S.A.P.; Gonzalez, A.; Kotov, R.; Luft, B.J. DSM-IV post-traumatic stress disorder among World Trade Center responders 11–13 years after the disaster of 11 September 2001 (9/11). *Psychol. Med.* **2016**, *46*, 771–783. [CrossRef]

8. Adams, R.E.; Boscarino, J.A.; Galea, S. Alcohol Use, Mental Health Status and Psychological Well-being 2 Years after the World Trade Center Attacks in New York City. *Am. J. Drug Alcohol Abuse* **2006**, *32*, 203–224. [CrossRef] [PubMed]

9. Cone, J.E.; Li, J.; Kornblith, E.; Gocheva, V.; Stellman, S.D.; Shaikh, A.; Schwarzer, R.; Bowler, R.M. Chronic probable ptsd in police responders in the world trade center health registry ten to eleven years after 9/11. *Am. J. Ind. Med.* **2015**, *58*, 483–493. [CrossRef]

10. Bowler, R.M.; Harris, M.; Li, J.; Gocheva, V.; Stellman, S.D.; Wilson, K.; Alper, H.; Schwarzer, R.; Cone, J.E. Longitudinal mental health impact among police responders to the 9/11 terrorist attack. *Am. J. Ind. Med.* **2012**, *55*, 297–312. [CrossRef]

11. Yip, J.; Zeig-Owens, R.; Webber, M.P.; Kablanian, A.; Hall, C.B.; Vossbrinck, M.; Liu, X.; Weakley, J.; Schwartz, T.; Kelly, K.J.; et al. World Trade Center-related physical and mental health burden among New York City Fire Department emergency medical service workers. *Occup. Environ. Med.* **2016**, *73*, 13–20. [CrossRef]

12. Wisnivesky, J.P.; Teitelbaum, S.L.; Todd, A.C.; Boffetta, P.; Crane, M.; Crowley, L.; de la Hoz, R.E.; Dellenbaugh, C.; Harrison, D.; Herbert, R.; et al. Persistence of multiple illnesses in World Trade Center rescue and recovery workers: A cohort study. *Lancet* **2011**, *378*, 888–897. [CrossRef]

13. Pietrzak, R.H.; Feder, A.; Singh, R.; Schechter, C.B.; Bromet, E.J.; Katz, C.L.; Reissman, D.B.; Ozbay, F.; Sharma, V.; Crane, M.; et al. Trajectories of PTSD risk and resilience in World Trade Center responders: An 8-year prospective cohort study. *Psychol. Med.* **2014**, *44*, 205–219. [CrossRef]

14. Adams, R.E.; Boscarino, J.A. Perievent Panic Attack and Depression after the World Trade Center Disaster: A Structural Equation Model Analysis. *Int. J. Emerg. Ment. Health* **2011**, *13*, 69–79.

15. Pietrzak, R.H.; Goldstein, R.B.; Southwick, S.M.; Grant, B.F. Prevalence and Axis I comorbidity of full and partial posttraumatic stress disorder in the United States: Results from Wave 2 of the National Epidemiologic Survey on Alcohol and Related Conditions. *J. Anxiety Disord.* **2011**, *25*, 456–465. [CrossRef]

16. Lowell, A.; Suarez-Jimenez, B.; Helpman, L.; Zhu, X.; Durosky, A.; Hilburn, A.; Schneier, F.; Gross, R.; Neria, Y. 9/11-related PTSD among highly exposed populations: A systematic review 15 years after the attack. *Psychol. Med.* **2018**, *48*, 537–553. [CrossRef]

17. Haugen, P.T.; Evces, M.; Weiss, D.S. Treating posttraumatic stress disorder in first responders: A systematic review. *Clin. Psychol. Rev.* **2012**, *32*, 370–380. [CrossRef] [PubMed]

18. Schneier, F.R.; Neria, Y.; Pavlicova, M.; Hembree, E.; Suh, E.J.; Amsel, L.; Marshall, R.D. Combined Prolonged Exposure Therapy and Paroxetine for PTSD Related to the World Trade Center Attack: A Randomized Controlled Trial. *AJP* **2012**, *169*, 80–88. [CrossRef]

19. Difede, J.; Malta, L.S.; Best, S.; Henn-Haase, C.; Metzler, T.; Bryant, R.; Marmar, C. A randomized controlled clinical treatment trial for World Trade Center attack-related PTSD in disaster workers. *J. Nerv. Ment. Dis.* **2007**, *195*, 861–865. [CrossRef] [PubMed]

20. Difede, J.; Cukor, J.; Jayasinghe, N.; Patt, I.; Jedel, S.; Spielman, L.; Giosan, C.; Hoffman, H.G. Virtual reality exposure therapy for the treatment of posttraumatic stress disorder following September 11, 2001. *J. Clin. Psychiatry* **2007**, *68*, 1639–1647. [CrossRef]

21. Watson, P.J.; Brymer, M.J.; Bonanno, G.A. Postdisaster psychological intervention since 9/11. *Am. Psychol.* **2011**, *66*, 482–494. [CrossRef]

22. Health Research and Analysis. *World Trade Center Health Program Evaluation Mental Health Utilization Final Report*; Health Research and Analysis: Bethesda, MD, USA, 2019.

23. Ganju, V. Mental health quality and accountability: The role of evidence-based practices and performance measurement. *Adm. Policy Ment. Health* **2006**, *33*, 659–665. [CrossRef] [PubMed]

24. Hermann, R.C.; Chan, J.A.; Zazzali, J.L.; Lerner, D. Aligning Measurement-based Quality Improvement with Implementation of Evidence-based Practices. *Adm. Policy Ment. Health* **2006**, *33*, 636–645. [CrossRef]

25. Charney, M.E.; Hellberg, S.N.; Bui, E.; Simon, N.M. Evidenced-Based Treatment of Posttraumatic Stress Disorder: An Updated Review of Validated Psychotherapeutic and Pharmacological Approaches. *Harv. Rev. Psychiatry* **2018**, *26*, 99–115. [CrossRef] [PubMed]

26. Watkins, L.E.; Sprang, K.R.; Rothbaum, B.O. Treating PTSD: A Review of Evidence-Based Psychotherapy Interventions. *Front. Behav. Neurosci.* **2018**, *12*, 258. [CrossRef]

27. Gyani, A.; Shafran, R.; Myles, P.; Rose, S. The Gap Between Science and Practice: How Therapists Make Their Clinical Decisions. *Behav. Ther.* **2014**, *45*, 199–211. [CrossRef] [PubMed]

28. Rosen, C.S.; Chow, H.C.; Finney, J.F.; Greenbaum, M.A.; Moos, R.H.; Sheikh, J.I.; Yesavage, J.A. VA practice patterns and practice guidelines for treating posttraumatic stress disorder. *J. Trauma. Stress* **2004**, *17*, 213–222. [CrossRef] [PubMed]

29. Rosen, C.S.; Matthieu, M.M.; Wiltsey Stirman, S.; Cook, J.M.; Landes, S.; Bernardy, N.C.; Chard, K.M.; Crowley, J.; Eftekhari, A.; Finley, E.P.; et al. A Review of Studies on the System-Wide Implementation of Evidence-Based Psychotherapies for Posttraumatic Stress Disorder in the Veterans Health Administration. *Adm. Policy Ment. Health* **2016**, *43*, 957–977. [CrossRef]

30. Maguen, S.; Madden, E.; Patterson, O.V.; DuVall, S.L.; Goldstein, L.A.; Burkman, K.; Shiner, B. Measuring Use of Evidence Based Psychotherapy for Posttraumatic Stress Disorder in a Large National Healthcare System. *Adm. Policy Ment. Health* **2018**, *45*, 519–529. [CrossRef]

31. Department of Veterans Affairs, Department of Defense. *VA/DOD Clinical Practice Guideline for the Management of Posttraumatic Stress Disorder and Acute Stress Disorder*; Department of Veterans Affairs, Department of Defense: Washington, DC, USA, 2017.

32. Clinical Practice Guideline for the Treatment of Posttraumatic Stress Disorder (PTSD). Available online: http://www.apa.org/ptsd-guideline/index.aspx (accessed on 3 December 2018).

33. National Institutes for Health and Care Excellence NICE Guidelines. Available online: https://www.nice.org.uk/about/what-we-do/our-programmes/nice-guidance/nice-guidelines (accessed on 28 February 2019).

34. Blevins, C.A.; Weathers, F.W.; Davis, M.T.; Witte, T.K.; Domino, J.L. The Posttraumatic Stress Disorder Checklist for DSM-5 (PCL-5): Development and Initial Psychometric Evaluation. *J. Trauma. Stress* **2015**, *28*, 489–498. [CrossRef]

35. Kroenke, K.; Spitzer, R.L.; Williams, J.B. The PHQ-9. *J. Gen. Intern. Med.* **2001**, *16*, 606–613. [CrossRef]

36. Löwe, B.; Decker, O.; Müller, S.; Brähler, E.; Schellberg, D.; Herzog, W.; Herzberg, P.Y. Validation and Standardization of the Generalized Anxiety Disorder Screener (GAD-7) in the General Population. *Med. Care* **2008**, *46*, 266–274. [CrossRef]

37. Ruggiero, K.J.; Del Ben, K.; Scotti, J.R.; Rabalais, A.E. Psychometric properties of the PTSD Checklist-Civilian Version. *J. Trauma. Stress* **2003**, *16*, 495–502. [CrossRef]

38. Monson, C.M.; Gradus, J.L.; Young-Xu, Y.; Schnurr, P.P.; Price, J.L.; Schumm, J.A. Change in posttraumatic stress disorder symptoms: Do clinicians and patients agree? *Psychol. Assess.* **2008**, *20*, 131–138. [CrossRef]

39. Kessler, R.C. Posttraumatic stress disorder: The burden to the individual and to society. *J. Clin. Psychiatry* **2000**, *61* (Suppl. 5), 4–12, discussion 13–14.

40. Substance Abuse and Mental Health Services Administration. *SAMHSA Strategic Plan FY2019-FY2023*; Substance Abuse and Mental Health Services Administration: Rockville, MD, USA, 2018.

41. National Quality Forum. *Behavioral Health Endorsement Maintenance 2014: Phase 3*; National Quality Forum: Washington, DC, USA, 2015.

42. National Committee for Quality Assurance Mental Health Utilization. Available online: https://www.ncqa.org/hedis/measures/mental-health-utilization/ (accessed on 28 February 2019).

43. Pedersen, M.S.; Landheim, A.; Møller, M.; Lien, L. Audit and feedback in mental healthcare: Staff experiences. *Int. J. Health Care Qual. Assur.* **2018**, *31*, 822–833. [CrossRef]

44. Stirman, S.W.; Gutner, C.A.; Langdon, K.; Graham, J.R. Bridging the Gap Between Research and Practice in Mental Health Service Settings: An Overview of Developments in Implementation Theory and Research. *Behav. Ther.* **2016**, *47*, 920–936. [CrossRef]

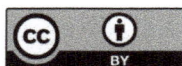

Article

International Journal of
Environmental Research and Public Health

MDPI

Molecular Study of Thyroid Cancer in World Trade Center Responders

Maaike A. G. van Gerwen [1], Stephanie Tuminello [1], Gregory J. Riggins [2], Thais B. Mendes [3],
Michael Donovan [4], Emma K.T. Benn [5], Eric Genden [6], Janete M. Cerutti [3] and
Emanuela Taioli [1,7,8,*]

[1] Institute for Translational Epidemiology and Department of Population Health Science and Policy,
     Icahn School of Medicine at Mount Sinai, New York, NY 10029, USA;
     maaike.vangerwen@icahn.mssm.edu (M.A.G.v.G.); stephanie.tuminello@mssm.edu (S.T.)
[2] Department of Neurosurgery, Johns Hopkins University School of Medicine, Baltimore, MD 21218, USA;
     griggin1@jhmi.edu
[3] Division of Genetics, Universidade Federal de São Paulo, São Paulo 04039-032, Brazil;
     thais_biude@hotmail.com (T.B.M.); j.cerutti@unifesp.br (J.M.C.)
[4] Department of Pathology, Icahn School of Medicine at Mount Sinai, New York, NY 10029, USA;
     michael.donovan@mssm.edu
[5] Department of Population Health Science and Policy, Center for Biostatistics, Icahn School of Medicine at
     Mount Sinai, New York, NY 10029, USA; emma.benn@mountsinai.org
[6] Department of Otolaryngology- Head and Neck Surgery, Icahn School of Medicine at Mount Sinai,
     New York, NY 10029, USA; Eric.Genden@mountsinai.org
[7] Department of Thoracic Surgery, Icahn School of Medicine at Mount Sinai, New York, NY 10029, USA
[8] Tisch Cancer Institute, Icahn School of Medicine at Mount Sinai, New York, NY 10029, USA
*   Correspondence: emanuela.taioli@mountsinai.org; Tel.: +1-212-659-9590

Received: 9 April 2019; Accepted: 2 May 2019; Published: 7 May 2019

Abstract: Thyroid cancer incidence is higher in World Trade Center (WTC) responders compared with the general population. It is unclear whether this excess in thyroid cancer is associated with WTC-related exposures or if instead there is an over-diagnosis of malignant thyroid cancer among WTC first responders due to enhanced surveillance and physician bias. To maximize diagnostic yield and determine the false positive rate for malignancy, the histological diagnoses of thyroid cancer tumors from WTC responders and age, gender, and histology matched non-WTC thyroid cancer cases were evaluated using biomarkers of malignancy. Using a highly accurate panel of four biomarkers that are able to distinguish benign from malignant thyroid cancer, our results suggest that over-diagnosis by virtue of misdiagnosis of a benign tumor as malignant does not explain the increased incidence of thyroid cancer observed in WTC responders. Therefore, rather than over-diagnosis due to physician bias, the yearly screening visits by the World Trade Center Health Program are identifying true cases of thyroid cancer. Continuing regular screening of this cohort is thus warranted.

Keywords: 9/11; screening; thyroid cancer; biomarkers

---

1. Introduction

A significantly increased risk of thyroid cancer has been reported in the Mount Sinai Health Program of World Trade Center (WTC) responders [1], WTC-exposed firefighters [2], and the New York City Department of Health exposed residents [3], with an excess risk in the range of 2–3 times the incidence reported by cancer registries.

The etiology behind this increased incidence of thyroid cancer remains unclear. Though multiple carcinogens were identified at Ground Zero, including soot, benzene, and other volatile organic compounds from the burning of the jet fuel, in addition to the asbestos, silica, and other fibers that were in the dust caused by the towers collapse, none are known to act as carcinogens on the thyroid [4]. Established risk factors for thyroid cancer, such as exposure to radiation or iodine-131, have not been reported in connection to Ground Zero [5].

Instead, overdiagnosis as a consequence of surveillance and physician biases has been suggested as a possible explanation of the excess risk of thyroid cancer in the WTC cohort [1]. Enhanced surveillance leading to heightened diagnosis is a well-recognized phenomenon in heavily screened populations [6]. This phenomenon has been suggested as an explanation for other cancers for which WTC responders have been observed to be at increased risk, such as prostate cancer [7]. Funded under the James Zadroga 9/11 Health and Compensation Act of 2010, the World Trade Center Health Program (WTCHP) monitors the health of WTC responders with yearly visits, including a physical examination, laboratory testing, spirometry, and chest radiography. Chest imaging is known to increase detection of incidental thyroid nodules [8], and WTC responders, many of whom report respiratory health problems [9], are referred for imaging at higher rates, thus making the chance of discovery of a thyroid nodule more likely. It is possible that some of these nodules would never have become clinically evident, and so would have never been discovered, if not for this heightened screening [7].

Physician's cognitive biases are known to lead to diagnostic inaccuracies [10]. Physicians treating WTC responders, including pathologists, may suspect a worse diagnosis for these patients compared with non-WTC responders due to implicit biases associated with knowledge of the patient's past WTC exposure. In addition, they may prefer risk aversion by a defensive diagnosing strategy to avoid missing any malignancies and classify a suspicious nodule as cancerous [10]. This, along with the increase in nodule detection due to enhanced screening through the WTCHP, may be leading to an over-diagnosis of malignant thyroid cancer among WTC first responders.

The goal of this study is to analyze pathologists' histological diagnosis of thyroid cancer in WTC first responders and, by doing so, determine the false positive rate for malignancy. We will examine the clinical characteristics and results of a cancer-detection four-biomarker panel of WTC tumors compared with non-WTC exposed age-, gender-, and histology-matched cases.

2. Methods

2.1. Selection and Enrollment of Study Participants

Eligible WTC responders who participated (as employees or volunteers) in rescue, recovery, and cleanup efforts at the WTC sites and who met established eligibility criteria [11] have been enrolled in the WTCHP at Mount Sinai. Over 27,000 responders have had at least one monitoring visit in the WTCHP and have consented to the aggregation of their data;20,984 of which have consented to have their records used for medical research [12].

Cancer cases are identified through periodical linkage with the cancer registries of New York, New Jersey, Pennsylvania, and Connecticut, as these states account for 98% of the responders' residencies at time of WTCHP enrollment. The full linkage methodology has been described elsewhere [1,12]. Only thyroid cancer cases validated by a cancer registry were eligible to participate in this study. Additionally, WTC responders were only eligible if their enrollment in the WTCHP predated their cancer diagnosis.

The full methodology used for patient recruitment and consent has been previously described [12]. In brief, eligible participants were contacted by phone, and those interested in participating were mailed a consent form. After a patient's consent, a cancer tissue sample was obtained from the hospital where the patient's thyroid surgery had taken place and clinical information related to their cancer was abstracted from the pathology reports. For each patient, a pathologist reviewed the tissue blocks to assure that cancer tissue was present, and 5 unstained slides of 4 μm thickness, in addition to 1 hematoxylin and eosin (H/E) stained slide, were cut from the chosen formalin-fixed paraffin-embedded (FFPE) tumor block. WTC cases were one-to-one matched by gender, histology, and age (+/- 5 years) to thyroid cancer samples obtained from the Mount Sinai Biorepository, with no known WTC exposure. For cases with rare histology (*n* = 3), such as columnar cell papillary carcinoma, it was not possible to match by histology, and matching was limited to age and gender. After de-identification, all samples were sent to John Hopkins University for analysis. This study protocol was approved by the Icahn School of Medicine at Mount Sinai's Institutional Review Board (IRB-17-01323).

2.2. Assessment of Clinical Characteristics

Pathology reports relating to the thyroid cancer surgeries of the WTC cases and Mount Sinai non-WTC exposed controls were obtained, and data pertaining to the patient's age, gender, tumor histology, and size was abstracted into an excel database. To ensure that the WTC thyroid cancer cases included in this study represented a random subset of the overall sample, characteristics of the study sample were compared with the overall WTCHP thyroid cancer cohort using clinical data provided by the WTCHP (Table 1).

Table 1. Characteristics of the study sample

Clinical–Pathological Features	WTC Thyroid Cancer Cases			Non-WTC Controls	
	Eligible (*n* = 43)	Included (*n* = 30)	*p* Value [a]	Included (*n* = 30)	*p* Value [b]
Age at Diagnosis (years)	48.5 (SD 7.7)	49.3 (SD 8.6)	0.65	47.8 (SD 11.3)	0.5652
Gender			0.16		1.00
Male	36 (83.7%)	21 (70%)		21 (70%)	
Female	7 (16.3%)	9 (30%)		9 (30%)	
Histology			0.74		1.00
Papillary thyroid carcinoma	27 (62.8%)	21 (70%)		21 (70%)	
Papillary thyroid carcinoma, follicular variant	12 (27.9%)	6 (20%)		6 (20%)	
Other	4 (9.3%)	3 (10%)		3 (10%)	
Tumor Size [c] (cm)		1.38 (SD 1.16)		1.46 (SD 0.93)	0.78
Microcarcinoma					
Yes [c]		14 (51.85%)		12 (40.0%)	0.37

[a] Eligible versus included WTC thyroid cancer cases; [b] Included WTC versus non-WTC thyroid cancer cases; [c] Tumor size unknown for 3 WTC cases; WTC: World Trade Center.

2.3. Immunohistochemistry Analysis

While diagnosis of papillary thyroid carcinoma (PTC), the most common subtype, can usually be achieved through cytology, diagnosis of other thyroid cancer histologies can prove to be more difficult [13], resulting in benign thyroid lesions being incorrectly classified as malignant. We have previously developed a panel of molecular markers to distinguish benign from malignant thyroid cancer, which can be used to cost-effectively identify the presence of over-diagnosis [14–16]. As seen in Figure 1, the panel of molecular markers includes DDIT3, ITM1, C1orf24, and PVALB antibodies, the utility of which has been described elsewhere [14–16], which can accurately discriminate between malignant and benign tumors with a sensitivity and specificity close to 100% (Figure 1).

FFPE WTC and non-WTC thyroid tumor tissues were analyzed using these carcinoma markers. Briefly, the FFPE sections (4 μm) were deparaffinized in xylene and rehydrated through a series of graded alcohols. The endogenous alkaline phosphatase activity was blocked with 15% (vol/vol) hydrogen peroxide in deionized water for 10 minutes. To expose the PVALB protein, permeabilization was performed with 0.5% Tween in phosphate-buffered saline (PBS: 10 mM phosphate buffer, pH 7.2, containing 0.15 M NaCl) at room temperature for 20 min. For PVALB and DDIT3, antigen retrieval was performed using 0.1 M Tris-HCl for 15 min in a steamer. For C1orf24, antigen retrieval was performed in a Tris-based solution pH 7.4 (AR-10; Biogenex Laboratories, San Ramon, CA) for 15 min in a pressure cooker. For ITM1, antigen retrieval was performed using 0.1 M Tris-HCl pH 7.4 for 5 min in a pressure cooker. After antigen retrieval, the slides were allowed to cool down for 30 min. Non-specific binding sites were blocked with 5% (C1orf24) or 10% (ITM1) normal goat serum 1 h or 5% bovine serum albumin (BSA) (DDIT3 and PVALB) for 30 min prior to incubation with primary antibodies. Polyclonal anti-C1orf24 and anti-ITM1 (custom produced) were used at 1:200 dilution. Monoclonal anti DDIT3 (Cat. 179823; Abcam, Cambridge) was used at 1:200 dilution, and anti-parvalbumin (clone PARV-19; Cat. P3088, Sigma-Aldrich, St. Louis, MO) was used at 1:1000 dilution. For all antibodies, incubation with primary antibodies was performed overnight in a moist chamber. Immunostaining was performed using the EnVisionTM Dual Link (Cat. K4061; Dako, Hamburg, Germany). The samples were stained with hematoxylin and eosin and analyzed using a light microscope.

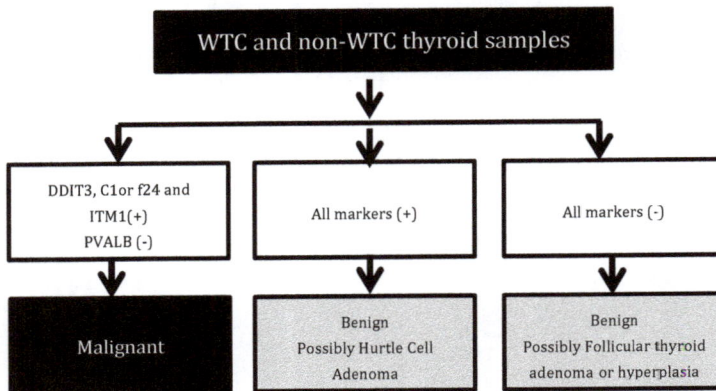

Figure 1. Antibody Assessment. WTC: World trade center.

2.4. Statistical Analysis

Continuous variables were summarized using mean ± standard deviation, whereas categorical variables were summarized as frequency (%). Bivariate hypothesis tests were conducted using two-sided t-tests or Wilcoxon Rank Sum tests for continuous variables and chi-square or Fisher's Exact tests for categorical variables. All statistical analyses were performed using SAS 9.4 (SAS Institute Inc., Cary, NC).

3. Results

There were 73 participants in the WTC cohort of responders who were eligible to be included in this study, four of whom had to be excluded as they did not speak English or because they had no viable contact information. Of the remaining 69 WTC thyroid cancer patients, 37 patients (54%) consented to participate. We were able to obtain FFPE thyroid tumor tissue samples for 30 WTC participants. The comparison of the 30 WTC thyroid cancer patients who consented and the 43 remaining WTC thyroid cancer patients showed that the groups were not significantly different for age at diagnosis, gender, and histology (Table 1).

After matching, the WTC- and the non-WTC thyroid patient groups were well balanced in terms of age at diagnosis ($p = 0.57$), gender ($p = 1.00$), and histology ($p = 1.00$) (Table 1). Evaluation of clinical and pathological characteristics showed that there was no statistically significant difference in terms of tumor size ($p = 0.77$). Microcarcinomas, defined as thyroid cancer ≤1cm, were found in 52% of the WTC thyroid cancer patients compared with 40% in the non-WTC thyroid cancer patients (Table 1). Antibody assessment correctly classified thyroid nodules in either group (Figure 2, Supplementary Table S1).

Except for three thyroid samples, all thyroid tumor tissue samples from thyroid tissue from the two groups and all histology types tested positive for malignancy with antibodies C1orf24, ITM1, and DDIT3 and negative PVALB (Supplementary Table S1). For the other three samples (two WTC cases and one control), it was not possible to detect actual tumor tissue in the slides used for immunohistochemistry, and therefore, these samples could not be confirmed as malignant in the antibody-based test; all three samples were taken from tumors originally less than 0.3 cm in size. Most of the tumors had a strong brown staining for three markers (DDIT3, ITM1, and C1orf24) and no staining for the benign Hurthle adenoma marker (PVALB) (Figure 2; Supplementary Table S1).

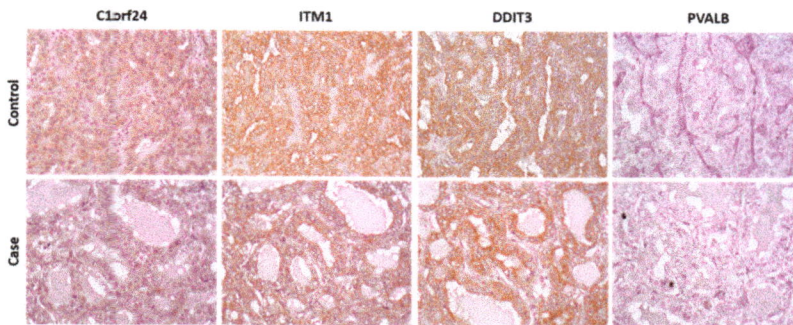

Figure 2. Representative results of molecular markers in WTC and non-WTC thyroid carcinomas (original magnification of ×40).

4. Discussion

The findings of the present study suggest that overdiagnosis by virtue of misdiagnosis of a benign tumor as malignant does not explain the increased incidence of thyroid cancer observed in WTC responders. If overdiagnosis were occurring, we would expect an excess of false-positive malignancies among WTC thyroid cancer cases; benign tumors would be detected because of enhanced screening efforts and diagnosed as malignant because of physician bias associated with knowing that the patient has a history of WTC exposure. However, there was not an excess of false-positive thyroid cancer diagnoses found among the WTC thyroid cancer cases. In fact, none of the WTC thyroid cancer tumors assessed were false-positives; instead, all samples tested using the antibody-based cancer panel were determined to be true malignant disease. Although it may still be that physicians treating WTC responders may have biases that make them more likely to defensively diagnose nodules as thyroid cancer to avoid missing malignancies, our results suggest that screening of WTC responders, at least in the case of thyroid cancer, may not be unwarranted.

It is important to note that surveillance bias may still be occurring in this cohort. Surveillance bias occurs when increased screening efforts result in nodules being detected that would otherwise have gone unnoticed given routine surveillance, thus inflating the actual incidence of disease in a heavily screened population. Smaller tumor size and younger age at diagnosis in the WTC cohort would generally be suggestive of surveillance bias, but the design of the present study does not allow any such conclusions to be drawn. For this study, WTC and non-WTC cases were matched by age, gender, and histology; thus, it is expected that age and tumor size are similar between the two groups. However, a descriptive study of the WTC thyroid cancer cases showed that these cases had similar clinical characteristics as thyroid cancer cases in the Mount Sinai registry in terms of age at diagnosis and tumor size, suggesting that surveillance bias alone cannot explain the excess risk of thyroid cancer in WTC responders [17].

Being that the increased risk of thyroid cancer in WTC responders does not appear to be an artifact due to physician bias, the results of this study leave open the possibility of an as-yet unknown carcinogenic mechanism through which WTC exposure is acting on thyroid cancer carcinogenesis. The biological basis of the tumors of WTC responders, including thyroid cancer tumors, warrants further research.

This is the first study to investigate the possible reasons for the increased incidence of thyroid cancer in the WTC population and the first to show that over-diagnosis due to physician bias does not appear to adequately explain the observed excess risk. The study is also novel in that it is the first to utilize biomarkers of malignancy in a WTC cohort. A further strength of this study is the high rate of compliance, with 54% of eligible WTC thyroid cancer patients agreeing to have their tumor sample molecularly analyzed.

This study is limited in that not all tumor samples could be retrieved from the institutions where the thyroid cancer surgery was performed and that, for a few samples, there was no tissue sample in the slides provided. However, this was a small portion of the samples (5%). In addition, a comparison of the characteristics of those patients for which we obtained a sample to the characteristics of the eligible patients does not show any difference in personal or tumor characteristics, thus reducing the possibility of selection bias.

Further analysis is needed to investigate a causal link between thyroid cancer in WTC-responders and high levels of exposure to potentially carcinogenic agents at Ground Zero, which may result in cancers with a shorter latency period, similar to that observed in individuals exposed to iodine-131 after the Chernobyl accident. It is well known that patients exposed to Chernobyl fallout demonstrated a linear dose–response association. Therefore, to define whether there is a correlation between the levels of exposure to the debris cloud and thyroid cancer, diagnosis is needed, as well as a longer follow-up. [18]

Additionally, the investigation of somatic events that drive thyroid cancer pathogenesis in this cohort, concomitant to longer follow-up and correlation with clinical-pathological features, will increase our knowledge of whether the molecular events in WTC responders differ from those not exposed to the dust cloud, as well as better define tumor aggressiveness [19,20].

5. Conclusions

In conclusion, rather than overdiagnosis of false-positives due to physician bias, it might instead be the case that the yearly screening visits by the WTCHP are identifying true cases of thyroid cancer earlier, increasing the possibility of a favorable prognosis, which warrants regular screening of this cohort.

Supplementary Materials: The following are available online at http://www.mdpi.com/1660-4601/16/9/1600/s1, Table S1: Antibody-based test results and final histology in WTC cases and non-WTC cases.

Author Contributions: Conceptualization: E.T., G.J.R., and J.M.C.; Methodology: J.M.C.; Software: J.M.C.; Validation: J.M.C. and T.B.M.; Formal Analysis: J.M.C. and T.B.M.; Data analysis: M.A.G.v.G.; Expertise for results preparation: E.T.; G.J.R.; J.M.C.; E.G.; Writing—Original Draft Preparation: M.A.G.v.G. and S.T.; Writing, Review, and Editing: M.A.G.v.G.; S.T.; G.J.R.; T.B.M.; M.D.; E.K.T.B.; E.G.; J.M.C.; and E.T.

Funding: This work was supported by the National Institute for Occupational Safety and Health- (1U01OH010984-01A1).

Acknowledgments: We thank the São Paulo State Research Foundation (FAPESP; grant number 2014/06570-6). JMC is a recipient of a scholarship of Research Productivity from Conselho Nacional de Desenvolvimento Científico e Tecnológico CNPq.

Conflicts of Interest: All authors declare no conflicts of interest.

References

1. Solan, S.; Wallenstein, S.; Shapiro, M.; Teitelbaum, S.L.; Stevenson, L.; Kochman, A.; Kaplan, J.; Dellenbaugh, C.; Kahn, A.; Biro, F.N.; et al. Cancer Incidence in World Trade Center Rescue and Recovery Workers, 2001–2008. *Environ. Health Perspect.* **2013**, *121*, 699–704. [CrossRef] [PubMed]

2. Zeig-Owens, R.; Webber, M.P.; Hall, C.B.; Schwartz, T.; Jaber, N.; Weakley, J.; Rohan, T.E.; Cohen, H.W.; Derman, O.; Aldrich, T.K.; et al. Early assessment of cancer outcomes in New York City firefighters after the 9/11 attacks: An observational cohort study. *Lancet* **2011**, *378*, 898–905. [CrossRef]

3. Jordan, H.T.; Brackbill, R.M.; Cone, J.E.; Debchoudhury, I.; Farfel, M.R.; Greene, C.M.; Hadler, J.L.; Kennedy, J.; Li, J.; Liff, J.; et al. Mortality among survivors of the Sept 11, 2001, World Trade Center disaster: Results from the World Trade Center Health Registry cohort. *Lancet* **2011**, *378*, 879–887. [CrossRef]

4. Lioy, P.J.; Georgopoulos, P. The Anatomy of the Exposures That Occurred around the World Trade Center Site. *Ann. N. Y. Acad. Sci.* **2006**, *1076*, 54–79. [CrossRef] [PubMed]

5. Siemiatycki, J.; Richardson, L.; Straif, K.; Latreille, B.; Lakhani, R.; Campbell, S.; Rousseau, M.-C.; Boffetta, P. Listing Occupational Carcinogens. *Environ. Health Perspect.* **2004**, *112*, 1447–1459. [CrossRef] [PubMed]

6. Davies, L.; Welch, H.G. Increasing incidence of thyroid cancer in the United States, 1973–2002. *JAMA* **2006**, *295*, 2164–2167. [CrossRef] [PubMed]

7. Brawley, O.W. Some Thoughts on Exposure to the World Trade Center Wreckage and Cancer. *JAMA Oncol.* **2018**, *4*, 775–776. [CrossRef]

8. Swensen, S.J.; Jett J.R.; Hartman, T.E.; Midthun, D.E.; Sloan, J.A.; Sykes, A.-M.; Aughenbaugh, G.L.; Clemens, M.A. Lung Cancer Screening with CT: Mayo Clinic Experience. *Radiology* **2003**, *226*, 756–761. [CrossRef]

9. Wisnivesky, J.P.; Teitelbaum, S.L.; Todd, A.C.; Boffetta, P.; Crane, M.; Crowley, L.; de la Hoz, R.E.; Dellenbaugh, C.; Harrison, D.; Herbert, R.; et al. Persistence of multiple illnesses in World Trade Center rescue and recovery workers: A cohort study. *Lancet* **2011**, *378*, 888–897. [CrossRef]

10. Saposnik, G.; Redelmeier, D.; Ruff, C.C.; Tobler, P.N. Cognitive biases associated with medical decisions: A systematic review. *BMC Med. Inform. Decis. Mak.* **2016**, *16*, 138. [CrossRef]

11. Herbert, R.; Moline, J.; Skloot, G.; Metzger, K.; Baron, S.; Luft, B.; Markowitz, S.; Udasin, I.; Harrison, D.; Stein, D.; et al. The World Trade Center disaster and the health of workers: Five-year assessment of a unique medical screening program. *Environ. Health Perspect.* **2006**, *114*, 1853–1858. [CrossRef] [PubMed]

12. Lieberman-Cribbin, W.; Tuminello, S.; Gillezeau, C.; van Gerwen, M.; Brody, R.; Donovan, M.; Taioli, E. The development of a Biobank of cancer tissue samples from World Trade Center responders. *J. Transl. Med.* **2018**, *16*, 280. [CrossRef] [PubMed]

13. Topliss, D. Thyroid incidentaloma: The ignorant in pursuit of the impalpable. *Clin. Endocrinol.* **2004**, *60*, 18–20. [CrossRef]

14. Cerutti, J.M.; Delcelo, R.; Amadei, M.J.; Nakabashi, C.; Maciel, R.M.B.; Peterson, B.; Shoemaker, J.; Riggins, G.J. A preoperative diagnostic test that distinguishes benign from malignant thyroid carcinoma based on gene expression. *J. Clin. Investig.* **2004**, *113*, 1234–1242. [CrossRef] [PubMed]

15. Cerutti, J.M.; Latini, F.R.M.; Nakabashi, C.; Delcelo, R.; Andrade, V.P.; Amadei, M.J.; Maciel, R.M.B.; Hojaij, F.C.; Hollis, D.; Shoemaker, J.; et al. Diagnosis of suspicious thyroid nodules using four protein biomarkers. *Clin. Cancer Res.* **2006**, *12*, 3311–3318. [CrossRef] [PubMed]

16. Cerutti, J.M.; Oler, G.; Delcelo, R.; Gerardt, R.; Michaluart, P.; de Souza, S.J.; Galante, P.A.F.; Huang, P.; Riggins, G.J. PVALB, a new Hürthle adenoma diagnostic marker identified through gene expression. *J. Clin. Endocrinol. Metab.* **2011**, *96*, E151–E160. [CrossRef] [PubMed]

17. Tuminello, S.; van Gerwen, M.A.G.; Genden, E.; Crane, M.; Lieberman-Cribbin, W.; Taioli, E. Increased incidence of thyroid cancer among World Trade Center first responders: A descriptive epidemiological assessment. *Int. J. Environ. Res. Public Health* **2019**, *16*, 1258. [CrossRef] [PubMed]

18. Cardis, E.; Kesminiene, A.; Ivanov, V.; Malakhova, I.; Shibata, Y.; Khrouch, V.; Drozdovitch, V.; Maceika, E.; Zvonova, I.; Vlassov, O.; et al. Risk of thyroid cancer after exposure to 131I in childhood. *J. Natl. Cancer Inst.* **2005**, *18*, 724–732. [CrossRef] [PubMed]

19. Liu, X.; Bishop, J.; Shan, Y.; Pai, S.; Liu, D.; Murugan, A.K.; Sun, H.; El-Naggar, A.K.; Xing, M. Highly prevalent TERT promoter mutations in aggressive thyroid tumors. *Endocr. Relat. Cancer* **2013**, *20*, 603–610. [CrossRef] [PubMed]

20. Shen, X.; Liu, R.; Xing, M. A six-type genetic prognostic model for papillary thyroid cancer. *Endocr. Relat. Cancer* **2017**, *24*, 41–52. [CrossRef] [PubMed]

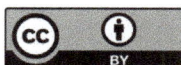

International Journal of
Environmental Research and Public Health

MDPI

Article

Abnormalities on Chest Computed Tomography and Lung Function Following an Intense Dust Exposure: A 17-Year Longitudinal Study

Charles Liu [1,†], Barbara Putman [1,2,3,†], Ankura Singh [2,4], Rachel Zeig-Owens [2,4,5], Charles B. Hall [6], Theresa Schwartz [2,4], Mayris P. Webber [2,5], Hillel W. Cohen [5], Melissa J. Fazzari [6], David J. Prezant [2,4] and Michael D. Weiden [1,2,*]

[1] Pulmonary, Critical Care and Sleep Medicine Division, Department of Medicine and Department of Environmental Medicine, New York University School of Medicine, New York, NY 10016, USA; Charles.Liu@nyulangone.org (C.L.); Barbara.Putman@nyulangone.org (B.P.)

[2] The Bureau of Health Services and the FDNY World Trade Center Health Program, Fire Department of the City of New York, Brooklyn, NY 11201, USA; Ankura.Singh@fdny.nyc.gov (A.S.); Rachel.Zeig-Owens@fdny.nyc.gov (R.Z.-O.); Theresa.Schwartz@fdny.nyc.gov (T.S.); Mayris.Webber@fdny.nyc.gov (M.P.W.); David.Prezant@fdny.nyc.gov (D.J.P.)

[3] Department of Bioanalysis, Faculty of Pharmaceutical Sciences, Ghent University, 9000 Ghent, Belgium

[4] Pulmonary Medicine Division, Department of Medicine, Montefiore Medical Center and Albert Einstein College of Medicine, Bronx, NY 10467, USA

[5] Division of Epidemiology, Department of Epidemiology and Population Health, Albert Einstein College of Medicine, Bronx, NY 10461, USA; Hillel.Cohen@einstein.yu.edu

[6] Division of Biostatistics, Department of Epidemiology and Population Health, Albert Einstein College of Medicine, Bronx, NY 10461, USA; Charles.Hall@einstein.yu.edu (C.B.H.); Melissa.Fazzari@einstein.yu.edu (M.J.F.)

[*] Correspondence: Michael.Weiden@nyulangone.org; Tel.: +1-718-999-1919

[†] Contributed equally to the investigation.

Received: 15 February 2019; Accepted: 9 May 2019; Published: 13 May 2019

Abstract: Fire Department of the City of New York (FDNY) firefighters experienced intense dust exposure working at the World Trade Center (WTC) site on and after 11/9/2001 (9/11). We hypothesized that high-intensity WTC exposure caused abnormalities found on chest computed tomography (CT). Between 11/9/2001–10/9/2018, 4277 firefighters underwent a clinically-indicated chest CT. Spirometric measurements and symptoms were recorded during routine medical examinations. High-intensity exposure, defined as initial arrival at the WTC on the morning of 9/11, increased the risk of bronchial wall thickening, emphysema, and air trapping. Early post-9/11 symptoms of wheeze and shortness of breath were associated with bronchial wall thickening, emphysema, and air trapping. The risk of accelerated forced expiratory volume at one second (FEV_1) decline (>64 mL/year decline) increased with bronchial wall thickening and emphysema, but decreased with air trapping. The risk of airflow obstruction also increased with bronchial wall thickening and emphysema but decreased with air trapping. In a previously healthy occupational cohort, high-intensity WTC exposure increased the risk for CT abnormalities. Bronchial wall thickening and emphysema were associated with respiratory symptoms, accelerated FEV_1 decline, and airflow obstruction. Air trapping was associated with respiratory symptoms, although lung function was preserved. Physiologic differences between CT abnormalities suggest that distinct types of airway injury may result from a common exposure.

Keywords: medical imaging; pulmonary function tests; lung injury; occupational exposure; epidemiological studies

1. Introduction

The collapse of the World Trade Center (WTC) on the morning of 11 September 2001 (9/11) produced a caustic dust plume containing more than 10,000,000 tons of irritating alkaline dust with pH > 10 [1]. Fire Department of the City of New York (FDNY) rescue and recovery workers who arrived at the site the morning of 9/11, were exposed to an extremely high concentration of dust that produced airway injury. Those who arrived in the afternoon and following days received a lower intensity, but substantial exposure, as rescue and recovery work resuspended the dust. WTC exposure produced an acute drop in forced expiratory volume at one second (FEV_1) and forced vital capacity (FVC) in FDNY workers present at the site prior to 24/9/2001 [2–4]. In the years following 9/11, WTC-exposed rescue/recovery workers had high rates of airway injury, including excessive loss of lung function [2], airflow obstruction [3], and airway hyper-reactivity [4]. A significant portion of the cohort experienced accelerated FEV_1 decline, defined as greater than 64 mL/year FEV_1 decline, a risk factor for chronic obstructive pulmonary disease (COPD) [5] and asthma/COPD overlap [6].

Computed tomography (CT) can detect structural lung abnormalities in individuals with respiratory symptoms and normal spirometry [7]. Self-report of exposure to vapors, gas, dust, or fumes was associated with an increase in emphysema, bronchial wall thickening, and air trapping on quantitative CT imaging in cohorts of smokers without WTC exposure [8,9]. Bronchial wall thickening was associated with FEV_1 decline in WTC-exposed cohorts [3,10,11]. Air trapping on expiratory CT imaging is a manifestation of small airway disease [12,13] and has been observed in a number of WTC-exposed cohorts [10,14]. The relationship between WTC dust exposure and these CT abnormalities, however, is still poorly defined.

The aim of this study was to determine predictors of WTC-related airway CT abnormalities on clinically-indicated chest CT (N = 4277). The main predictor of interest was high-intensity WTC dust exposure, defined as initial arrival at the WTC site during the morning of 9/11. We also examined the associations of emphysema, bronchial wall thickening and air trapping with early respiratory symptoms and longitudinal lung function in order to understand the clinical correlates of radiographic airway abnormalities in this population.

2. Methods

2.1. Study Population

The source population consisted of 9638 male firefighters who were actively employed by the FDNY on 9/11, first arrived at the WTC site between 11/9–24/9/2001, and had ≥3 post-9/11 routine medical monitoring spirometries taken at FDNY [5]. A subset of this population received at least one clinically-indicated chest CT at a hospital-based radiology facility between 11/9/2001 and 10/9/2018. The final study population included 4277 firefighters (Figure 1). Participants provided written informed consent. The Montefiore Medical Center (FWA #00002558)/Albert Einstein College of Medicine (FWA #00023382) Institutional Review Board approved this study.

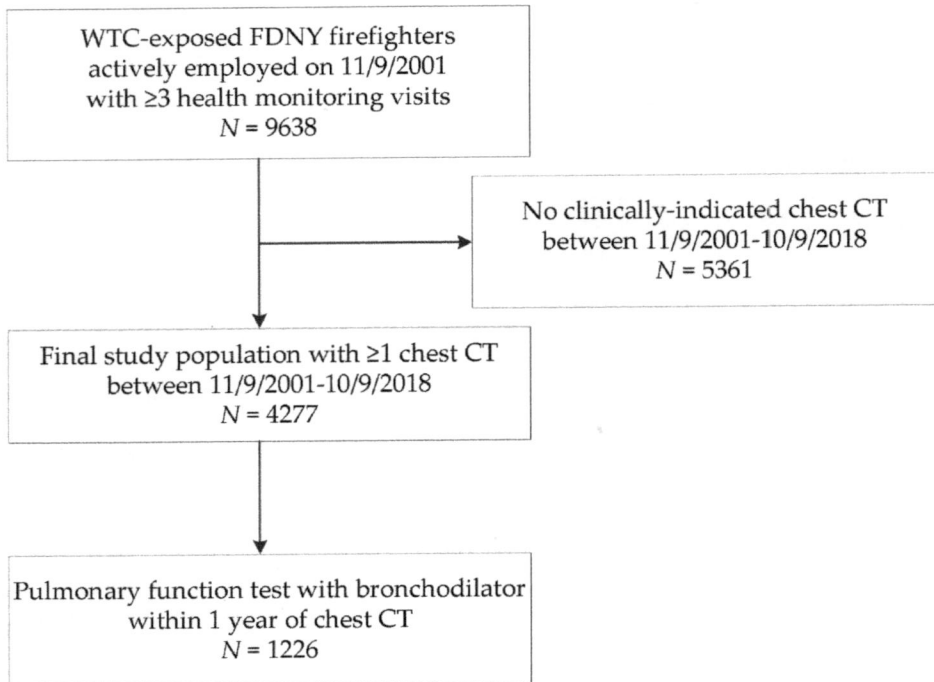

Figure 1. Firefighters who participated in the chest computed tomography (CT) study. Shown is the source population of male firefighters who were employed by the Fire Department of the City of New York (FDNY) on 11/9/2001, present at the World Trade Center (WTC) site between 11/9/2001 and 24/9/2001, and had at least three monitoring pulmonary function tests (PFTs) between 11/9/2001–10/9/2018 to assess longitudinal forced expiratory volume at one second (FEV_1) and FEV_1/FVC (forced vital capacity). The final study population included those who had received a clinically-indicated chest CT scan between 11/9/2001 and 10/9/2018. A subgroup had a clinically-indicated bronchodilator PFT within one year of the chest CT.

2.2. CT Scans

Inspiratory and expiratory noncontrast chest CTs were performed at a hospital-based radiology facility. Clinical indications for chest CT included symptoms or reductions in spirometry. All CT scans received standard radiologic evaluation. Radiologists were unaware of intensity of WTC exposure, and radiologist reports were entered into the FDNY medical record in real-time. The findings of emphysema, bronchial wall thickening, and air trapping were abstracted and entered into the FDNY medical record. The first post-9/11 CT scan report was used for analysis.

2.3. Participant Characteristics

Demographic data (age and race) were obtained from the FDNY employee database. Participants' height, weight, and self-reported smoking status (ever or never-smoker) were assessed during routine medical monitoring examinations at FDNY, scheduled once every 12–18 months. Those who consistently self-reported no cigarette smoking were classified as never-smokers. Those who ever reported current or former smoking on medical monitoring exams were defined as ever-smokers.

2.4. World Trade Center Dust Exposure

Participants' time of initial arrival at the WTC site was determined during the first medical monitoring examination. We classified individuals who arrived at the site on the morning of 9/11 as having high-intensity WTC exposure [4].

2.5. Longitudinal Respiratory Symptoms

A total of 44,832 medical monitoring exams, which included administration of health questionnaires and spirometry, were performed in the study population between 2/10/2001 and 10/9/2018 (median per individual: 11, interquartile range: 9–12). Reports of lower respiratory symptoms were collected via the self-administered physical health questionnaires [15]. For the respiratory symptoms within 6 months post 9/11, the first monitoring exam was used.

2.6. Longitudinal Screening Spirometry

FEV_1 and FVC measurements were obtained from spirometry performed during the monitoring examinations. Spirometry was carried out as described in our previous studies [2,4]. Post-9/11 rates of FEV_1 decline (FEV_1 slopes) were estimated for each participant using the first post-9/11 FEV_1 and all subsequent FEV_1 measurements in linear regression analyses that modeled FEV_1 as a linear function of time since 9/11. An FEV_1 slope of more than 64 mL/year was defined as accelerated FEV_1 decline. Airflow obstruction was defined as two consecutive FEV_1/FVC ratios less than 0.70; we required that measurements be at least one year apart [5].

2.7. Complete Pulmonary Function Testing

A subset of participants underwent complete pulmonary function tests (PFTs), which were performed according to American Thoracic Society standards [16] at a hospital-based pulmonary function laboratory. Because the Global Initiative for Chronic Obstructive Lung Disease definition of airflow limitation requires a postbronchodilator FEV_1/FVC ratio < 0.70, we conducted a sensitivity analysis within the participants who had had a complete PFT, which included pre- and postbronchodilator flow rates [17]. Total lung capacity, functional residual capacity (FRC) and residual volume (RV) measurements were also available from the complete PFT data; these were measured prior to bronchodilator administration and were used to calculate expiratory reserve volume (FRC minus RV).

2.8. Statistical Analyses

Demographic and other characteristics of the study population were assessed as n (%) and means (±SD). Chi-square tests were used to evaluate associations between bronchial wall-thickening, emphysema, and air-trapping. Hierarchic cluster analysis of the CT abnormalities was performed and a dendrogram was generated using SAS proc varclus with centroid method. We performed log-rank Mantel–Cox tests to examine the univariable associations of WTC exposure with the CT diagnoses of air trapping, emphysema, and bronchial wall thickening. Three separate multivariable Cox regression models assessed the associations of WTC exposure intensity with the outcomes emphysema, bronchial wall thickening, and air trapping. These analyses were repeated in the subset of the cohort that underwent medical monitoring in the first six months after 9/11 in order to investigate the relationship between early post-9/11 respiratory symptoms and abnormalities on chest CT ($N = 3610$). Follow-up time for these Cox models started at 9/11 and ended at the date of the CT scan. Parametric interval-censored survival models were used as sensitivity analyses, as the date of incidence of abnormalities would necessarily be prior to the CT on which they are identified. As a secondary analysis we performed a logistic regression to estimate associations between CT abnormalities and respiratory symptoms throughout the follow-up period, adjusting confidence intervals and p-values for potential overdispersion using the Pearson goodness-of-fit statistic. We then used logistic regression models to estimate associations of CT abnormalities with accelerated FEV_1 decline and airflow obstruction. We first used minimally-adjusted models, with age on 9/11 and race as the only covariates, and later added the covariates smoking status at the end of follow-up, first post-9/11 FEV_1, first post-9/11 BMI, and WTC exposure level. Covariates were selected based on previously known factors that affect lung physiology.

Linear mixed models with random intercepts were used to examine longitudinal FEV_1 % predicted and FEV_1/FVC ratio trajectories in those who had CT abnormalities. Participants' age on 9/11, height, and race were included as fixed effects in the models with FEV_1/FVC ratio as the outcome. Mean FEV_1 % predicted and FEV_1/FVC ratio were estimated for each 1-year period between 11/9/2000 and 10/9/2018 for four separate groups based on the following CT outcomes: no CT diagnosis, isolated air trapping, isolated emphysema, and isolated bronchial wall thickening. For these analyses, we excluded 403 participants with more than one CT abnormality.

Two analyses were performed in the subset of study participants with complete PFTs ($N = 1226$). A multivariable logistic regression model assessed the associations between the CT abnormalities and airflow obstruction (post-bronchodilator FEV_1/FVC ratio < 0.70), and multivariable linear regression models were used to assess the associations between CT abnormalities and prebronchodilator lung volumes. Age on 9/11, race, BMI, smoking status at the end of follow-up, WTC exposure level and first post-9/11 FEV_1 were included as covariates. As stated above, covariates were selected based on previously known factors that affect lung physiology.

Reported *p*-values are two-sided and considered significant at the < 0.05 level. Data analyses and dendrogram were performed using SAS version 9.4 (SAS Institute, Inc., Cary, NC, USA). Cumulative incidence curves and lung function figures were created with Prism 8 (GraphPad Software, Inc., San Diego, CA, USA).

3. Results

3.1. Population Characteristics

The final study population, with clinically-indicated inspiratory and expiratory chest CT, was 37% of the source population. The CT scans were performed throughout the entire follow-up period, with a peak at year six post-9/11; this was due to increased outreach to recently retired WTC-exposed firefighters at that time (Figure S1 in Supplementary Materials). Demographic and other characteristics of the 4277 firefighters in the final study population (Figure 1) and those without chest CT scans are presented in Table 1. Fewer than 1% of study participants had missing covariate data. Compared with WTC-exposed firefighters who did not have a clinically indicated chest CT, the study population with a clinically indicated chest CT was slightly different in that it was older, had a greater proportion of ever-smokers, higher intensity WTC exposure (arrival at the WTC site on the morning of 9/11), lower postexposure lung function, and had a higher proportion of reports of shortness of breath and wheeze within six months of 9/11.

Table 1. Population characteristics *.

Variable	Population without Chest CT $N = 5361$	Chest CT Study Population $N = 4277$
Age on 9/11	39.4 ± 7.5	41.2 ± 7.2
BMI ‡	28.7 ± 3.4	29.0 ± 3.5
	Smoking Status, *N* (%)	
Never	3804 (71.0)	2653 (62.0)
Ever	1557 (29.0)	1624 (38.0)
	Race, *N* (%)	
White	5026 (93.8)	4053 (94.8)
Black	139 (2.6)	86 (2.0)
Hispanic	180 (3.4)	128 (3.0)
Other	16 (0.3)	10 (0.2)

Table 1. Cont.

Variable	Population without Chest CT N = 5361	Chest CT Study Population N = 4277
World Trade Center exposure, N (%)		
Morning of 9/11	463 (8.6)	1113 (26.0)
Afternoon on 9/11–9/12	4125 (76.9)	2781 (65.0)
9/13–9/24	773 (14.4)	383 (9.0)
First Post-9/11 Spirometry		
FEV_1 % predicted	98.3 ± 13.1	95.4 ± 14.2
FVC % predicted	93.4 ± 11.8	91.1± 12.3
FEV_1/FVC	0.84 ± 0.05	0.83 ± 0.06
Post-9/11: FEV_1 slope (mL/year)	−34.6 ± 25.6	−38.9 ± 30.5
Report of respiratory symptoms within 6 months of 9/11		
Shortness of breath	1004 (22.3) [§]	1289 (35.7) [‖]
Wheeze	797 (17.7) [§]	989 (27.4) [‖]

* All values are mean ± standard deviation unless otherwise stated. [‡] Body Mass Index. [§] N = 4500. [‖] N = 3610.

3.2. CT Abnormalities and WTC Exposure

Inspiratory and expiratory chest CTs diagnosed bronchial wall thickening in 837 individuals (20%) and air trapping in 894 (21%). Nodules greater than or equal to 5 mm and ground glass opacities were less common but present in over 10% of participants (Table 2). Emphysema, pleural thickening, and bronchiectasis were present in between 3% and 6% of participants. Pulmonary fibrosis was rare, present in just 0.6% of individuals with a CT. Bronchial wall thickening was correlated with air trapping and emphysema ($p < 0.001$ and $p < 0.001$, respectively), but air trapping and emphysema were not correlated with one another ($p = 0.72$). Hierarchical clustering demonstrated that bronchial wall thickening clustered with air trapping (Figure 2). Bronchiectasis and emphysema clustered but were distantly related to bronchial wall thickening and air trapping. The parenchymal abnormalities of pleural thickening and pulmonary nodules clustered as did ground glass opacities and pulmonary fibrosis.

Table 2. Prevalence of CT abnormality.

CT Abnormality	Percentage of Chest CT Scans with Abnormality
Air Trapping	20.9
Bronchial Wall Thickening	19.6
Nodules ≥ 5 mm	14.6
Ground Glass Opacities	12.2
Emphysema	5.9
Bronchiectasis	3.6
Pleural Thickening	3.0
Pulmonary Fibrosis	0.6

Note: abnormalities are not mutually exclusive.

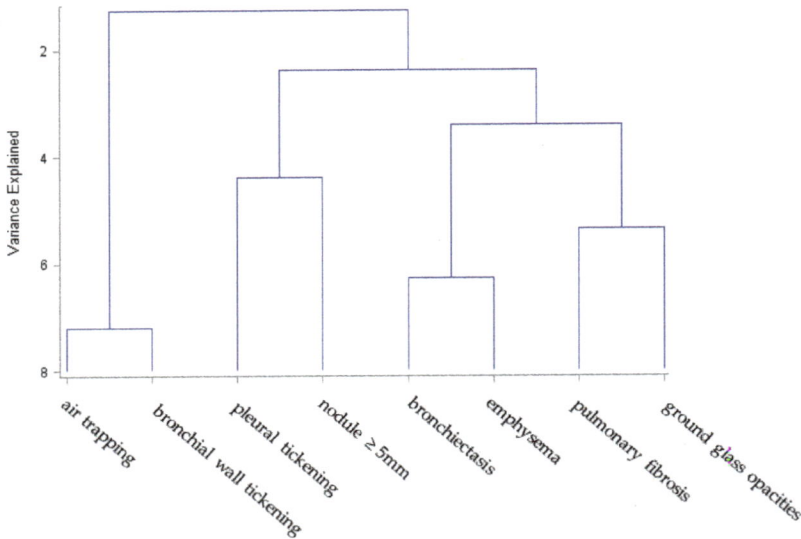

Figure 2. Chest CT abnormalities in WTC-exposed firefighters. The dendrogram demonstrates clustering of abnormalities on chest CTs.

Univariable analyses showed that high-intensity WTC exposure is associated with a 2.2-fold increased risk of air trapping, a 1.6-fold increased risk of emphysema, and a 2.2-fold increase in the risk of bronchial wall thickening Figure 3. The associations between high-intensity WTC exposure and chest CT diagnoses persisted in a multivariable Cox regression model (Table 3). Emphysema was strongly associated with ever-smoking. Bronchial wall thickening was also associated with ever-smoking, though the magnitude of association was lower.

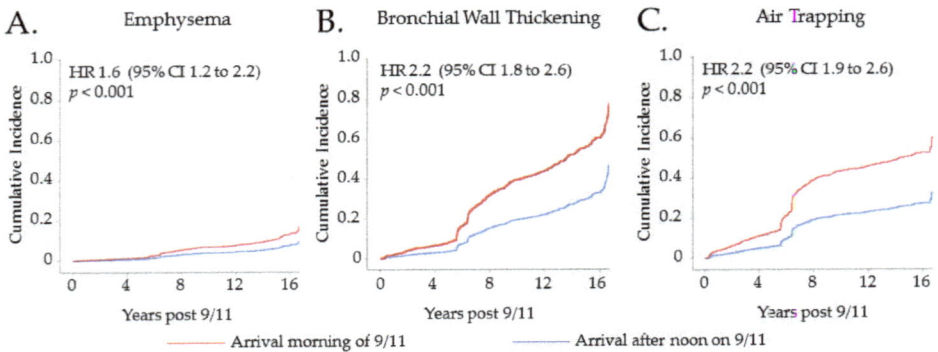

Figure 3. Cumulative incidence of chest CT diagnosis according to WTC exposure intensity. (**A**) shows the cumulative incidence of emphysema in participants who arrived morning of 9/11 at the WTC site (red line) compared with those who arrived between the afternoon of 9/11 and 24/9/2001 (blue line). (**B**) shows the cumulative incidence of bronchial wall thickening in those who arrived morning of 9/11 (red) and those who arrived later (blue). (**C**) shows the cumulative incidence of air trapping in participants who arrived morning of 9/11 (red) and those who arrived later (blue).

Table 3. Cox regression models predicting three Chest CT abnormalities [a,b].

Variables	Emphysema			Bronchial Wall Thickening			Air Trapping		
	HR	95% CI	p	HR	95% CI	p	HR	95% CI	p
WTC exposure morning of 9/11	1.83	1.36–2.45	<0.001	2.33	2.00–2.72	<0.001	2.34	1.95–2.80	<0.001
Ever-smoker [c]	7.04	4.94–10.04	<0.001	1.25	1.08–1.44	0.003	0.73	0.61–0.88	0.001

[a] $N = 4277$. [b] Adjusted for age, race, BMI and first post-9/11 FEV_1. [c] Reference is never-smoker.

3.3. CT Abnormalities and Respiratory Symptoms

Respiratory symptoms of shortness of breath and wheezing were common during the first six months after 9/11; 28.2% (1,018/3,610) reported a single symptom of either shortness of breath or wheezing, and 17.5% (630/3,610) reported both shortness of breath and wheezing. Early respiratory symptoms increased the risk of air trapping, emphysema, and bronchial wall thickening according to a Cox model adjusted for age, race, BMI, smoking status, WTC exposure and first post-9/11 FEV_1. Having both shortness of breath and wheezing was a greater risk factor for each of the CT abnormalities than having either symptom by itself (Table 4). We also assessed persistence of symptoms in longitudinal follow-up. Participants with air trapping, emphysema, or bronchial wall thickening on chest CT reported shortness of breath and/or wheeze more frequently during medical monitoring exams between 11/9/2001 and 10/9/2018 than those without one of those abnormalities on chest CT. (data not shown).

Table 4. Subpopulation with respiratory symptoms reported within six months of exposure [a,b].

Variables	Emphysema			Bronchial Wall Thickening			Air Trapping		
	HR	95% CI	p	HR	95% CI	p	HR	95% CI	p
Either shortness of breath or wheeze	1.43	1.04–1.97	0.03	1.38	1.16–1.63	<0.001	1.27	1.08–1.49	0.005
Both shortness of breath and wheeze	1.62	1.12–2.33	0.01	1.49	1.22–1.83	<0.001	1.41	1.16–1.70	<0.001

[a] $N = 3610$. [b] Adjusted for age, race, BMI, smoking status, WTC exposure and first post-9/11 FEV_1.

3.4. CT Abnormalities and Longitudinal Spirometry

To assess spirometric correlates of CT abnormalities, we tested the associations of emphysema, bronchial wall thickening, and air trapping with accelerated FEV_1 decline. A minimally-adjusted logistic regression model, adjusted for only age and race, showed similar results as Table 5 (data not shown). Emphysema and bronchial wall thickening were associated with increased risk of accelerated FEV_1 decline in a multivariable-adjusted logistic model (Table 5), and air trapping was associated with reduced odds of accelerated FEV_1 decline.

Table 5. Multivariable logistic regression model assessing associations of CT diagnoses with accelerated FEV_1 decline [*,†].

CT Diagnosis	OR	95% CI
Emphysema	1.89	1.37–2.60
Bronchial Wall Thickening	1.55	1.25–1.92
Air Trapping	0.77	0.61–0.97

[*] $N = 4277$; [†] Adjusted for age, race, BMI, smoking status, WTC exposure and first post 9/11 FEV_1.

We then examined how airway abnormalities on CT were associated with longitudinal FEV_1 and FEV_1/FVC ratio using stratified mixed effect linear models (Figure 4). Isolated emphysema was associated with the most rapid longitudinal FEV_1 decline, while FEV_1 decline in those with isolated bronchial wall thickening was intermediate between the isolated emphysema and air trapping subgroups (Figure 4A).

A different pattern emerged when examining longitudinal FEV$_1$/FVC ratio (Figure 4B). When compared with individuals with no airway abnormalities on CT, isolated air trapping was associated with increased FEV$_1$/FVC ratio both before and after 9/11. FEV$_1$/ FVC ratio was lowest in the isolated emphysema subgroup, and intermediate in those with isolated bronchial wall thickening.

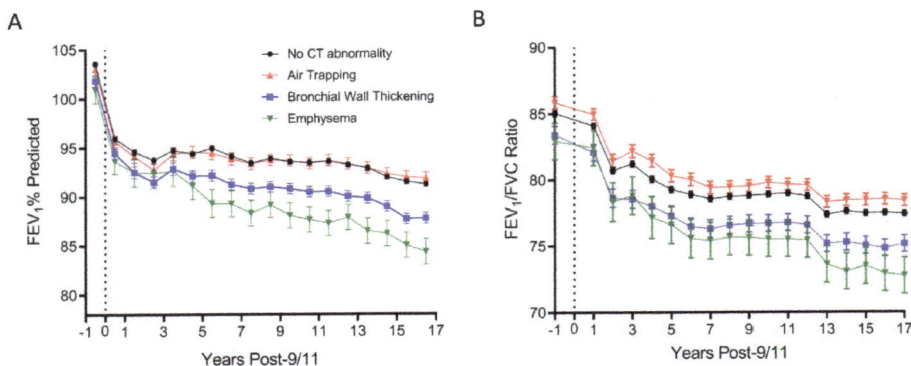

Figure 4. Longitudinal lung function according to CT abnormality. (**A**) shows mean FEV$_1$ % predicted (± SEM) in each year between 11/9/2000 and 10/9/2018 in the no chest CT diagnosis (black circles), isolated air trapping (blue triangles), isolated bronchial wall thickening (brown squares), and isolated emphysema (red inverted triangle) groups. (**B**) shows mean (± SEM) FEV$_1$/FVC ratio in each year in the aforementioned groups, adjusted for age, race and height. Number of subjects in each nonoverlapping group is shown. The vertical line at 0 represents 11/9/2001.

We then tested whether having airway abnormalities on CT was associated with airflow obstruction, defined as either two consecutive FEV$_1$/FVC ratios < 0.70 on screening spirometry (N = 4277) or as postbronchodilator FEV$_1$/FVC ratio <0.70 in the subgroup with complete PFTs (N = 1226). Minimally-adjusted logistic regression, adjusting for age and race only, showed that both emphysema and bronchial wall thickening increased the odds of airflow obstruction (OR: 3.34, 95% CI: 2.47–4.51 and OR: 2.19, 95% CI: 1.04–1.07), but air trapping was associated with a reduced odds of this outcome (OR: 0.46, 95% CI: 0.34–0.62). Emphysema and bronchial wall thickening were also associated with an elevated odds of airflow obstruction in multivariable logistic regression analyses that included age, race, BMI, smoking status, first post-9/11 FEV$_1$, and WTC exposure level (Table 6). Air rapping was still associated with a lower odds of airflow obstruction after adjusting for these additional covariates. Analyses performed in the subpopulation with complete PFTs showed similar results.

Table 6. Multivariable logistic regression models assessing association of CT diagnosis with two definitions of airflow obstruction*.

CT Diagnosis	Two Consecutive Screening Spirometric FEV$_1$/FVC < 0.70 N = 4277		Post-BD $ FEV$_1$/FVC < 0.70 N = 1225	
	OR	95% CI	OR	95% CI
Emphysema	2.03	1.44–2.88	2.63	1.56–4.42
Bronchial Wall Thickening	2.25	1.77–2.87	2.67	1.84–3.88
Air Trapping	0.40	0.29–0.55	0.36	0.22–0.58

* Adjusted for age, race, BMI, smoking status, WTC exposure and first post-9/11 FEV$_1$. $ Post-bronchodilator.

3.5. CT Abnormalities and Lung Volumes

We evaluated the associations of emphysema, bronchial wall thickening, and air trapping with lung volumes in the subgroup with complete PFTs. In multivariable linear regression analyses, emphysema, bronchial wall thickening, and air trapping were associated with greater total lung capacity. Emphysema and bronchial wall thickening were also associated with increased functional residual capacity, while air trapping was associated with reduced expiratory reserve volume (Table 7).

Table 7. Multivariable linear models assessing the association of CT abnormalities with lung volumes [a,b].

CT Abnormality	Total Lung Capacity [c]			Functional Residual Capacity [c]			Expiratory Reserve Volume [c]		
	Beta	95% CI	*p*	Beta	95% CI	*p*	Beta	95% CI	*p*
Air Trapping	57	−76, 189	0.40	−71	−169, 27	0.16	−205	−281, −129	<0.001
Emphysema	571	357, 786	<0.001	478	319, 637	<0.001	161	38, 285	0.01
Bronchial Wall Thickening	300	169, 432	<0.001	236	139, 334	<0.001	−46	−122, 30	0.23

[a] Adjusted for age, race, BMI, smoking status, WTC exposure and first post-9/11 FEV$_1$. [b] mL. [c] N = 1226 due to missing covariates. [d] N = 1224 due to missing covariates.

4. Discussion

This study documented that firefighters who arrived at the WTC site on the morning of 9/11 (high-intensity exposure) had a higher risk of subsequent airway abnormalities on chest CT than those with lesser WTC exposure. This supports the hypothesis that WTC exposure contributed to the development of these airway abnormalities. Those with the highest dust exposure had an increased odds of subsequent emphysema, bronchial wall thickening and air trapping after controlling for potential confounders. The increased risk of CT abnormalities following high-intensity WTC exposure suggests that a massive but brief irritant contact is a risk factor for radiographic abnormalities even years after the exposure. Because both the high and low WTC exposure groups share the non-WTC occupational exposure of firefighting, the increased risk of CT abnormalities in the high exposure group is therefore attributable to WTC exposure. These data are consistent with prior case-control studies in WTC-exposed cohorts [10] and in occupational cohorts with high smoking prevalence [8,9].

The airway abnormalities on CT were associated with early respiratory symptoms in this cohort. Large cohort studies in the general population have demonstrated associations between respiratory symptoms and CT abnormalities including emphysema, bronchial wall thickening, and air trapping [7,18–20]. In our population, those with CT abnormalities had elevated functional residual capacity. Similar elevated lung volumes have been observed in other WTC cohorts [14], suggesting that dynamic hyperinflation could contribute to respiratory symptoms even in individuals with normal FEV$_1$ and FEV$_1$/FVC ratio [21].

Unlike other dust-exposed occupational cohorts, WTC exposed firefighters were a health occupational cohort prior to WTC exposure with normal lung function [2]. This could be a reason why certain CT abnormalities were rare. Pulmonary fibrosis was present in only 0.6% of the first post-9/11 clinically indicated chest CTs. Similarly, ground glass opacities, pulmonary nodules, and pleural thickening were uncommon present in only 3 to 15%.

Only 6% of the study population had emphysema, likely due to the healthy worker effect of a physically demanding occupation, and the fact that there were fewer smokers than in the general population. As expected, emphysema was strongly associated with cigarette smoking, accelerated FEV$_1$ decline, and airflow obstruction. Importantly, those with the most intense dust exposure had an increased risk of emphysema when compared with those with less intense exposure after adjusting for potential confounders. This suggests that those caught in the dust cloud on the morning of 9/11, especially ever-smokers, will continue to be at a higher risk for developing emphysema than those with less intense WTC dust exposure.

While bronchial wall thickening and air trapping cluster closely together, air trapping is a physiologically distinct manifestation of dust-induced small airway injury. Unlike bronchial wall thickening, small airways disease leading to air trapping was associated with reduced odds of airflow obstruction in this cohort. Reduction of expiratory reserve volume associated with air trapping likely contributes to the observed reduction of FVC. This could account for the elevated longitudinal FEV_1/FVC ratio. The preservation of FEV_1 in those with air trapping suggests the disease process spares the larger airways that limit forced expiratory airflow. In our cohort, the impact of high-intensity exposure on subsequent air trapping was stronger in never-smokers than ever-smokers. In non-WTC cohorts, excessive FEV_1 decline was observed in those with smoking-associated and age-related air trapping [12,13,22]. Furthermore, in smokers, air trapping may be a transition state to emphysema [23]. In our cohort with preserved lung function and low smoking prevalence, air trapping was not associated with smoking or emphysema, suggesting that the mechanism of small airway injury or stage of disease may influence the relationships between CT abnormalities and FEV_1 decline. This highlights the need to use different measures of distal airway function, such as impulse oscillometry, to assess and follow the physiology of small airway abnormalities associated with air trapping on CT [24–26]. Further research is needed to define effective treatments in those who have air trapping-associated symptoms, but preserved FEV_1 and FEV_1/FVC ratio.

Firefighters with bronchial wall thickening had greater longitudinal FEV_1 decline and airflow obstruction when compared with those having no airway abnormalities or air trapping. Bronchial wall thickening had a phenotype that was similar to but less severe than emphysema, with increased total lung capacity, functional residual capacity, and increased risk of accelerated FEV_1 decline and airflow obstruction. Greater FEV_1 decline observed on serial spirometry is a strong risk factor for airflow obstruction [5]. The increased risk of airflow obstruction associated with bronchial wall thickening was similar regardless of whether obstruction was determined by $FEV_1/FVC < 0.70$ in the entire study group (serial spirometry) or in the subgroup with postbronchodilator measurements. This suggests that misclassification or selection bias associated with the different definitions of obstruction did not change the associations with CT abnormalities. The association of bronchial wall thickening with accelerated FEV_1 decline highlights the utility of CT in risk assessment of symptomatic patients with preserved lung function [7]. Future investigation of longitudinal CT scans is needed to assess if bronchial wall thickening is a risk factor for developing emphysema, especially in never-smokers.

There are several limitations to this investigation. FDNY firefighters are overwhelmingly white, male, and previously healthy workers, potentially limiting generalizability of these findings; however, most findings from the FDNY cohort have been replicated in other WTC-exposed cohorts [10,11,14]. The reported CT abnormalities were real world data defined by clinical radiologists without quantitative image analysis or inter-reader reliability measures. Nonetheless, there were strong correlations between CT abnormalities and exposure intensity. CT airway abnormalities also correlated with PFT measurements, including lung volumes, suggesting validity of the clinical CT interpretation. Lastly, since the CT scans were clinically indicated, this study was vulnerable to selection bias. The study population differed from those without chest CTs, with more intense WTC exposure, more respiratory symptoms and worse postexposure lung function. This precludes assessment of the incidence of abnormal CTs in the entire cohort, since undiagnosed cases are likely. Nevertheless, analyses within the CT population provide a valid assessment of risk factors for specific diagnoses within a symptomatic subgroup.

5. Conclusions

In WTC-exposed firefighters, high-intensity dust exposure was associated with subsequent bronchial wall thickening, air trapping, and emphysema, a causal link between WTC exposure and these CT abnormalities. Emphysema and bronchial wall thickening were associated with airflow obstruction and an accelerated rate of longitudinal FEV_1 loss. Isolated air trapping identifies a symptomatic subgroup without excessive FEV_1 decline or airflow obstruction.

The findings from this study are a valuable resource for understanding irritant-induced airways disease in a previously healthy population. In those with radiographic abnormalities, the 17-year decline in lung function is still mild enough that the potential exists for interventions, such as tobacco cessation or pharmacologic targeting of specific inflammatory pathways, to improve lung function trajectory and respiratory symptoms.

Supplementary Materials: The following are available online at http://www.mdpi.com/1660-4601/16/9/1655/s1, Figure S1: Distribution of the timing of chest CT. The histogram is showing the number of chest CT scans used for this study, grouped by year post-9/11. There is a peak at year 6–7 post-9/11, with 1049/4277 (25%) CT scans performed that year.

Author Contributions: Conceptualization, M.D.W.; Data curation, A.S. and T.S.; Formal analysis, B.P.; Methodology, R.Z.-C., C.B.H. and M.J.F.; Supervision, R.Z.-O., D.J.P. and M.D.W.; Visualization, C.L., B.P. and M.D.W.; Writing—original draft, C.L., B.P. and M.D.W.; Writing—review & editing, A.S., R.Z.-O., C.B.H., M.P.W., H.W.C., M.J.F and D.J.P.

Funding: This research was funded by National Institute for Occupational Safety and Health, grant number U01 OH011302 and contracts #200-2011-39383, #200-2011-39378, #200-2017-93426 and #200-2017-93326. The APC was funded by U01 OH011302.

Acknowledgments: Role of sponsors: The sponsors had no role in the design and conduct of the study, the collection, management, analysis, and interpretation of the data, the preparation, review, and approval of the manuscript, or the decision to submit the manuscript for publication.

Conflicts of Interest: The authors declare no conflicts of interest.

References

1. Lioy, P.J.; Weisel, C.P.; Millette, J.R.; Eisenreich, S.; Vallero, D.; Offenberg, J.; Buckley, B.; Turpin, B.; Zhong, M.; Cohen, M.D.; et al. Characterization of the dust/smoke aerosol that settled east of the world trade center (wtc) in lower manhattan after the collapse of the wtc 11 september 2001. *Environ. Health Perspect* **2002**, *110*, 703–714. [CrossRef]

2. Aldrich, T.K.; Gustave, J.; Hall, C.B.; Cohen, H.W.; Webber, M.P.; Zeig-Owens, R.; Cosenza, K.; Christodoulou, V.; Glass, L.; Al-Othman, F.; et al. Lung function in rescue workers at the world trade center after 7 years. *N. Engl. J. Med.* **2010**, *362*, 1263–1272. [CrossRef] [PubMed]

3. Weiden, M.D.; Ferrier, N.; Nolan, A.; Rom, W.N.; Comfort, A.; Gustave, J.; Zeig-Owens, R.; Zheng, S.; Goldring, R.M.; Berger, K.I.; et al. Obstructive airways disease with air trapping among firefighters exposed to world trade center dust. *Chest* **2010**, *137*, 566–574. [CrossRef] [PubMed]

4. Aldrich, T.K.; Vossbrinck, M.; Zeig-Owens, R.; Hall, C.B.; Schwartz, T.M.; Moir, W.; Webber, M.P.; Cohen, H.W.; Nolan, A.; Weiden, M.D.; et al. Lung function trajectories in world trade center-exposed new york city firefighters over 13 years: The roles of smoking and smoking cessation. *Chest* **2016**, *149*, 1419–1427. [CrossRef] [PubMed]

5. Zeig-Owens, R.; Singh, A.; Aldrich, T.K.; Hall, C.B.; Schwartz, T.; Webber, M.P.; Cohen, H.W.; Kelly, K.J.; Nolan, A.; Prezant, D.J.; et al. Blood leukocyte concentrations, fev1 decline, and airflow limitation. A 15-year longitudinal study of world trade center-exposed firefighters. *Ann. Am. Thorac. Soc.* **2018**, *15*, 173–183. [CrossRef] [PubMed]

6. Singh, A.; Liu, C.; Putman, B.; Zeig-Owens, R.; Hall, C.B.; Schwartz, T.; Webber, M.P.; Cohen, H.W.; Berger, K.I.; Nolan, A.; et al. Predictors of asthma/copd overlap in fdny firefighters with world trade center dust exposure: A longitudinal study. *Chest* **2018**, *154*, 1301–1310. [CrossRef] [PubMed]

7. Regan, E.A.; Lynch, D.A.; Curran-Everett, D.; Curtis, J.L.; Austin, J.H.; Grenier, P.A.; Kauczor, H.U.; Bailey, W.C.; DeMeo, D.L.; Casaburi, R.H.; et al. Clinical and radiologic disease in smokers with normal spirometry. *JAMA Intern. Med.* **2015**, *175*, 1539–1549. [CrossRef] [PubMed]

8. Paulin, L.M.; Smith, B.M.; Koch, A.; Han, M.; Hoffman, E.A.; Martinez, C.; Ejike, C.; Blanc, P.D.; Rous, J.; Barr, R.G.; et al. Occupational exposures and computed tomographic imaging characteristics in the spiromics cohort. *Ann. Am. Thorac. Soc.* **2018**, *15*, 1411–1419. [CrossRef]

9. Marchetti, N.; Garshick, E.; Kinney, G.L.; McKenzie, A.; Stinson, D.; Lutz, S.M.; Lynch, D.A.; Criner, G.J.; Silverman, E.K.; Crapo, J.D.; et al. Association between occupational exposure and lung function, respiratory symptoms, and high-resolution computed tomography imaging in copdgene. *Am. J. Respir. Crit. Care Med.* **2014**, *190*, 756–762. [CrossRef]

10. Mendelson, D.S.; Roggeveen, M.; Levin, S.M.; Herbert, R.; de la Hoz, R.E. Air trapping detected on end-expiratory high-resolution computed tomography in symptomatic world trade center rescue and recovery workers. *J. Occup. Env. Med.* **2007**, *49*, 840–845. [CrossRef]

11. de la Hoz, R.E.; Liu, X.; Doucette, J.T.; Reeves, A.P.; Bienenfeld, L.A.; Wisnivesky, J.P.; Celedon, J.C.; Lynch, D.A.; San Jose Estepar, R. Increased airway wall thickness is associated with adverse longitudinal first-second forced expiratory volume trajectories of former world trade center workers. *Lung* **2018**, *196*, 481–489. [CrossRef] [PubMed]

12. Galban, C.J.; Han, M.K.; Boes, J.L.; Chughtai, K.A.; Meyer, C.R.; Johnson, T.D.; Galban, S.; Rehemtulla, A.; Kazerooni, E.A.; Martinez, F.J.; et al. Computed tomography-based biomarker provides unique signature for diagnosis of copd phenotypes and disease progression. *Nat. Med.* **2012**, *18*, 1711–1715. [CrossRef]

13. Martinez, C.H.; Diaz, A.A.; Meldrum, C.; Curtis, J.L.; Cooper, C.B.; Pirozzi, C.; Kanner, R.E.; Paine, R., 3rd; Woodruff, P.G.; Bleecker, E.R.; et al. Age and small airway imaging abnormalities in subjects with and without airflow obstruction in spiromics. *Am. J. Respir. Crit. Care Med.* **2017**, *195*, 464–472. [CrossRef] [PubMed]

14. Berger, K.I.; Reibman, J.; Oppenheimer, B.W.; Vlahos, I.; Harrison, D.; Goldring, R M. Lessons from the world trade center disaster: Airway disease presenting as restrictive dysfunction. *Chest* **2013**, *144*, 249–257. [CrossRef] [PubMed]

15. Weakley, J.; Webber, M.P.; Gustave, J.; Kelly, K.; Cohen, H.W.; Hall, C.B.; Prezant, D.J. Trends in respiratory diagnoses and symptoms of firefighters exposed to the world trade center disaster: 2005–2010. *Prev. Med.* **2011**, *53*, 364–369. [CrossRef]

16. Miller, M.R.; Hankinson, J.; Brusasco, V.; Burgos, F.; Casaburi, R.; Coates, A.; Crapo, R.; Enright, P.; van der Grinten, C.P.; Gustafsson, P.; et al. Standardisation of spirometry. *Eur. Respir. J.* **2005**, *25*, 319–338. [CrossRef]

17. Vogelmeier, C.F.; Criner, G.J.; Martinez, F.J.; Anzueto, A.; Barnes, P.J.; Bourbeau, J.; Celli, B.R.; Chen, R.; Decramer, M.; Fabbri, L.M.; et al. Global strategy for the diagnosis, management, and prevention of chronic obstructive lung disease 2017 report. Gold executive summary. *Am. J. Respir. Crit. Care Med.* **2017**, *195*, 557–582. [CrossRef]

18. Tan, W.C.; Hague, C.J.; Leipsic, J.; Bourbeau, J.; Zheng, L.; Li, P.Z.; Sin, D.D.; Coxson, H.O.; Kirby, M.; Hogg, J.C.; et al. Findings on thoracic computed tomography scans and respiratory outcomes in persons with and without chronic obstructive pulmonary disease: A population-based cohort study. *PLoS ONE* **2016**, *11*, e0166745. [CrossRef]

19. Woodruff, P.G.; Barr, R.G.; Bleecker, E.; Christenson, S.A.; Couper, D.; Curtis, J.L.; Gouskova, N.A.; Hansel, N.N.; Hoffman, E.A.; Kanner, R.E.; et al. Clinical significance of symptoms in smokers with preserved pulmonary function. *N. Engl. J. Med.* **2016**, *374*, 1811–1821. [CrossRef]

20. Nambu, A.; Zach, J.; Schroeder, J.; Jin, G.; Kim, S.S.; Kim, Y.I.; Schnell, C.; Bowler, R.; Lynch, D.A. Quantitative computed tomography measurements to evaluate airway disease in chronic obstructive pulmonary disease: Relationship to physiological measurements, clinical index and visual assessment of airway disease. *Eur. J. Radiol.* **2016**, *85*, 2144–2151. [CrossRef]

21. Elbehairy, A.F.; Ciavaglia, C.E.; Webb, K.A.; Guenette, J.A.; Jensen, D.; Mourad, S.M.; Neder, J.A.; O'Donnell, D.E.; Canadian Respiratory Research Network. Pulmonary gas exchange abnormalities in mild chronic obstructive pulmonary disease. Implications for dyspnea and exercise intolerance. *Am. J. Respir. Crit. Care Med.* **2015**, *191*, 1384–1394. [CrossRef]

22. Bhatt, S.P.; Soler, X.; Wang, X.; Murray, S.; Anzueto, A.R.; Beaty, T.H.; Boriek, A.M.; Casaburi, R.; Criner, G.J.; Diaz, A.A.; et al. Association between functional small airway disease and fev1 decline in chronic obstructive pulmonary disease. *Am. J. Respir. Crit. Care Med.* **2016**, *194*, 178–184. [CrossRef] [PubMed]

23. Boes, J.L.; Hoff, B.A.; Bule, M.; Johnson, T.D.; Rehemtulla, A.; Chamberlain, R.; Hoffman, E.A.; Kazerooni, E.A.; Martinez, F.J.; Han, M.K.; et al. Parametric response mapping monitors temporal changes on lung ct scans in the subpopulations and intermediate outcome measures in copd study (spiromics). *Acad. Radiol.* **2015**, *22*, 186–194. [CrossRef]

24. Friedman, S.M.; Maslow, C.B.; Reibman, J.; Pillai, P.S.; Goldring, R.M.; Farfel, M.R.; Stellman, S.D.; Berger, K.I. Case-control study of lung function in world trade center health registry area residents and workers. *Am. J. Respir. Crit. Care Med.* **2011**, *184*, 582–589. [CrossRef] [PubMed]
25. Jordan, H.T.; Friedman, S.M.; Reibman, J.; Goldring, R.M.; Miller Archie, S.A.; Ortega, F.; Alper, H.; Shao, Y.; Maslow, C.B.; Cone, J.E.; et al. Risk factors for persistence of lower respiratory symptoms among community members exposed to the 2001 world trade center terrorist attacks. *Occup. Env. Med.* **2017**, *74*, 449–455. [CrossRef]
26. Crisafulli, E.; Pisi, R.; Aiello, M.; Vigna, M.; Tzani, P.; Torres, A.; Bertorelli, G.; Chetta, A. Prevalence of small-airway dysfunction among copd patients with different gold stages and its role in the impact of disease. *Respiration* **2017** *93*, 32–41. [CrossRef] [PubMed]

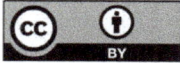

International Journal of
Environmental Research and Public Health

MDPI

Article

Post-9/11 Peripheral Neuropathy Symptoms among World Trade Center-Exposed Firefighters and Emergency Medical Service Workers

Hilary L. Colbeth [1,2], Rachel Zeig-Owens [1,2,3,*], Mayris P. Webber [1,3,4], David G. Goldfarb [1,2], Theresa M. Schwartz [1,2], Charles B. Hall [3,5] and David J. Prezant [1,6]

[1]   Fire Department of the City of New York, Bureau of Health Services, 9 Metrotech Center,
      Brooklyn, NY 11201, USA; Hilary.Colbeth@fdny.nyc.gov (H.L.C.); Mayris.Webber@fdny.nyc.gov (M.P.W.);
      David.Goldfarb@fdny.nyc.gov (D.G.G.); Theresa.Schwartz@fdny.nyc.gov (T.M.S.);
      David.Prezant@fdny.nyc.gov (D.J.P.)
[2]   Department of Medicine, Pulmonology Division, Montefiore Medical Center, Bronx, NY 10467, USA
[3]   Department of Epidemiology and Population Health, Albert Einstein College of Medicine,
      Bronx, NY 10461, USA; charles.hall@einstein.yu.edu
[4]   Department of Epidemiology and Population Health, Montefiore Medical Center,
      Department of Epidemiology and Population Health, Bronx, New York, NY 10467, USA
[5]   Saul R. Korey Department of Neurology, Albert Einstein College of Medicine, Bronx, NY 10461, USA
[6]   Department of Medicine, Pulmonology Division, Albert Einstein College of Medicine, Bronx, NY 10461, USA
*   Correspondence: rachel.zeig-owens@fdny.nyc.gov; Tel.: +1-718-403-4416

Received: 26 April 2019; Accepted: 14 May 2019; Published: 16 May 2019

Abstract: Peripheral neuropathy can result from numerous conditions including metabolic disorders, inflammatory disease, or exposure to environmental or biological toxins. We analyzed questionnaire data from 9239 Fire Department of the City of New York (FDNY) World Trade Center (WTC)-exposed firefighters and emergency medical service workers (EMS) to evaluate the association between work at the WTC site and subsequent peripheral neuropathy symptoms using the validated Diabetic Neuropathy Symptom (DNS) score. We grouped the population into an "Indicated" group with conditions known to be associated with paresthesia ($N = 2059$) and a "Non-Indicated" group without conditions known to be associated ($N = 7180$). The level of WTC exposure was categorized by time of arrival to the WTC. Overall, 25% of workers aged 40 and older reported peripheral neuropathy symptoms: 30.6% in the Indicated and 23.8% in the Non-Indicated groups, respectively. Multivariable logistic models performed on the Non-Indicated group, and on the Non-Indicated in comparison with non-WTC exposed National Health and Nutrition Examination Survey (NHANES), found that the highest level of WTC-exposure was significantly associated with DNS positive outcomes, after controlling for potential confounders. In conclusion, this study suggests that symptoms of peripheral neuropathy and paresthesias are common and are associated with WTC-exposure intensity.

Keywords: peripheral neuropathy; prevalence; World Trade Center; rescue/recovery workers; occupational exposure

---

1. Introduction

The collapse of the World Trade Center (WTC) buildings in New York City after the terrorist attacks on 11 September, 2001 (9/11) resulted in high volumes of aerosolized dust and gases including neurotoxins such as lead, aluminum, cadmium, manganese, tin, and complex hydrocarbons, specifically polychlorinated biphenyl (PCB), dioxins, and polycyclic aromatic hydrocarbons (PAHs) [1,2]. Additionally, the 10-month rescue/recovery effort may have exposed workers to organic solvents [3] and pesticides [4], which are known causes of peripheral neuropathy and neurodegenerative diseases [1].

The peripheral nervous system may be particularly vulnerable to environmental and metabolic insult that can result in peripheral neuropathy (PN), which can take axonal, demyelinating, or mixed forms [5]. Diabetic neuropathy is most common [6,7], but there are other types, such as inflammatory and toxic. Inflammatory neuropathies include those that are infectious, for example, those of autoimmune origin like sarcoidosis and Gullian–Barré syndrome [5,8]. Toxic neuropathies are often related to chemotherapeutic agents (chemotherapy-induced toxic peripheral neuropathy) [9,10], chronic alcohol abuse [11,12], or exposure to heavy metals and other environmental toxins [13], which result in primary axonal damage. Toxins may also include industrial solvents due to their use of hexacarbons [14], a group of chemical compounds shown to cause length-dependent distal sensory loss, weakness, atrophy, reduced distal reflexes, and autonomic dysfunction.

To date, three previous questionnaire-based studies have investigated the prevalence and risk factors for peripheral neuropathy in smaller WTC-exposed populations and reported that neuropathy symptoms were commonly associated with WTC-related exposure or WTC cleaning work [15–17]. The purpose of the current study is to investigate the prevalence of self-reported peripheral neuropathic symptoms and paresthesias among more than 9000 WTC-exposed Fire Department of the City of New York (FDNY) firefighters and emergency medical workers (EMS) between 7 June 2017, when the Diabetic Neuropathy Symptom (DNS) score was added to FDNY monitoring questionnaires, and 6 April 2019. The DNS score was developed by an expert panel consisting of a diabetologist, a vascular internist, a neurologist, and a physician for rehabilitation medicine seeking a validated, rapid, and easy to preform screening tool. The score demonstrates good inter-rater agreement (Cohen's weighted κ for both raters was 0.89 and 0.78), reliability (0.64) and sound screening properties due, in particular, to its high sensitivity (79%) and specificity (78%) [18]. We hypothesized that WTC exposure, overall, and specifically, arrival time to the disaster site would be associated with a higher prevalence of neuropathic symptoms both as measured by the DNS and by paresthesias of the lower and upper extremities. Further, we included as a comparison population, data from non-WTC individuals who participated in the 2003–2004 National Health and Nutrition Examination Survey (NHANES) survey [19].

2. Materials and Methods

2.1. Data Collection

The FDNY WTC Health Program performs periodic health evaluations on all active FDNY members, and on WTC-exposed retired members, both firefighters and EMS, every 12–18 months. Since 2001, self-administered health questionnaires have been used to collect information about WTC exposure, health behaviors such as smoking history, and physician diagnoses.

2.2. Description of the Study Population

The source population consisted of 14,185 WTC-exposed firefighters and EMS enrolled in FDNY WTC Health Program (WTCHP) who provided written consent for research. The inclusion criteria for this study were: (1) having arrived at the disaster site between the morning of 11 September, 2001 (9/11) and 24 September, 2001; (2) being an active FDNY firefighter or EMS on 9/11; (3) having taken at least one post-9/11 health questionnaire within the study period; and, (4) being 40 years or older at the time of their most recent questionnaire. The final study population included 9239 firefighters and EMS; this population was separated into two groups. The first, hereafter called the 'Indicated' group, was comprised of those with conditions that are known to be linked to peripheral neuropathy (N = 2059), which include those with: diabetes (glucose ≥140 mg/dL on the most recent FDNY blood test), a history of confirmed cancer (not including in situ cancers or non-melanoma skin cancers) [20–22], or a history of a confirmed autoimmune disease (including phospholipid, aplastic, myositis, lupus, sclerosis, myasthenia, psoria, rheum, sarcoidosis, Sjögren's, thrombocytopenia, and Wegener's) [23,24]. The second, hereafter called the 'Non-Indicated' group, was comprised of those without such conditions (N = 7180). These groups are mutually exclusive.

The Montefiore Medical Center/Albert Einstein College of Medicine's Institutional Review Board approved this study (IRB: 07-09-320).

2.3. Defining WTC Exposure Intensity

WTC exposure is defined from the earliest post-9/11 health questionnaire. We categorized exposure based on the FDNY-WTC exposure intensity index [25] as being high (arrived on the morning of 9/11), moderate (arrived afternoon of 9/11 or on 9/12/2001), or low (arrived between 9/13/2001 and 9/24/2001) [25,26].

2.4. Defining FDNY Peripheral Neuropathy Symptoms

Self-administered health questionnaires completed by all FDNY firefighters and EMS at their monitoring exams captured self-reported, physician-diagnosed peripheral neuropathy, and beginning in 2017, the validated four-item DNS score was used for diagnosing distal diabetic polyneuropathy [18]. Each DNS item scores one point, a score of 1 or greater signals the presence of polyneuropathy. Additionally, FDNY added the following two questions: "Considering any time in the last two weeks (excluding during exercise), do you have prickling, pins and needles, burning, aching pain or tenderness in your legs or feet?" followed by the same question regarding the arms or hands. Answer choices were "never, occasional, often, or almost continuously". All analyses used information from each participant's most recent questionnaire within the study period.

2.5. Defining NHANES Peripheral Neuropathy Symptoms

The 2003–2004 National Health and Nutrition Examination Survey (NHANES) [19] ($N = 3299$) asked participants 40 years and older about numbness, loss of feeling, painful sensation, or tingling in the hands or feet, other than from the hands or feet falling asleep, in the past three months. Survey participants who confirmed such experiences in their feet or both their hands and feet were identified as having symptoms of peripheral neuropathy. We excluded 519 who reported that a health professional had ever diagnosed them with "diabetes" or "sugar diabetes", and 62 who reported either "borderline" or "don't know" for diagnosed diabetes. The final population consisted of 2718 non-diabetic NHANES survey participants.

2.6. Statistical Methods

First, prevalences of self-reported peripheral neuropathy and symptoms were calculated among the Indicated and Non-Indicated groups, and a weighted prevalence was calculated for NHANES (via SAS PROC SURVEYMEANS) using the two-year interviewed sample weights provided in the NHANES data file.

Then we conducted two phases of analyses exclusively on the Non-Indicated group: (1) the association of WTC exposure and peripheral neuropathy and (2) the estimation of the likelihood of symptoms in the FDNY cohort relative to NHANES.

(1) Odds ratios (ORs) and 95% confidence intervals (CIs) were used to explore associations between peripheral neuropathic symptoms and various risk factors. Multivariable logistic regression was used to analyze the association between the level of WTC exposure and peripheral neuropathy as defined by the DNS. Further, we investigated the association with the frequency of paresthesia (often or almost continuously vs never or occasional) separately in the lower and upper extremities, and in the extremities compiled. Additionally, we tested linear trends in the exposure–response relationship of each model by including WTC exposure as an ordinal predictor. All multivariable models controlled for work assignment on 9/11 (EMS, firefighter), sex, race (non-Hispanic white, non-white (non-Hispanic black, Hispanic, other)), smoking history at the time of the questionnaire (ever, never), chronic alcohol abuse (yes, no), and age at exam. Chronic alcohol abuse, based on the Alcohol Use Disorders Identification Test (AUDIT) [27], was defined as positive for alcohol abuse on every questionnaire after the first ever indication.

(2) Using the analytic technique employed by Myers et al. [28], we created a combined analytic file for multivariable logistic regression estimation by normalizing variable names and variable coding for the NHANES and FDNY Non-Indicated datasets and appending the two data files. In the combined file, two-year interviewed sample weights formed the frequency weights for NHANES records, and FDNY records received a frequency weight of one. An indicator variable identified records that were NHANES or FDNY. In this way, the NHANES cohort is used as a national reference population to standardize the FDNY Non-Indicated group. Our models compared the association of peripheral neuropathic symptoms with the FDNY cohort overall and to each level of WTC exposure (via SAS PROC SURVEYLOGISTIC), adjusting for sex, race (non-Hispanic white, non-white (non-Hispanic black, Hispanic, other)), and age at exam. As a secondary analysis, a WTC exposure test for trend was conducted. In order to compare the DNS questions to NHANES, we removed the first DNS item which asks if a person is suffering from unsteadiness in walking; thus, a positive score on the DNS was restricted to a score of 1 or higher using only the other three items.

All analyses were conducted using SAS 9.4 (SAS Institute, Inc., Cary, NC, USA).

3. Results

3.1. Baseline Characteristics

The study cohort (N = 9239) was 97.6% male, 89.7% non-Hispanic white, and 88.2% were firefighters on 9/11. Most of the cohort (69.3%) was moderately-exposed to the WTC disaster. The mean (SD) age on 9/11 was 39.7 (7.5) years, and 25.3% (N = 2341) of the study cohort scored positive on the DNS. These demographic characteristics are reflected in the Indicated and Non-Indicated groups presented in Table 1. Compared with the Indicated, the Non-Indicated group was younger, on average, included a slightly higher percentage of non-Hispanic whites and firefighters, and had a greater proportion of never smokers.

Table 1. Demographic characteristics among individuals 40 years and older (7 June, 2017–6 April, 2019).

Variable	Indicated [†] (N = 2059)	Non-Indicated (N = 7180)
Age on 9/11, y [a]	42.1 ± 7.6	39.0 ± 7.3
Age at exam, y [a]	59.0 ± 7.6	56.0 ± 7.3
Sex, N (%)		
Male	1997 (97.0)	7022 (97.8)
Female	62 (3.0)	158 (2.2)
Race, N (%)		
Non-Hispanic white	1778 (86.4)	6512 (90.7)
Non-Hispanic black	120 (5.8)	264 (3.7)
Hispanic	141 (6.9)	372 (5.2)
Other	20 (1.0)	32 (0.5)
Work assignment on 9/11, N (%)		
Firefighter	1666 (80.9)	6484 (90.3)
EMS	393 (19.1)	696 (9.7)
Smoking status, N (%) [b]		
Never	1453 (70.6)	5625 (78.3)
Former	519 (25.2)	1342 (18.7)
Current	87 (4.2)	213 (3.0)
WTC exposure level, N (%)		
High	383 (18.6)	1155 (16.1)
Moderate	1356 (65.9)	5047 (70.3)
Low	320 (15.5)	978 (13.6)

Table 1. *Cont.*

Variable	Indicated [†] (N = 2059)	Non-Indicated (N = 7180)
Chronic Alcohol Abuse [c]		
Yes	0 (0.0)	107 (1.5)
No	2059 (100.0)	7073 (98.5)
PN Risk Factor		
Diabetes (glucose ≥ 140 mg/dL)	1147 (55.7)	-
Cancer (not 'in situ')	886 (43.0)	-
Autoimmune Disease	184 (8.9)	-

PN = peripheral neuropathic symptoms; 9/11 = 11 September, 2001; WTC = World Trade Center. [†] Rescue/recovery workers with any of the following conditions: diabetes, cancer (not including in situ cancers or non-melanoma skin cancers), or an autoimmune disease. [a] Mean ± SD. [b] Value at the time of the physical health questionnaire. [c] Scored positive on the Alcohol Use Disorders Identification Test (AUDIT) on all questionnaires after the first indication.

3.2. Prevalence of Neuropathic Symptoms

The prevalence of scoring positive on the DNS among the Indicated group was 30.6% while the Non-Indicated group scored 23.8% (Table 2). Both groups, with 20.2% of the Indicated group and 15.2% of the Non-Indicated group, commonly reported symptoms of burning, aching pain or tenderness in the legs or feet. The greatest proportion of overlap between items in the Indicated group and Non-Indicated group, respectively, was by those who answered positively to questions 2–4 (19.8%; 16.1%); additionally, 72 (11.4%) of the Indicated group and 146 (8.5%) of the Non-Indicated group answered positively to all four questions. The Indicated group reported a greater prevalence of paresthesia in the legs or feet (11.7%, N = 240) than in the arms or hands (8.1%, N = 167), as did the Non-Indicated group (8.5%, N = 613; 7.1%, N = 509). Physician-diagnosed peripheral neuropathy was very rare: approximately 2% of the Indicated group and 1% of the Non-Indicated group.

Table 2. The Diabetic Neuropathy Symptom (DNS) score prevalence among the Indicated and Non-Indicated peripheral neuropathy groups.

DNS Item	Indicated [†], N = 2059 (%)	Non-Indicated, N = 7180 (%)
1. Considering any time in the last two weeks (excluding during exercise), are you suffering of unsteadiness in walking?	184 (8.9)	419 (5.8)
2. Considering any time in the last two weeks (excluding during exercise), do you have a burning, aching pain or tenderness at your legs or feet?	416 (20.2)	1091 (15.2)
3. Considering any time in the last two weeks (excluding during exercise), do you have prickling sensations at your legs and feet?	344 (16.7)	817 (11.4)
4. Considering any time in the last two weeks (excluding during exercise), do you have places of numbness on your legs or feet?	372 (18.1)	954 (13.3)
5. Any of the Above	630 (30.6)	1711 (23.8)

[†] Rescue/recovery workers with any of the following conditions: diabetes, cancer (not including in situ cancers or non-melanoma skin cancers), or an autoimmune disease.

3.3. Associations of 9/11-Related Exposures with Peripheral Neuropathy Symptoms

Final logistic regression models used the following outcomes: positive on the DNS; and often/almost continuously experiencing paresthesias in the legs or feet, in the arms or hands, or in both (Table 3). Those with the highest exposure to the WTC disaster (arriving the morning of 9/11) were more likely to score positive on the DNS (OR 1.35, 95% CI 1.10–1.65) than those in the lowest exposure group (P test for trend $P = 0.004$). This signal became stronger when assessing paresthesias, except for paresthesias of the legs or feet where the association was not significant. Trend tests between WTC exposure level and paresthesias of the arms and the extremities compiled, respectively, were significant (P test for trend $P = 0.036$; 0.006). There were no significant associations with work assignment on 9/11 (EMS vs Fire). Sex, older age, a history of smoking, and chronic alcohol abuse were associated with almost every outcome.

Table 3. Reports of DNS positive scores and paresthesias of the upper and lower extremities in World Trade Center-exposed workers from 7 June, 2017 to 4 April, 2019.

Variable	DNS Positive OR (95% CI)	Paresthesias [†]		
		Legs/Feet OR (95% CI)	Arms/Hands OR (95% CI)	Legs/Feet and Arms/Hands OR (95% CI)
WTC exposure level				
High	1.35 (1.10, 1.65)	1.36 (0.99, 1.87)	1.47 (1.04, 2.08)	2.47 (1.35, 4.53)
Moderate	1.17 (0.99, 1.38)	1.30 (1.00, 1.70)	1.33 (0.99, 1.78)	2.18 (1.27, 3.75)
Low	Ref.	Ref.	Ref.	Ref.
Age at exam	1.04 (1.03, 1.04)	1.03 (1.02, 1.04)	1.02 (1.00, 1.03)	1.03 (1.01, 1.05)
Race				
Non-Hispanic white	0.97 (0.78, 1.19)	1.03 (0.74, 1.42)	0.93 (0.66, 1.32)	0.77 (0.47, 1.26)
Non-white	Ref.	Ref.	Ref.	Ref.
Sex				
Male	0.64 (0.44, 0.95)	0.41 (0.24, 0.70)	0.46 (0.26, 0.84)	0.36 (0.17, 0.77)
Female	Ref.	Ref.	Ref.	Ref.
Work assignment on 9/11				
EMS	1.05 (0.84, 1.33)	0.91 (0.63, 1.33)	0.81 (0.54, 1.22)	1.14 (0.63, 2.03)
Firefighter	Ref.	Ref.	Ref.	Ref.
Smoking status [a]				
Ever	1.22 (1.07, 1.39)	1.20 (0.99, 1.46)	1.02 (0.82, 1.28)	1.16 (0.83, 1.61)
Never	Ref.	Ref.	Ref.	Ref.
Chronic Alcohol Abuse [b]				
Yes	2.32 (1.57, 3.42)	1.48 (0.84, 2.63)	1.43 (0.76, 2.69)	1.99 (0.86, 4.62)
No	Ref.	Ref.	Ref.	Ref.

OR = odds ratio; CI = confidence interval; EMS = emergency medical service worker; Ref. = reference group; DNS = Diabetic Neuropathy Symptom score; 9/11 = 11 September, 2001. [†] Often/almost continuously experiencing prickling, pins and needles, burning, aching pain or tenderness in the area defined. [a] At the time the questionnaire was taken. [b] Scored positive on the Alcohol Use Disorders Identification Test (AUDIT) on all questionnaires after the first indication.

3.4. U.S. Population Prevalence and Comparison to FDNY Cohort

Among the 2003–2004 non-diabetic NHANES population, a weighted estimate of 13% (95% CI 11.2–15.1) reported experiencing symptoms of peripheral neuropathy, as compared with the estimated 23% (95% CI 19.0–27.1%) of the 519 diabetic survey participants. Our restricted DNS definition (DNS scored excluding the first question) reduced the prevalence of reported symptoms to 22.3% among the Non-Indicated group. The multivariable logistic regressions (Table 4) found that any exposure to the WTC increased the odds of reporting symptoms (OR 2.06, 95% CI 1.65–2.57). An exposure response gradient became apparent when each level of WTC exposure was compared to the NHANES population (*P* test for trend *P* < 0.0001) (Table 4).

Table 4. Multivariable logistic regression using the NHANES 2003–2004 non-diabetic cohort as a national referent population.

Title	OR (95% CI) [†]
Model 1: WTC exposure overall	
Exposed	2.06 (1.65, 2.57)
Unexposed NHANES	Ref.
Model 2: WTC exposure level	
High	2.36 (1.84, 3.04)
Moderate	2.04 (1.62, 2.56)
Low	1.82 (1.41, 2.35)
Unexposed NHANES	Ref.

NHANES = National Health and Nutrition Examination Survey; WTC = World Trade Center; 9/11 = 11 September, 2001; Ref. = reference. [†] Exposure measurements adjusted for age at exam, sex, and race (non-Hispanic white, other).

4. Discussion

Our study uniquely examines peripheral neuropathy symptoms reported about 15 years after the inhalation and dermal absorption of WTC particulates and gases in a cohort of exposed firefighters and EMS. Nearly one-quarter of the Non-Indicated group reported one or more symptoms of peripheral neuropathy, compared with 31% of those with a comorbid condition known to be associated with paresthesias, specifically diabetes, cancer, or autoimmune disease. The prevalence of reported DNS symptoms was lower in the Non-Indicated than in the Indicated group, but not by half, a prevalence difference that has been demonstrated between non-diabetic and diabetic groups in the general population [19,29,30]. Not only does this result demonstrate the applicability of the DNS in our cohort, it also indicates a potential for WTC-exposed workers, other than those typically at risk, to be experiencing peripheral nerve damage. Our findings illustrated moderate associations between the most highly exposed workers (rescue/recovery workers most exposed to massive volumes of aerosolized particulates and pulverized building materials) and a positive DNS score and with paresthesias of the upper extremities. As expected, we found stronger associations with those who reported paresthesias of both the upper and lower extremities.

Unlike the previous two WTC-associated studies of paresthesia, we used peripheral neuropathic symptom data from the 2003–2004 NHANES non-exposed, non-diabetic population as a comparison. NHANES prevalence data from this period suggested that any WTC exposure, whether the most or the least exposed, increased by two-fold the likelihood of reporting neuropathic symptoms. This standardization to NHANES bolsters the connection between WTC exposure and paresthesia symptoms also found in previous neuropathy symptom studies [15–17]. Moreover, we used a validated screening questionnaire, the DNS, in addition to questions on paresthesias of the upper and lower extremities, similar to the questions used by Marmor et al. [16], to examine prevalence in our population using multiple measures; therefore, giving our findings a more robust framework. Further support for our findings can also be found in a 2016 study of 16 WTC-exposed responders and survivors, which concluded that there was a higher probability of a neuropathy diagnosis in patients who were WTC-exposed as compared with others referred for electromyography (EMG) testing [31].

Our study has some limitations. Since the FDNY WTCHP did not add questions about peripheral neuropathy symptoms to the monitoring questionnaires until 2017, we are not yet able to assess longitudinal persistence of paresthesias, which could help elucidate the long-term effects of the WTC on neurodegeneration in the peripheral nervous system. And, while we adjusted for work assignment on 9/11, sex, race, smoking history, chronic alcohol abuse, and age, our logistic models may not have fully controlled for unmeasured confounding. Additionally, during the second phase of analysis, we were unable to remove those who had a history of cancer or autoimmune disease from the NHANES dataset. We can assume, therefore, that the already strong association between WTC exposure and peripheral neuropathy symptoms was biased toward the null. We acknowledge that NHANES does not represent an exact counterfactual for our WTC-exposed cohort and, instead, a comparison group comprised exclusively of firefighters with no exposure to the disaster or a truly random sample of the U.S. population would be most desirable; nevertheless, no such cohort data were available at this time. Finally, the use of cross-sectional questionnaire data cannot establish causality, we cannot account for the specific impacts of career firefighting versus WTC-specific particulate exposures, and very few rescue/recovery workers reported a physician diagnosis of peripheral neuropathy. However, the high prevalence of symptoms in the Non-Indicated group and significant associations with WTC exposure intensity and as compared to the general population underscore the need for further investigation.

5. Conclusions

EMG, skin punch biopsy, and nerve conduction velocity testing will provide confirmation of neuropathies and determine the specific types of nerve injuries that may be associated with WTC exposure. The mechanism by which WTC exposure results in neuropathy will require further investigation by others. Such research has been started by Stecker et al.'s 2014 study on rat sciatic nerves [32], which provided biological plausibility for the effect of WTC exposure mediated by a methanol-soluble element in WTC dust, leading to an increased risk of neuropathy. Furthermore, recent studies of neurodegeneration, in the military and populations exposed to terrorist attacks other than the WTC, have begun to stress the relevance of toxic neuropathy [33–35]. In conclusion, our study suggests that WTC exposure may result in an increased risk of peripheral neuropathy in rescue/recovery workers, especially those who were most highly exposed to the dust cloud. This risk appears to be independent of the illnesses and conditions generally related to neuropathic symptoms. Treatment for peripheral neuropathy is not currently covered under the James Zadroga 9/11 Health and Compensation Act. Therefore, if confirmed by future studies, our research may have policy implications for consideration of neuropathy as an addition to the list of covered conditions.

Author Contributions: R.Z.-O. and D.J.P. had full access to all of the data in the study and take responsibility for the integrity of the data and the accuracy of the data analysis. Conceptualization: H.L.C., R.Z.-O., and D.J.P.; methodology: H.L.C., R.Z.-O., and D.J.P.; data curation: H.L.C. and T.M.S.; formal analysis: H.L.C.; validation: D.G.G.; writing—original draft preparation: H.L.C.; writing—review and editing: All authors; supervision: R.Z.-O.; funding acquisition: D.J.P.

Funding: This research was supported through the National Institute for Occupational Safety and Health (NIOSH) contract numbers 200-2011-39378, 200-2011-39383, 200-2017-93326, 200-2017-93426; NIOSH had no role in study design; collection, analysis, and/or interpretation of data; writing the report; and the decision to submit the report for publication.

Conflicts of Interest: The authors declare no conflicts of interest.

References

1. Lioy, P.J.; Weisel, C.P.; Millette, J.R.; Eisenreich, S. Characterization of the dust/smoke aerosol that settled east of the World Trade Center (WTC) in lower Manhattan after the collapse of the WTC 11 September 2001. *Environ. Health Perspect.* **2002**, *110*, 703–714. [CrossRef] [PubMed]
2. Kahn, L.G.; Han, X.; Koshy, T.T.; Shao, Y.; Chu, D.B.; Kannan, K.; Trasande, L. Adolescents exposed to the World Trade Center collapse have elevated serum dioxin and furan concentrations more than 12 years later. *Environ. Int.* **2018**, *111*, 268–278. [CrossRef]
3. Dick, F.D. Solvent neurotoxicity. *Occup. Environ. Med.* **2006**, *63*, 221–226. [CrossRef] [PubMed]
4. Rao, D.B.; Jortner, B.S.; Sills, R.C. Animal models of peripheral neuropathy due to environmental toxicants. *Ilar J.* **2014**, *54*, 315–323. [CrossRef] [PubMed]
5. Katona, I.; Weis, J. Diseases of the peripheral nerves. *Handb. Clin. Neurol.* **2017**, *145*, 453–474.
6. Singleton, J.R.; Smith, A.G.; Bromberg, M.B. Increased prevalence of impaired glucose tolerance in patients with painful sensory neuropathy. *Diabetes Care* **2001**, *24*, 1448–1453. [CrossRef] [PubMed]
7. Jolivalt, C.G.; Frizzi, K.E.; Guernsey, L.; Marquez, A.; Ochoa, J.; Rodriguez, M.; Calcutt, N.A. Peripheral Neuropathy in Mouse Models of Diabetes. *Curr. Protoc. Mouse. Biol.* **2016**, *6*, 223–255. [PubMed]
8. Bourque, P.R.; Chardon, J.W.; Massie, R. Autoimmune peripheral neuropathies. *Clin. Chim. Acta* **2015**, *449*, 37–42. [CrossRef]

9. Diezi, M.; Buclin, T.; Kuntzer, T. Toxic and drug-induced peripheral neuropathies: Updates on causes, mechanisms and management. *Curr. Opin. Neurol.* **2013**, *26*, 481–488. [CrossRef] [PubMed]

10. Staff, N.P.; Grisold, A.; Grisold, W.; Windebank, A.J. Chemotherapy-induced peripheral neuropathy: A current review. *Ann. Neurol.* **2017**, *81*, 772–781. [CrossRef]

11. Hanewinckel, R.; van Oijen, M.; Ikram, M.A.; van Doorn, P.A. The epidemiology and risk factors of chronic polyneuropathy. *Eur. J. Epidemiol.* **2016**, *31*, 5–20. [CrossRef]

12. Chopra, K.; Tiwari, V. Alcoholic neuropathy: Possible mechanisms and future treatment possibilities. *Br. J. Clin. Pharmacol.* **2012**, *73*, 348–362. [CrossRef]

13. Caito, S.; Aschner, M. Neurotoxicity of metals. *Handb. Clin. Neurol.* **2015**, *131*, 169–189.

14. London, Z.; Albers, J.W. Toxic neuropathies associated with pharmaceutic and industrial agents. *Neurol. Clin.* **2007**, *25*, 257–276. [CrossRef]

15. Wilkenfeld, M.; Fazzari, M.; Segelnick, J.; Stecker, M. Neuropathic Symptoms in World Trade Center Disaster Survivors and Responders. *J. Occup. Environ. Med.* **2016**, *58*, 83–86. [CrossRef]

16. Marmor, M.; Shao, Y.; Bhatt, D.H.; Stecker, M.M.; Berger, K.I.; Goldring, R.M.; Wilkenfeld, M. Paresthesias Among Community Members Exposed to the World Trade Center Disaster. *J. Occup. Environ. Med.* **2017**, *59*, 389–396. [CrossRef] [PubMed]

17. Thawani, S.; Wang, B.; Shao, Y.; Reibman, J.; Marmor, M. Time to Onset of Paresthesia Among Community Members Exposed to the World Trade Center Disaster. *Int. J. Environ. Res. Public. Health.* **2019**, *16*, 1429. [CrossRef] [PubMed]

18. Meijer, J.W.G.; Smit, A.J.; Sonderen, E.V.; Groothoff, J.W.; Eisma, W.H.; Links, T.P. Symptom scoring systems to diagnose distal polyneuropathy in diabetes: The Diabetic Neuropathy Symptom score. *Diabet. Med.* **2002**, *19*, 962–965. [CrossRef]

19. National Health and Nutrition Examination Survey: NHANES 2003–2004. U.S. Centers for Disease Control and Prevention. Available online: https://wwwn.cdc.gov/Nchs/Nhanes/2003-2004/DIQ_C.htm (accessed on 12 April 2019).

20. Zeig-Owens, R.; Webber, M.P.; Hall, C.B.; Schwartz, T.; Jaber, N.; Weakley, J.; Kelly, K. Early assessment of cancer outcomes in New York City firefighters after the 9/11 attacks: An observational cohort study. *Lancet* **2011**, *378*, 898–905. [CrossRef]

21. Moir, W.; Zeig-Owens, R.; Daniels, R.D.; Hall, C.B.; Webber, M.P.; Jaber, N.; Kelly, K. Post-9/11 cancer incidence in World Trade Center-exposed New York City firefighters as compared to a pooled cohort of firefighters from San Francisco, Chicago and Philadelphia (9/11/2001-2009). *Am. J. Ind. Med.* **2016**, *59*, 722–730. [CrossRef]

22. Singh, A.; Zeig-Owens, R.; Moir, W.; Hall, C.B.; Schwartz, T.; Vossbrinck, M.; Koffler, E. Estimation of Future Cancer Burden Among Rescue and Recovery Workers Exposed to the World Trade Center Disaster. *JAMA Oncol.* **2018**, *4*, 828–831. [CrossRef]

23. Webber, M.P.; Moir, W.; Zeig-Owens, R.; Glaser, M.S.; Jaber, N.; Hall, C.; Prezant, D.J. Nested case-control study of selected systemic autoimmune diseases in World Trade Center rescue/recovery workers. *Arthr. Rheumatol.* **2015**, *67*, 1369–1376. [CrossRef]

24. Webber, M.P.; Yip, J.; Zeig-Owens, R.; Moir, W.; Ungprasert, P.; Crowson, C.S.; Prezant, D.J. Post-9/11 sarcoidosis in WTC-exposed firefighters and emergency medical service workers. *Respir. Med.* **2017**, *132*, 232–237. [CrossRef]

25. Prezant, D.J.; Weiden, M.; Banauch, G.I.; McGuinness, G.; Rom, W.N.; Aldrich, T.K.; Kelly, K.J. Cough and bronchial responsiveness in firefighters at the World Trade Center site. *N.Engl. J. Med.* **2002**, *347*, 806–815. [CrossRef]

26. Weakley, J.; Hall, C.B.; Liu, X.; Zeig-Owens, R.; Webber, M.P.; Schwartz, T.; Prezant, D. The effect of World Trade Center exposure on the latency of chronic rhinosinusitis diagnoses in New York City firefighters: 2001–2011. *Occup. Environ. Med.* **2016**, *73*, 280–283. [CrossRef]

27. Reinert, D.F.; Allen, J.P. The Alcohol Use Disorders Identification Test (AUDIT): A review of recent research. *Alcohol. Clin. Exp. Res.* **2002**, *26*, 272–279. [CrossRef]

28. Myers, O.B.; Pankratz, V.S.; Norris, K.C.; Vassalotti, J.A.; Unruh, M.L.; Argyropoulos, C. Surveillance of CKD epidemiology in the US—A joint analysis of NHANES and KEEP. *Sci. Rep.* **2018**, *8*, 15900. [CrossRef]

29. Gregg, E.W.; Sorlie, P.; Paulose-Ram, R.; Gu, Q.; Eberhardt, M.S.; Wolz, M.; Geiss, L. Prevalence of lower-extremity disease in the U.S. adult population ≥40 years of age with and without diabetes: 1999–2000 national health and nutrition examination survey. *Diabetes Care* **2004**, *27*, 1591–1597. [CrossRef]

30. Gregg, E.W.; Gu, Q.; Williams, D.; De Rekeneire, N.; Cheng, Y.J.; Geiss, L.; Engelgau, M. Prevalence of lower extremity diseases associated with normal glucose levels, impaired fasting glucose, and diabetes among U.S. adults aged 40 or older. *Diabetes Res. Clin. Pract.* **2007**, *77*, 485–488. [CrossRef]

31. Stecker, M.M.; Yu, H.; Barlev, R.; Marmor, M.; Wilkenfeld, M. Neurologic Evaluations of Patients Exposed to the World Trade Center Disaster. *J. Occup. Environ. Med.* **2016**, *58*, 1150–1154. [CrossRef]

32. Stecker, M.; Segelnick, J.; Wilkenfeld, M. Analysis of short-term effects of World Trade Center dust on rat sciatic nerve. *J. Occup. Environ. Med.* **2014**, *56*, 1024–1028. [CrossRef] [PubMed]

33. De Cauwer, H.; Somville, F. Neurological disease in the aftermath of terrorism: A review. *Acta. Neurol. Belg.* **2018**, *118*, 193–199. [CrossRef] [PubMed]

34. Miyaki, K.; Nishiwaki, Y.; Maekawa, K.; Ogawa, Y.; Asukai, N.; Yoshimura, K.; Omae, K. Effects of sarin on the nervous system of subway workers seven years after the Tokyo subway sarin attack. *J. Occup. Health* **2005**, *47*, 299–304. [CrossRef] [PubMed]

35. Beard, J.D.; Kamel, F. Military service, deployments, and exposures in relation to amyotrophic lateral sclerosis etiology and survival. *Epidemiol. Rev.* **2015**, *37*, 55–70. [CrossRef] [PubMed]

International Journal of
Environmental Research and Public Health

MDPI

Article

Genetic Variants Associated with FDNY WTC-Related Sarcoidosis

Krystal L. Cleven [1,2,*,†], **Kenny Ye** [3,*,†], **Rachel Zeig-Owens** [1,3,4], **Kerry M. Hena** [5], **Cristina Montagna** [6,7,8], **Jidong Shan** [6,8], **H. Dean Hosgood III** [3], **Nadia Jaber** [4], **Michael D. Weiden** [4,5], **Hilary L. Colbeth** [1,4], **David G. Goldfarb** [1,4], **Simon D. Spivack** [1,3,5,6,†] and **David J. Prezant** [1,4,5,†]

1   Pulmonology Division, Department of Medicine, Montefiore Medical Center, Bronx, NY 10467, USA;
    rachel.zeig-owens@fdny.nyc.gov (R.Z.-O.); hilary.colbeth@fdny.nyc.gov (H.L.C.);
    david.goldfarb@fdny.nyc.gov (D.G.G.); simon.spivack@einstein.yu.edu (S.D.S.);
    david.prezant@fdny.nyc.gov (D.J.P.)
2   Pulmonology Division, Department of Medicine, Albert Einstein College of Medicine, Bronx, NY 10467, USA
3   Department of Epidemiology and Population Health, Albert Einstein College of Medicine, Bronx, NY 10461,
    USA; dean.hosgood@einstein.yu.edu
4   Fire Department of the City of New York, Bureau of Health Services, Brooklyn, NY 11201, USA;
    nadia.jaber@fdny.nyc.gov (N.J.); michael.weiden@nyulangone.org (M.D.W.)
5   Pulmonary & Critical Care Division, Department of Medicine, NYU School of Medicine, New York,
    NY 10016, USA; kerry.hena@nyulangone.org
6   Department of Genetics, Albert Einstein College of Medicine, Bronx, NY 10461, USA;
    cristina.montagna@einstein.yu.edu (C.M.); jidong.shan@einstein.yu.edu (J.S.)
7   Department of Pathology, Albert Einstein College of Medicine, Bronx, NY 10461, USA
8   Molecular Cytogenetic Core, Albert Einstein College of Medicine, Bronx, NY 10461, USA
*   Correspondence: kcleven@montefiore.org (K.L.C.); kenny.ye@einstein.yu.edu (K.Y.);
    Tel.: +1-718-920-6054 (K.L.C.); +1-718-430-2590 (K.Y.)
†   These authors share equal authorship.

Received: 15 February 2019; Accepted: 19 May 2019; Published: 23 May 2019

Abstract: Sarcoidosis is a systemic granulomatous disease of unknown etiology. It may develop in response to an exposure or inflammatory trigger in the background of a genetically primed abnormal immune response. Thus, genetic studies are potentially important to our understanding of the pathogenesis of sarcoidosis. We developed a case-control study which explored the genetic variations between firefighters in the Fire Department of the City of New York (FDNY) with World Trade Center (WTC)-related sarcoidosis and those with WTC exposure, but without sarcoidosis. The loci of fifty-one candidate genes related to granuloma formation, inflammation, immune response, and/or sarcoidosis were sequenced at high density in enhancer/promoter, exonic, and 5′ untranslated regions. Seventeen allele variants of human leukocyte antigen (HLA) and non-HLA genes were found to be associated with sarcoidosis, and all were within chromosomes 1 and 6. Our results also suggest an association between extrathoracic involvement and allele variants of HLA and non-HLA genes found not only on chromosomes 1 and 6, but also on chromosomes 16 and 17. We found similarities between genetic variants with WTC-related sarcoidosis and those reported previously in sporadic sarcoidosis cases within the general population. In addition, we identified several allele variants never previously reported in association with sarcoidosis. If confirmed in larger studies with known environmental exposures, these novel findings may provide insight into the gene-environment interactions key to the development of sarcoidosis.

Keywords: sarcoidosis; World Trade Center; 9/11; genetics; firefighters; FDNY

1. Introduction

Sarcoidosis is a multisystem granulomatous disease that presents with pulmonary involvement in 90% of cases and extrapulmonary manifestations, mostly skin, in 10% of patients [1]. The annual age-adjusted incidence in the United States (U.S.) between 1946–2013, in a mostly Caucasian cohort, was 10 per 100,000 (9.4 in males and 10.5 in females) [2]. Between 1985 and 1998, firefighters in the Fire Department of the City of New York (FDNY) had an annual incidence of sarcoidosis somewhat higher than the white male general population at 12.9 per 100,000 and many-fold higher than an internal control group of emergency service workers [3]. The incidence doubled following the World Trade Center (WTC) attacks on September 11, 2001 (9/11), giving an age-adjusted incidence rate of 25 per 100,000 in mostly Caucasian male WTC-exposed FDNY firefighters between 2002–2015 [4].

Since the disorder clusters in families, genetic factors are thought to play an important role in sarcoidosis pathogenesis, presumably through mechanisms of immunologic response to antigenic or other triggering exposures. A recent population-based study suggests a genetic risk factor for sarcoidosis in a large Swedish cohort, where a 3.7-fold increase in risk of sarcoidosis was observed in those with first-degree relatives with the disease. The risk further increased in those with relatives with Lofgren's syndrome or with ≥1 relative with sarcoidosis [5]. A case-control etiologic study of sarcoidosis (ACCESS) found a five-fold increase in siblings of those with sarcoidosis [6].

We selected several candidate genes for genetic analysis based on their function encoding proteins involved in granuloma formation, innate and immune recognition, and inflammation. Several have been implicated in genetic studies of sarcoidosis such as the highly polymorphic human leukocyte antigen (HLA) genes. HLA genes encode the major histocompatibility complex (MHC) in humans and are involved in immunologic recognition and regulation. Within various racial groups, allele variations within HLA genes are associated with sarcoidosis. Examples include the HLA-DRB1*1101 allele in both Caucasians and African Americans [7], HLA-DRB1*1501, -*03 and -*0402 specifically in European Americans [7–9], HLA-DRB1*1201 and -*0302 in African-Americans [7,10]. The HLA-DQB1 alleles HLA-DQB1-*0402, and -*0503 are associated in Asian Indians [7] and HLA-DQB1-*0602 in a Dutch cohort [8]. Several other non-HLA genes have been associated with sarcoidosis, such as prostaglandin G/H synthase/cyclooxygenase (PTGS2/COX2), neurogenic locus notch homolog 4 (NOTCH4), nucleotide-binding oligomerization domain-containing protein 2 (NOD2), and Butyrophilin-like 2 (BTNL2) [11–15].

The current case-control study is the first to examine genetic features associated with WTC-related sarcoidosis. Compared to other genetics studies of sarcoidosis, our study uniquely includes a baseline sarcoidosis rate, a known time point of exposure (9/11), and extensive, systematized clinical follow-up for over 14 years. The objective of this study is to explore the genetic characteristics of WTC-associated sarcoidosis and understand its similarities to and differences from sporadic sarcoidosis cases without a clear environmental exposure.

2. Materials and Methods

2.1. Study Population

The source population for the cases and controls was WTC-exposed firefighters. Recruitment of sarcoidosis cases for this study was part of a larger study that explored the clinical course of firefighters with post-9/11 sarcoidosis between the time of diagnosis and 14 years after 9/11 [16]. As outlined in Hena, et al (2018), cases were identified as WTC-exposed firefighters with WTC-related sarcoidosis if they had normal chest imaging prior to 9/11 and then post-9/11 radiographic findings consistent with sarcoidosis [16]. Extra-pulmonary organ involvement was determined from study questionnaires and medical records and was defined according to the World Association of Sarcoidosis and Other Granulomatous Diseases (WASOG) criteria [17].

Controls were randomly selected from the source population and were matched to cases based on race, age on 9/11, smoking history, and WTC-exposure history. WTC-exposure history was determined by arrival time to the WTC site: arrival group 1 (arriving the morning of 9/11) being the group with the highest dust cloud exposure and arrival group 4 (arriving between 9/13–9/24) having the least dust cloud exposure [18]. Controls also had normal chest radiographs at the time of the study.

The final study population included 55 cases and 100 controls. All cases and controls had peripheral blood drawn in 2015–2016 and completed a questionnaire at the time of blood draw to aid with matching on clinical characteristics and WTC-exposure history. The study was approved by the Montefiore Medical Center/Albert Einstein Institutional Review Board (2014-4291). All study participants provided written informed consent.

2.2. Genotyping

Peripheral blood mononuclear cells were obtained from cases and controls for sequencing analysis. A panel of 51 candidate genes were pre-selected based on their function encoding proteins involved in granuloma formation, innate and immune recognition, inflammation, and sarcoidosis. The loci of targeted candidate genes were sequenced using a custom designed sequencing panel for IonTorrent Ampliseq technology. The custom sequencing panel contained 1193 amplicons spanning all known exons, splice junctions and promoter regions of the genes. Promoter regions were defined as 2 kb upstream from the transcriptional start site. The panel overall coverage was over 90% for 422 exons (Supplementary Table S1). One exception was HLA-A, which had 41% coverage, but is known to be associated with low coverage in prior design assays as well. The sequencing panel was designed for the analysis of amplicons of 125–375 bp using the Ion AmpliSeq technology and was suitable for sequencing using the Ion Proton Sequencer as previously reported [19].

DNA was extracted using the QuickGene 610 system and the whole blood kit (Kurabo #DB-L), and quality verified and quantitated by the NanoDrop^{TM} 1000 Spectrophotometer (Thermo Fischer Scientific, Waltham, MA, USA). The Qubit® dsDNA HS Assay Kit (Life Technologies, Carlsbad, CA, USA) was used to determine the concentration of each sample. Approximately 20 ng of DNA was used to generate libraries for sequencing. When not in use, samples were stored at −20 °C. For each sample, a PCR reaction was set up according to the manufacturer's protocol using 20 ng of genomic DNA, two separate primer pools, and 16 amplification cycles. Following amplification, each sample was treated with FuPa reagent and ligated to a uniquely barcoded adapter to enable sample multiplexing. Libraries were then purified using the 1.5X Agencourt AMPure XP (Beckman Coulter Inc, Brea, CA, USA) kit. Amplification products from each primer pool were quantified individually using the KAPA Library Quantitation kit (Roche, Mannheim, Germany) and then pooled together. Template preparation was performed using the Ion OneTouch 2 system and the Ion PI Template OT2 200 kit v2 (Thermo Fisher Scientific, Waltham, MA, USA), according to the manufacturer's protocol. All libraries were sequenced on the Ion Proton sequencer using the Ion PI chip and the Ion PI Sequencing 200 kit v2 (Thermo Fisher Scientific, Waltham, MA, USA) to generate 200bp single ended sequencing.

For the identification and reporting of germline variants, we used a custom validated bioinformatic pipeline for the identification of SNPs as well as insertions and deletions (INDELs) included in the target panels [20–22]. The sequence reads obtained from the samples were aligned to the human reference genome (hg19-Genome Reference Consortium GRCh37) using the Ion Torrent Suite and then processed by the Torrent Variant Caller for variant calling. The generated BAM files were next imported into the Ion Reporter Software^{TM} (Thermo Fisher Scientific, Waltham, MA, USA) for filtering and annotation.

2.3. Statistical Analysis

2.3.1. Common Variants

We identified 909 variants (SNPs or INDELs) with minor allele frequency (MAF) ≥ 0.05 and p-value for Hardy-Weinberg Equilibrium Test > 0.0001. The variants were classified by their genomic locations to four categories: exon, intron (likely intron/exon boundaries), upstream, and 5'untranslated region

(5′UTR). For those in an exonic region, they were further classified by their function as synonymous, nonsense, missense, or frameshift (Supplementary Tables S2 and S3). For each of these common variants, Pearson Chi-square test was used to compare the genotype frequencies between the 55 cases and 100 controls that were successfully sequenced (see Supplementary Table S4). To verify the robustness of our results, Fisher's Exact Tests were also performed. For each of the variants, odds ratios were estimated using unconditional logistic regression under the co-dominant model.

We conducted two secondary analyses. First, we explored the interaction between each common variant and degree of WTC exposure, measured as arrival time to the WTC site. For each variant, we applied unconditional logistic regression under the co-dominant model with sarcoidosis as the outcome and the genotypes, WTC exposure group and their interaction term, as the explanatory variables. Likelihood ratio tests are applied to compare two models with and without the interaction term between the genotype and degree of WTC exposure. We also conducted a secondary analysis in which we associate the genetic variants with extrathoracic sarcoidosis. In these analyses, for each variant we applied unconditional logistic regression under the co-dominant model with extrathoracic sarcoidosis as the outcome and the genotypes as the explanatory variable.

2.3.2. Rare Variants

For variants whose MAF < 0.05, for each individual, the total number of rare alleles located in each gene were counted. We then compared the number of rare alleles between the cases and controls for each gene by each genomic location category (exon, intron, upstream, or 5′untranslated region) using two-sample T-tests. Furthermore, we counted rare variants with MAF < 0.01 across all target genes by the above-mentioned categories by genomic location and function, and then performed two-sample t-tests comparing the cases and controls for each of the categories.

3. Results

Final genetics analyses were completed on 55 cases and 100 controls. All but one case (54/55) and one control (99/100) self-identified as Caucasian, the remaining one case and one control self-identified as African American. The cases and controls were well matched, with at least one control for each case (Table 1).

Table 1. Demographics of WTC Study Population.

Demographics	Case Characteristics		Control Characteristics		*p*-Value
	N	%	N	%	
Total	55	100	100	100	
Arrival group					0.99
Morning of 9/11	12	21.8	22	22	
Afternoon of 9/11	24	43.6	46	46	
Day 9/12	15	27.3	25	25	
Day 9/13–9/24	4	7.3	7	7	
Race					1.00
White	54	98.2	99	99	
African-American	1	1.8	1	1	
Smoking status at time of blood draw					0.66
Never	40	72.7	72	72	
Former	14	25.5	23	23	
Current	1	1.8	5	5	
Age on 9/11, years, median [IQR]	36.8 [32.7–39.0]		35.4 [30.2–39.3]		0.29
Age at sarcoidosis diagnosis, median [IQR]	43.0 [38.2–46.6]				–
Time to diagnosis post 9/11, median [IQR]	6.7 [3.3–9.6]				–

IQR: interquartile range.

Organ involvement for the 55 cases included 47/55 (85.5%) with biopsy proven sarcoidosis. The 8/55 (14.5%) without biopsy results had their imaging and organ involvement reviewed by two pulmonologists to confirm consistency with sarcoidosis [16]. As outlined in Table 2, there was a decrease in intrathoracic involvement from the time of diagnosis to the time of the blood draw (mean eight-years post diagnosis) from 95% to 47% and an increase in extrathoracic involvement, especially cardiac and joint.

Table 2. Sarcoidosis organ involvement in WTC genetics study population.

Organ Involvement	Study Cases (N = 55)	
	At Diagnosis	Time of Blood Draw [a]
Bone marrow	0	0
Bone/joint	3	8
Calcium	0	0
Cardiac	0	9
Ear/nose/throat	0	1
Extrathoracic lymph nodes	0	0
Eyes	3	3
Intrathoracic involvement by CT Imaging	52	26
Kidney	1	0
Liver	1	1
Muscle	0	0
Nervous system	0	1
Other organs	0	0
Salivary	0	0
Skin	1	1
Spleen	2	2

[a] All cases had complete data regarding organ involvement at diagnosis and blood draw with the following exceptions: chest CT scan at diagnosis (N = 52), and at blood draw (N = 53); muscle at diagnosis (N = 54), and at blood draw (N = 54); spleen at diagnosis (N = 54), and at blood draw (N = 53); cardiac at blood draw (N = 53); and ear/nose/throat at diagnosis (N = 51), and at blood draw (N = 53).

Within the 51 candidate genes analyzed, we identified 3619 total number of variants. A total of seventeen common variants were found to be associated with sarcoidosis with Chi-Squared p-value < 0.01 (Table 3). All of the 17 variants were within chromosomes 1 and 6. Multiple variants were in HLA genes such as HLA-C, HLA-DRB1, HLA-DQB1, HLA-DPA1, and HLA-DPB1. There was a strong association with sarcoidosis within exonic regions of the HLA-DQB1 gene, represented by rs1049133 and rs1049130, two SNPs 12bp apart (ORs = 2.56 and 1.90, respectively). Two variants upstream from an intronic/exonic border region of HLA-DQB1 were also significantly associated with sarcoidosis, rs4516985 and rs9274614 (ORs = 1.74 and 2.49, respectively). In addition, several genetic variants within or near non-HLA genes were also significantly associated with sarcoidosis: BTNL2, PTGS2/COX2, and PACERR (PTGS2 Antisense NFKB1 Complex-Mediated Expression Regulator RNA). SNPs in a non-coding region of BTNL2, rs2076525 and rs2076524, were significantly associated with sarcoidosis (OR = 1.71). In addition, rs2076523, representing a missense mutation within a BTNL2 coding region was associated (OR = 1.97). Upstream from PTGS2/COX2 gene, rs20417 was also associated with sarcoidosis cases in our cohort (OR = 1.79).

In our secondary analysis, we did not find statistical evidence of an interaction between common variants and the degree of WTC exposure. We also found no statistical significance when we compared the number of rare variants between the cases and controls.

Our results also suggest an association between extrathoracic involvement and genetic variants within several HLA and non-HLA genes: HLA-B, PTGS2/COX2, PACERR, NOTCH4, NOD2, and ITGAE (Integrin Subunit Alpha E) (Table 4). Genetic variants associated with extrathoracic cases were found on chromosomes 1 and 6, similar to the loci associated with all sarcoidosis cases, and were also found on chromosomes 16 and 17. On chromosome 1, rs2066826 represents an intronic region/exonic border of PTGS2/COX2 associated with sarcoidosis, and specifically, extrathoracic disease in this cohort (OR 1.88 and 1.45, respectively). As seen in all sarcoidosis cases with rs20417, another variant only a few hundred base pairs away and downstream from PACERR, is rs689466, for which the allele C was more common in those with extrathoracic disease. A genetic variant within an HLA-B, rs2276448, was also associated with extrathoracic sarcoidosis. In addition, on chromosome 6, a locus upstream from NOTCH4, rs3134929, was associated with extrathoracic disease. And in chromosome 16 and 17, three variants were associated with extrathoracic involvement: two SNPs within chromosome 16, rs2066843 and rs2066842, both within exonic regions of NOD2; and one within chromosome 17, rs220465, representing a genetic variant within the intronic region/exonic border of ITGAE. As shown in Table 2, cardiac and joint involvement were common, but our cohort size was too small to identify genetic variants associated with any specific extrathoracic organ manifestation. We also found no association between the degree of exposure and extrathoracic organ involvement.

Table 3. Genetic variants most associated with sarcoidosis.

Gene	Position(hg19)	dbSNP	Alleles *	Risk Allele	Chi-sq p-Value	Fisher's p-value	OR **
PTGS2/COX2	chr1:186645927	rs2066826	T/C	C	0.002	0.001	1.88
PTGS2|PACERR ‡	chr1:186650321	rs20417	G/C	C	0.003	0.001	1.79
HLA-C	chr6:31239681	rs9264669	T/A	A	0.004	0.003	1.75
BTNL2	chr6:32370616	rs2076525	C/T	T	0.006	0.003	1.71
BTNL2	chr6:32370684	rs2076524	G/A	A	0.006	0.003	1.71
BTNL2	chr6:32370835	rs2076523	C/T	T	0.005	0.002	1.97
HLA-DRB1	chr6:32549424	rs112116022	T/C	C	0.003	0.002	5.21
HLA-DQB1	chr6:32629847	rs1049133	G/A	A	0.004	0.003	2.56
HLA-DQB1	chr6:32629859	rs1049130	G/A	A	0.006	0.004	1.90
HLA-DQB1	chr6:32635632	rs4516985	G/A	A	0.004	0.005	1.74
HLA-DQB1	chr6:32635846	rs9274614	G/C	C	0.005	0.004	2.49
HLA-DPA1|HLA-DP31 ‡	chr6:33048457	rs386699868 rs1126504 rs386699869	G/C	G	0.007	0.006	1.80 †
HLA-DPA1|HLA-DP31 ‡	chr6:33048466	rs1126511 rs1126513	TT/GG	TT	0.007	0.007	1.66 †
HLA-DPA1|HLA-DP31 ‡	chr6:33049211	rs928976	T/C	T	0.007	0.008	1.74 †

‡ indicates that SNP overlaps part of both genes; * listed as alternative allele/reference allele; ** ORs are calculated under the co-dominant model and are relative to the alternative allele unless specified with † which is in relation to the reference allele. This was done to maintain the OR as a comparison between the risk allele and non-risk allele.

Table 4. Genetic variants associated with extrathoracic organ involvement.

Gene	Position(hg19)	dbSNP	Alleles *	Risk Allele	Chi-sq p-Value	Fisher's p-Value	OR **
PTGS2	chr1:186645927	rs2066826	T/C	C	0.009	0.012	1.45
PACERR	chr1:186650751	rs689466	C/T	C	0.006	0.016	2.33 †
HLA-B	chr6:31323020	rs2276448	C/T	T	0.008	0.003	2.13
NOTCH4	chr6:32192107	rs3134929	G/C	G	0.009	0.012	2.39 †
NOD2	chr16:50744624	rs2066842	T/C	T	0.010	0.019	2.00 †
NOD2	chr16:50745199	rs2066843	T/C	T	0.010	0.019	2.21 †
ITGAE	chr17:3637915	rs220465	T/C	T	0.005	0.006	1.08 †

* listed as alternative allele/reference allele; ** ORs are calculated under the co-dominant model and are relative to the alternative allele unless specified with † which is in relation to the reference allele. This was done to maintain the OR as a comparison between the risk allele and non-risk allele.

4. Discussion

Sarcoidosis has been identified in all WTC cohorts (FDNY, general responders other than FDNY, the survivor population and the WTC Registry), the most extensively described being that from FDNY [4,16,23–26]. In our current FDNY case-control study, we examine genetic characteristics in our cases as compared with our WTC-exposed controls without sarcoidosis. Seventeen allele variants of HLA and non-HLA genes were found to be associated with sarcoidosis with p-value < 0.01 and all were within chromosomes 1 and 6. Our results also suggest an association between extrathoracic involvement and allele variants of HLA and non-HLA genes found not only on chromosomes 1 and

6, but also on chromosomes 16 and 17. Comparing our findings to published studies of sporadic sarcoidosis, we found similarities between genetic variants with WTC-related sarcoidosis and those reported in studies of sarcoidosis without known environmental exposures. In addition, we identified several allele variants not previously reported to be in association with sarcoidosis. If confirmed in larger studies with known environmental exposures, these novel findings may provide insight into the gene-environment interactions key to the development of sarcoidosis.

For example, our data are consistent with a prior study showing an association between SNP rs20417, in a non-coding region of the PTGS2/COX2 gene on chromosome 1, and sarcoidosis in a UK and Austrian Caucasian cohort without known environmental exposure [11]. This allele variant, described using prior nomenclature -765C (-765 is the nucleotide base pair position and C is the base pair), was found to be more often present in sarcoidosis subjects with severe pulmonary disease (poor lung function or extensive fibrosis). The authors also created lung fibroblast cell lines that were stimulated by transforming growth factor (TGF)-β1. They found that the cell lines with the -765C (currently named rs20147) produced little to no prostaglandin E2 (PGE2), an important inhibitor of the proliferation of fibroblasts. The loss of this lung protective inflammatory mediator could explain its relationship to more severe forms of pulmonary sarcoidosis. As eloquently described by Valentonyte and colleagues (2005), allele variations in BTNL2 impact the negative T-cell regulation function of BTNL2 [14]. Thus, the dysregulation of T-cell function from some BTNL2 mutations may explain its relationship to sarcoidosis. Interestingly, Akers and colleagues (2011) determined there was strong linkage disequilibrium between rs9274614, an allele significantly associated with sarcoidosis in our cohort, and several HLA-DQB1*06 alleles [27]. Another study found an association between the HLA-DQB1*0601 allele and cardiac sarcoidosis in a Japanese cohort [28]. Although our sample size was too small to identify specific alleles associated with cardiac sarcoidosis, the known association between the SNP rs9274614 and an allele associated with cardiac sarcoidosis, HLA-DQB1*0601, is one of interest in this cohort given the significant number of participants with cardiac sarcoidosis.

Except as noted above, the genetic variants associated with sarcoidosis in our WTC-exposed cohort have not previously been reported. Several of the SNPs identified in our cohort as associated with WTC-related sarcoidosis have been associated with other diseases in cohorts without known environmental exposures. Perhaps the most frequently investigated is rs20417 in PTGS2/COX2. Studies have identified its association with carotid-calcified plaque in those with diabetes [29], protection against myocardial infarction and stroke [30], as well as asthma [31]. In addition, SNP rs1126513, significantly associated with WTC-related sarcoidosis in our cohort, was found to be associated with ankylosing spondylitis [32].

The main strength of this study was its reliance on a rigorously characterized prospective cohort, with a clearly defined time of exposure (9/11). One limitation of this study is that it was focused on candidate genes already identified in sarcoidosis studies from the general population without WTC exposure. Additionally, the identification of novel SNPs may be partially due to our high-density sequencing which evaluated almost every base pair of these candidate genes. The main limitation, however, is that this study includes a relatively small sample size. Our statistical power was limited to detect only sizable effects. At significance level 0.01, we had 0.8 power to detect an odds ratio of 2.3 at variants with MAF = 0.5 and an odds ratio of 4 at variants with MAF = 0.05; we had 0.2 power to detect an odds ratio of 1.5 at variants with MAF = 0.5 and an odds ratio of 2 at variants with MAF = 0.05. Additional power would be obtained if this study was expanded to include all of the various WTC health program cohorts to allow for both replication of the main effects observed, and to allow for gene-environment analyses. This could potentially allow for more robust causal inferences to be made regarding the etiology of sarcoidosis, and whether there are unique differences in those with extrathoracic disease, particularly cardiac and joint involvement.

5. Conclusions

The incidence of sarcoidosis was increased after the collapse of the WTC towers and this is best demonstrated in the FDNY cohort where there was clear evidence that these cases were new in onset after 9/11 [4,16]. Our findings suggest that the genetic characteristics of WTC-related sarcoidosis are similar to the sporadic cases found in the general population without known environmental exposures. These data suggest the granulomatous disease observed post-9/11 and originally termed "Sarcoid-Like" Granulomatous Disease (SLGD) is better described as WTC-related Sarcoidosis. Our findings, however, suggest that there are several novel allele variants (SNPs) which may be uniquely associated with WTC-related sarcoidosis and with extrathoracic disease. These novel findings may provide some insights into the unique gene-environment interactions key to the development of sarcoidosis in this population, among others. Future studies should focus on increasing the power of our findings by combining sarcoidosis cases from all WTC health program cohorts and comparing them to matched controls with non-WTC associated sarcoidosis.

Supplementary Materials: The following are available online at http://www.mdpi.com/1660-4601/16/10/1830/s1, Table S1: Candidate genes and exon coverage, Table S2: Location and function of gene variants associated with sarcoidosis, Table S3: Location and function of gene variants associated with extrathoracic organ involvement, Table S4: Genotype frequencies.

Author Contributions: Conceptualization, K.Y., R.Z.-O., K.M.H., C.M., J.S., S.D.S. and D.J.P.; Data curation, K.L.C., R.Z.-O., K.M.H., C.M., J.S., N.J. and D.G.G.; Formal analysis, K.Y., R.Z.-O. and H.L.C.; Funding acquisition, K.M.H., S.D.S. and D.J.P.; Investigation, K.L.C., K.M.H., N.J. and D.G.G.; Methodology, K.Y., R.Z.-O., K.M.H., C.M., S.D.S. and D.J.P.; Project administration, R.Z.-O., K.M.H., C.M., S.D.S. and D.J.P.; Resources, C.M., S.D.S. and D.J.P.; Software, K.Y., C.M. and J.S.; Supervision, S.D.S. and D.J.P.; Validation, K.L.C. and K.Y.; Visualization, K.L.C. and H.L.C.; Writing—original draft, K.L.C., K.Y., C.M. and S.D.S.; Writing—review & editing, K.L.C., K.Y., H.D.H.III, M.D.W., H.L.C., S.D.S. and D.J.P.

Funding: This research was funded by the National Institute of Occupational Safety and Health (NIOSH), Grant U01-OH010993 and contracts #200-2011-39383, #200-2011-39378, #200-2017-93326 and #200-2017-93426.

Acknowledgments: We would like to acknowledge Thomas K. Aldrich, for his significant contribution to project design, supervision, and funding acquisition and was the original PI on this study. He sadly died of pancreatic cancer while this project was underway. Aldrich's work was guided by his desire to understand the health impacts of 9/11 in order to improve the lives of those affected. He was a mentor and personal friend to many of us and is deeply missed. We would also like to thank Miao Kevin Shi for technical support in Spivack's lab.

Conflicts of Interest: The authors declare no conflict of interest.

References

1. Baughman, R.P.; Teirstein, A.S.; Judson, M.A.; Rossman, M.D.; Yeager, H., Jr.; Bresnitz, E.A.; DePalo, L.; Hunninghake, G.; Iannuzzi, M.C.; Johns, C.J.; et al. Clinical characteristics of patients in a case control study of sarcoidosis. *Am. J. Respir. Crit. Care Med.* **2001**, *164*, 1885–1889. [CrossRef] [PubMed]

2. Ungprasert, P.; Carmona, E.M.; Utz, J.P.; Ryu, J.H.; Crowson, C.S.; Matteson, E.L. Epidemiology of Sarcoidosis 1946–2013: A Population-Based Study. *Mayo Clin. Proc.* **2016**, *91*, 183–188. [CrossRef]

3. Prezant, D.J.; Dhala, A.; Goldstein, A.; Janus, D.; Ortiz, F.; Aldrich, T.K.; Kelly, K.J. The incidence, prevalence, and severity of sarcoidosis in New York City firefighters. *Chest* **1999**, *116*, 1183–1193. [CrossRef] [PubMed]

4. Webber, M.P.; Yip, J.; Zeig-Owens, R.; Moir, W.; Ungprasert, P.; Crowson, C.S.; Hall, C.B.; Jaber, N.; Weiden, M.D.; Matteson, E.L.; et al. Post-9/11 sarcoidosis in WTC-exposed firefighters and emergency medical service workers. *Respir. Med.* **2017**, *132*, 232–237. [CrossRef]

5. Rossides, M.; Grunewald, J.; Eklund, A.; Kullberg, S.; Di Giuseppe, D.; Askling, J.; Arkema, E.V. Familial aggregation and heritability of sarcoidosis: A Swedish nested case-control study. *Eur. Respir. J.* **2018**, *52*. [CrossRef] [PubMed]

6. Rybicki, B.A.; Iannuzzi, M.C.; Frederick, M.M.; Thompson, B.W.; Rossman, M.D.; Bresnitz, E.A.; Terrin, M.L.; Moller, D.R.; Barnard, J.; Baughman, R.P.; et al. Familial aggregation of sarcoidosis. A case-control etiologic study of sarcoidosis (ACCESS). *Am. J. Respir. Crit. Care Med.* **2001**, *164*, 2085–2091. [CrossRef] [PubMed]

7. Rossman, M.D.; Thompson, B.; Frederick, M.; Maliarik, M.; Iannuzzi, M.C.; Rybicki, B.A.; Pandey, J.P.; Newman, L.S.; Magira, E.; Beznik-Cizman, B.; et al. HLA-DRB1*1101: A significant risk factor for sarcoidosis in blacks and whites. *Am. J. Hum. Genet.* **2003**, *73*, 720–735. [CrossRef] [PubMed]

8. Voorter, C.E.; Drent, M.; van den Berg-Loonen, E.M. Severe pulmonary sarcoidosis is strongly associated with the haplotype HLA-DQB1*0602-DRB1*150101. *Hum. Immunol.* **2005**, *66*, 826–835. [CrossRef] [PubMed]

9. Swider, C.; Schnittger, L.; Bogunia-Kubik, K.; Gerdes, J.; Flad, H.; Lange, A.; Seitzer, U. TNF-alpha and HLA-DR genotyping as potential prognostic markers in pulmonary sarcoidosis. *Eur. Cytokine Netw.* **1999**, *10*, 143–146. [PubMed]

10. Levin, A.M.; Adrianto, I.; Datta, I.; Iannuzzi, M.C.; Trudeau, S.; Li, J.; Drake, W.P.; Montgomery, C.G.; Rybicki, B.A. Association of HLA-DRB1 with Sarcoidosis Susceptibility and Progression in African Americans. *Am. J. Respir. Cell Mol. Biol.* **2015**, *53*, 206–216. [CrossRef]

11. Hill, M.R.; Papafili, A.; Booth, H.; Lawson, P.; Hubner, M.; Beynon, H.; Read, C.; Lindahl, G.; Marshall, R.P.; McAnulty, R.J.; et al. Functional prostaglandin-endoperoxide synthase 2 polymorphism predicts poor outcome in sarcoidosis. *Am. J. Respir. Crit. Care Med.* **2006**, *174*, 915–922. [CrossRef]

12. Adrianto, I.; Lin, C.P.; Hale, J.J.; Levin, A.M.; Datta, I.; Parker, R.; Adler, A.; Kelly, J.A.; Kaufman, K.M.; Lessard, C.J.; et al. Genome-wide association study of African and European Americans implicates multiple shared and ethnic specific loci in sarcoidosis susceptibility. *PLoS ONE* **2012**, *7*, e43907. [CrossRef]

13. Sato, H.; Williams, H.R.; Spagnolo, P.; Abdallah, A.; Ahmad, T.; Orchard, T.R.; Copley, S.J.; Desai, S.R.; Wells, A.U.; du Bois, R.M.; et al. CARD15/NOD2 polymorphisms are associated with severe pulmonary sarcoidosis. *Eur. Respir. J.* **2010**, *35*, 324–330. [CrossRef]

14. Valentonyte, R.; Hampe, J.; Huse, K.; Rosenstiel, P.; Albrecht, M.; Stenzel, A.; Nagy, M.; Gaede, K.I.; Franke, A.; Haesler, R.; et al. Sarcoidosis is associated with a truncating splice site mutation in BTNL2. *Nat. Genet.* **2005**, *37*, 357–364. [CrossRef]

15. Rybicki, B.A.; Walewski, J.L.; Maliarik, M.J.; Kian, H.; Iannuzzi, M.C. The BTNL2 gene and sarcoidosis susceptibility in African Americans and Whites. *Am. J. Hum. Genet.* **2005**, *77*, 491–499. [CrossRef]

16. Hena, K.M.; Yip, J.; Jaber, N.; Goldfarb, D.; Fullam, K.; Cleven, K.; Moir, W.; Zeig-Owens, R.; Webber, M.P.; Spevack, D.M.; et al. Clinical Course of Sarcoidosis in World Trade Center-Exposed Firefighters. *Chest* **2018**, *153*, 114–123. [CrossRef]

17. Judson, M.A.; Costabel, U.; Drent, M.; Wells, A.; Maier, L.; Koth, L.; Shigemitsu, H.; Culver, D.A.; Gelfand, J.; Valeyre, D.; et al. The WASOG Sarcoidosis Organ Assessment Instrument: An update of a previous clinical tool. *Sarcoidosis Vasc. Diffus. Lung Dis. Off. J. WASOG* **2014**, *31*, 19–27.

18. Prezant, D.J.; Weiden, M.; Banauch, G.I.; McGuinness, G.; Rom, W.N.; Aldrich, T.K.; Kelly, K.J. Cough and bronchial responsiveness in firefighters at the World Trade Center site. *New Engl. J. Med.* **2002**, *347*, 806–815. [CrossRef]

19. Miller, E.M.; Patterson, N.E.; Zechmeister, J.M.; Bejerano-Sagie, M.; Delio, M.; Patel, K.; Ravi, N.; Quispe-Tintaya, W.; Maslov, A.; Simmons, N.; et al. Development and validation of a targeted next generation DNA sequencing panel outperforming whole exome sequencing for the identification of clinically relevant genetic variants. *Oncotarget* **2017**, *8*, 102033–102045. [CrossRef]

20. Delio, M.; Patel, K.; Maslov, A.; Marion, R.W.; McDonald, T.V.; Cadoff, E.M.; Golden, A.; Greally, J.M.; Vijg, J.; Morrow, B.; et al. Development of a Targeted Multi-Disorder High-Throughput Sequencing Assay for the Effective Identification of Disease-Causing Variants. *PLoS ONE* **2015**, *10*, e0133742. [CrossRef]

21. Shastri, A.; Msaouel, P.; Montagna, C.; White, S.; Delio, M.; Patel, K.; Alexis, K.; Strakhan, M.; Elrafei, T.N.; Reed, L.J. Primary Hepatic Small Cell Carcinoma: Two Case Reports, Molecular Characterization and Pooled Analysis of Known Clinical Data. *Anticancer Res.* **2016**, *36*, 271–277.

22. Josephs, K.; Patel, K.; Janson, C.M.; Montagna, C.; McDonald, T.V. Compound heterozygous CASQ2 mutations and long-term course of catecholaminergic polymorphic ventricular tachycardia. *Mol. Genet. Genom. Med.* **2017**, *5*, 788–794. [CrossRef] [PubMed]

23. Izbicki, G.; Chavko, R.; Banauch, G.I.; Weiden, M.D.; Berger, K.I.; Aldrich, T.K.; Hall, C.; Kelly, K.J.; Prezant, D.J. World Trade Center "sarcoid-like" granulomatous pulmonary disease in New York City Fire Department rescue workers. *Chest* **2007**, *131*, 1414–1423. [CrossRef]

24. Crowley, L.E.; Herbert, R.; Moline, J.M.; Wallenstein, S.; Shukla, G.; Schechter, C.; Skloot, G.S.; Udasin, I.; Luft, B.J.; Harrison, D.; et al. "Sarcoid like" granulomatous pulmonary disease in World Trade Center disaster responders. *Am. J. Ind. Med.* **2011**, *54*, 175–184. [CrossRef] [PubMed]

25. Parsia, S.S.; Yee. H.; Young, S.; Turetz, M.L.; Marmor, M.; Wilkenfeld, M.; Kazeros, A.; Caplan-Shaw, C.E.; Reibman, J. Characteristics of sarcoidosis in residents and workers exposed to World Trade Center (WTC) dust, gas and fumes presenting for medical care. *Am. J. Respir. Crit. Care Med.* **2010**, *181*, A1740.

26. Jordan, H.T.; Stellman, S.D.; Prezant, D.; Teirstein, A.; Osahan, S.S.; Cone, J.E. Sarcoidosis diagnosed after September 11, 2001, among adults exposed to the World Trade Center disaster. *J. Occup. Environ. Med.* **2011**, *53*, 966–974. [CrossRef] [PubMed]

27. Akers, N.K.; Curry, J.D.; Conde, L.; Bracci, P.M.; Smith, M.T.; Skibola, C.F. Association of HLA-DQB1 alleles with risk of follicular lymphoma. *Leuk. Lymphoma* **2011**, *52*, 53–58. [CrossRef] [PubMed]

28. Naruse, T.K.; Matsuzawa, Y.; Ota, M.; Katsuyama, Y.; Matsumori, A.; Hara, M.; Nagai, S.; Morimoto, S.; Sasayama, S.; Inoko, H. HLA-DQB1*0601 is primarily associated with the susceptibility to cardiac sarcoidosis. *Tissue Antigens* **2000**, *56*, 52–57. [CrossRef]

29. Rudock, M.E.; Liu, Y.; Ziegler, J.T.; Allen, S.G.; Lehtinen, A.B.; Freedman, B.I.; Carr, J.J.; Langefeld, C.D.; Bowden, D.W. Association of polymorphisms in cyclooxygenase (COX)-2 with coronary and carotid calcium in the Diabetes Heart Study. *Atherosclerosis* **2009**, *203*, 459–465. [CrossRef]

30. Cipollone, F.; Toniato, E.; Martinotti, S.; Fazia, M.; Iezzi, A.; Cuccurullo, C.; Pini, B.; Ursi, S.; Vitullo, G.; Averna, M.; et al. A polymorphism in the cyclooxygenase 2 gene as an inherited protective factor against myocardial infarction and stroke. *JAMA* **2004**, *291*, 2221–2228. [CrossRef]

31. Szczeklik, W.; Sanak, M.; Szczeklik, A. Functional effects and gender association of COX-2 gene polymorphism G-765C in bronchial asthma. *J. Allergy Clin. Immunol.* **2004**, *114*, 248–253. [CrossRef] [PubMed]

32. Cortes, A.; Pulit, S.L.; Leo, P.J.; Pointon, J.J.; Robinson, P.C.; Weisman, M.H.; Ward, M.; Gensler, L.S.; Zhou, X.; Garchon, H.J.; et al. Major histocompatibility complex associations of ankylosing spondylitis are complex and involve further epistasis with ERAP1. *Nat. Commun.* **2015**, *6*, 7146. [CrossRef] [PubMed]

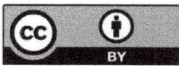

International Journal of
Environmental Research and Public Health

MDPI

Article

Air Pollution/Irritants, Asthma Control, and Health-Related Quality of Life among 9/11-Exposed Individuals with Asthma

Janette Yung *, Sukhminder Osahan, Stephen M. Friedman, Jiehui Li and James E. Cone

New York City Department of Health and Mental Hygiene, World Trade Center Health Registry,
New York, NY 10013, USA; osukhmin@health.nyc.gov (S.O.); sfriedm2@health.nyc.gov (S.M.F.);
jli3@health.nyc.gov (J.L.); jcone@health.nyc.gov (J.E.C.)
* Correspondence: jyung@health.nyc.gov; Tel.: +1-646-632-6688

Received: 25 April 2019; Accepted: 25 May 2019; Published: 30 May 2019

Abstract: Asthma control is suboptimal among World Trade Center Health Registry (WTCHR) enrollees. Air pollution/irritants have been reported as the most prevalent trigger among World Trade Center responders. We examined the relationship between air pollution/irritants and asthma control. We also evaluated the association of asthma control with health-related quality of life (HRQoL). We included 6202 enrollees age ≥18 with a history of asthma who completed the WTCHR asthma survey between 2015 and 2016. Based on modified National Asthma Education and Prevention Program criteria, asthma was categorized as controlled, poorly-controlled, or very poorly-controlled. HRQoL indicators include ≥14 unhealthy days, ≥14 activity limitation days, and self-rated general health. We used multinomial logistic regression for asthma control, and unconditional logistic regression for HRQoL, adjusting for covariates. Overall, 27.1% had poorly-controlled and 32.2% had very poorly-controlled asthma. Air pollution/irritants were associated with poorly-controlled (adjusted odds ratio (AOR) = 1.70; 95% CI = 1.45–1.99) and very poorly-controlled asthma (AOR = 2.15; 95% CI = 1.83–2.53). Poor asthma control in turn worsened the HRQoL of asthmatic patients. Very poorly-controlled asthma was significantly associated with ≥14 unhealthy days (AOR = 3.60; 95% CI = 3.02–4.30), ≥14 activity limitation days (AOR = 4.37; 95% CI = 3.48–5.50), and poor/fair general health status (AOR = 4.92; 95% CI = 4.11–5.89). Minimizing World Trade Center (WTC) asthmatic patients' exposure to air pollution/irritants may improve their disease management and overall well-being.

Keywords: 9/11 disaster; asthma; trigger(s); air pollution; irritant(s); health-related quality of life

1. Introduction

The prevalence of asthma has increased in the last decade and placed a significant economic burden on the United States and globally. Asthma is a chronic disease characterized by inflammation of the airways, reversible airflow obstruction, and bronchial hyper-responsiveness, with symptoms including wheezing, coughing, tightness of the chest, shortness of breath, and sleep awakening. These symptoms can greatly affect daily activities and quality of life. In the United States, asthma was responsible for $3 billion in losses due to missed work and school days, $29 billion due to asthma-related mortality, and $50.3 billion in medical costs during 2008–2013 [1]. A previous World Trade Center (WTC) study reported that asthma control was poor or very poor in over 68% of World Trade Center Health Registry (WTCHR) enrollees diagnosed after 9/11 [2], likely affecting their quality of life.

The presence of asthma triggers that are difficult to avoid may be responsible for some of this lack of asthma control in many patients. Part of the difficulty in asthma medical management is explicitly defining triggers that contribute to exacerbations [3,4]. A higher number of triggers experienced [3] and a wide array of asthma triggers have been identified and perceived by patients as contributing to the severity and frequency of asthma exacerbations [3,5,6].

Air pollution/irritants are materials in the indoor or outdoor air that can have adverse effects on humans and the ecosystem. These substances can be in the form of particulates, liquid droplets, or gases, and can be of natural origin or man-made. They induce airway inflammation or an allergen-induced response by causing direct cellular injury or by inducing intracellular signaling pathways and transcription factors that are known to be sensitive to oxidative stress [6]. The subsequent mucosal damage and impaired mucociliary clearance may facilitate access of inhaled allergens to the cells of the immune system [6]. Air pollutants/irritants were the most prevalent type of asthma triggers reported in previous studies [7,8]. The most abundant components of air pollution in urban areas are particulate matter (PM), nitrogen dioxide (NO_2), and ozone (O_3). PM is a mixture of organic and inorganic solid and liquid particles of different origin and size. NO_2 can enhance the allergic response to inhaled allergens, and its concentration in ambient air is reportedly associated with cough, wheezing, and shortness of breath in atopic patients. O_3 is thought to increase asthma morbidity by enhancing airway inflammation and epithelial permeability [6]. High ambient concentrations of these materials are associated with an increased rate of asthma exacerbations [6,9], and were associated with increased post-9/11 asthma-related hospital admissions [9].

Health-related quality of life (HRQoL) has been increasingly recognized as an important endpoint and measure for interventions [10–12]. It is regarded as a measure of the effect of the disease on a patient's life. A previous study reported that greater severity and frequency of exacerbations were significantly associated with decreases in asthma-related quality of life [13]. Poorly-controlled asthma were also found to be related to poorer HRQoL in the United Kingdom [14]. Moreover, asthmatic patients had worse indicators of quality of life compared to the general population regardless of whether symptoms were clinically controlled [15].

To better understand the relationship between asthma triggers, asthma control, and HRQoL among asthmatic enrollees who were exposed to the WTC disaster, the current study consists of two parts. The first part aims to supplement existing knowledge regarding the various triggers in an effort to determine whether air pollution/irritants are an important trigger reported by individuals exposed to 9/11. The second part of this study assesses two objectives: (1) to examine the association of self-reported air pollution/irritants trigger with asthma control among all asthmatic enrollees who were exposed to WTC disaster; and (2) to examine the association of different level of asthma control with three domains of impaired HRQoL: self-reported mental or physical unhealthy days, self-reported activity limitation days, and self-reported general health. We hypothesized that reporting air pollution/irritants as an asthma trigger is associated with poorer asthma control, and that poorer asthma control is associated with lower HRQoL among 9/11-exposed individuals with asthma.

2. Materials and Methods

The WTCHR has been described in detail elsewhere [16,17]. Briefly, this is a longitudinal cohort study including rescue/recovery workers and volunteers (RRW) and community members not involved in rescue/recovery (lower Manhattan area residents, students, and workers; passersby and commuters on 9/11). Participants were recruited through Lower Manhattan area building or employer lists, or encouraged to enroll via a toll-free telephone number or website [17]. Between 12 September 2003 and 24 November 2004, 71,431 people completed a computer-assisted (95%) or in-person (5%) enrollment interview on demographics, exposures incurred during and after the WTC disaster and health information. Since that baseline enrollment (Wave 1), the Registry has conducted three follow-up surveys (Waves 2 to 4) via mail, website, or telephone interview to collect updated health information. The response rates for Wave 2 (2006–2007), Wave 3 (2011–2012), and Wave 4 (2015–2016) were 65.2%, 60.4%, and 51.6%, respectively. All surveys inquired about enrollees' medical history and physical and mental health status. The Wave 4 asthma survey began on 3 September 2015 and continued through 20 March 2016, and was administered as a supplement to the Wave 4 Core (Wave 4) survey. We sent out the Wave 4 asthma survey to 14,983 eligible enrollees age ≥18 who reported ever being diagnosed with asthma in any of the three prior wave surveys, either before or after 9/11/2001. Asthma survey data were collected via the internet or through paper mailings and entailed disease management questions, including triggers, asthma control and exacerbation. The Registry's protocol was approved by the institutional review boards of the US Centers for Disease Control and Prevention and the New York City Department of Health and Mental Hygiene (#02-058).

2.1. Study Sample

Of the 14,983 eligible enrollees who were sent the Wave 4 asthma survey, 8482 responded to the survey either fully or partially. Of these, 4653 (55%) were completed by web and 3829 (45%) were completed by paper. In our study, we only included those who reported "yes" to the gate question of "Have you ever been told by a doctor or other health professional that you had asthma?" on the Wave 4 asthma survey ($N = 7129$), though we only mailed the Wave 4 asthma survey to enrollees who had reported an asthma diagnosis on at least one of the three prior Registry surveys (Waves 1 through 3). We excluded enrollees who had missing age ($N = 3$), and those who did not respond to the Wave 4 survey ($N = 830$) since we used the sociodemographic and health variables from Wave 4. We also excluded additional persons who had missing value for the asthma control variable ($N = 94$). The final study sample was 6202 for data analyses.

2.2. Study Outcomes and Variables

2.2.1. Determining Air Pollution/Irritants as Trigger

We derived this variable by analyzing asthma triggers following the method of Ritz [4]. Briefly, open-ended responses to the asthma triggers question "Please list up to six of the strongest triggers of your asthma" were grouped into 11 main categories: air pollution/irritants, exercise, infection, allergens (pollen), allergens (animal), allergens (general), air temperature, psychological, allergens (food), medications, and other. Similar to findings in previous studies [7,8], air pollution/irritants was the most prevalent type of trigger, reported by over 50% of the participants. We therefore derived a dichotomous variable of air pollution/irritants.

2.2.2. Asthma Control and HRQoL

We focused on two main outcomes in the second part of the study. The first outcome was asthma control and the second outcome was HRQoL. We categorized asthma control for study participants as having controlled, poorly-controlled, or very poorly-controlled asthma reported in the Wave 4 asthma survey, based on criteria modified from the National Asthma Education and Prevention Program's Third Expert Panel Report 3 (EPR 3). Briefly, the criteria consist of four components: shortness of breath, wheezing, and/or cough; nighttime awakenings; interference with normal activity; and use of a rescue inhaler or nebulizer. The level of asthma control category was determined by frequency of experience on each component. Participants were assigned to the most severe category in which any component was reported. In our slightly modified criteria, for interference with normal activity, we specified none/a little of the time to well-controlled, some/most of the time to poorly-controlled, all of the time to very poorly-controlled asthma, versus no interference with normal activity, some limitation, and extreme limitation for well-controlled, poorly-controlled, and very poorly-controlled asthma, respectively, based on EPR 3 definition. We also slightly modified use of a rescue inhaler or nebulizer. We specified inhaler use of <3 times/week to well-controlled, 1–2 times/d to poorly-controlled, and >2 times/d to very poorly-controlled asthma, versus ≤2 days/week, >2 days/week, and several times per day for well-controlled, poorly-controlled, and very poorly-controlled asthma, respectively, based on EPR 3 definition [2,18]. In the second analysis, asthma control was treated as predictor variable, and we assessed three dichotomous outcome variables for HRQoL: ≥14 physically or mentally unhealthy days; ≥14 days of poor physical or mental health that keep you from doing your usual activities (activity limitation); and self-rated general health status (excellent, very good, or good versus fair or poor) [19,20].

2.3. Covariates

In both analyses, we adjusted for age, gender, race/ethnicity, marital status, education, social integration, smoking status, depression, probable post-traumatic stress disorder (PTSD), gastroesophageal reflux symptoms (GERS), obstructive sleep apnea (OSA), body mass index (BMI), having at least one regular healthcare provider, and WTC dust/debris cloud exposure. WTC dust/debris exposure was a dichotomous variable obtained from the Wave 1 survey. Those who reported having been caught in the dust and debris cloud on 9/11/2001 were considered to have had dust cloud exposure. Comorbid conditions were assessed at Wave 4 survey. The Wave 4 survey began in 20 March 2015 and continued through 31 January 2016, while the Wave 4 asthma survey began on 3 September 2015 and continued through 20 March 2016. The mean time interval between the Wave 4 and Wave 4 asthma surveys was 132 days, with a range from 0 to 323 days. Probable PTSD, depression, and generalized anxiety disorder (GAD) were defined using validated scales. Participants with a score ≥44 on the PTSD Checklist, Stressor-Specific Version, a 17-item scale that inquired about 9/11-related psychological symptoms during the 30 day before Wave 4, were considered to have probable PTSD [21,22]. Depression within the two weeks before completion of Wave 4 was defined as a score ≥10 on the 8-item Patient Health Questionnaire depression scale [23]. Probable GAD during the two weeks before Wave 4 was defined as a score ≥10 on the 7-item GAD scale [24]. Self-reported GERS and history of OSA were also obtained from Wave 4 questionnaire responses. Participants who reported having heartburn at least once a week during the 12 months preceding Wave 4 were considered to have GERS. Smoking history was taken from the most recent questionnaire where smoking data were available. Social integration was defined as either low or high based on participants' responses to the four questions that assess the components of social integration construct [25]: "In the last 30 days, have you visited, talked, or e-mailed with friends at least twice?", "In the last 30 days, have you attended a religious service at least twice?", "In the last 30 days, have you been actively involved in a volunteer organization or club?", and "About how many close friends or relatives do you have now? Include people you feel at ease with and can talk with about what is on your mind." Each of these questions received a score of 1 if the response was yes or more than zero. Participants were considered as having lower social integration if the total score was less than two, higher social integration if the total score was two or higher. BMI at Wave 4 was calculated from self-reported height and weight data; a BMI <25 was considered under or normal weight, 25–29.9 was considered overweight and ≥30 was obese.

2.4. Statistical Analyses

We used a multinomial logistic regression model to examine the association of self-reported air pollution/irritants as trigger with poor and very poor asthma control, adjusting for covariates. We also used multiple logistic regression model to examine the association between asthma control and three health-related quality of life indicators: ≥14 days of poor physical or mental health, ≥14 days of activity limitation, and self-rated general health, adjusting for the same covariates as analysis 1. In both analyses, we used two-sided tests of significance and assumed a type 1 error of 5%. We used SAS software (Version 9.4, SAS Institute Inc., Cary, NC, USA) for all analyses.

3. Results

3.1. Asthma Trigger

The frequencies of different self-reported asthma triggers are shown in Figure 1. Half of the WTCHR enrollees with asthma reported air pollution/irritants as their asthma trigger. It was the most prevalent trigger, followed by physical activity and general allergens.

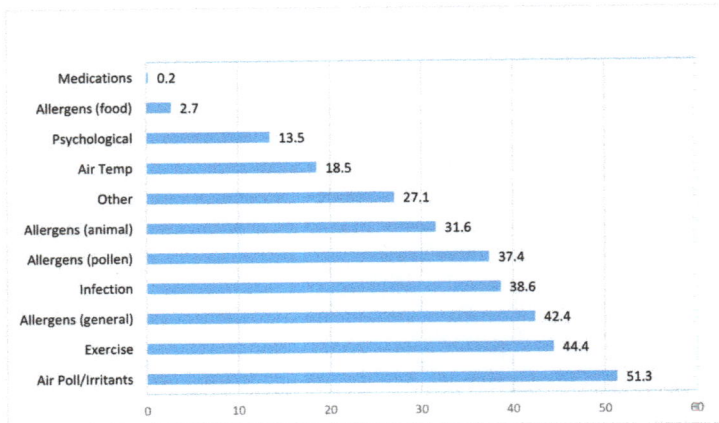

Figure 1. Percentage of each self-reported asthma trigger among World Trade Center Health Registry enrollees with asthma (not mutually exclusive).

Asthma control status by sociodemographic characteristics, comorbid conditions, reporting air pollution/irritants as an asthma trigger, and WTC dust exposure are shown in Table 1. The overall prevalence of poorly-controlled and very poorly-controlled asthma were 27.1% and 32.2%, respectively. We also observed an increase in prevalence of very poorly-controlled asthma among those with self-reported air pollution/irritants trigger (39.8%), depression (55.8%), and probable PTSD (58.1%).

Table 1. Prevalence of asthma control by sociodemographic, air pollution/irritants, and World Trade Center (WTC) dust cloud exposure among 9/11-exposed individuals with asthma (N = 6202).

Characteristics at Wave 4 *	Total *	% Controlled	% Poorly-Controlled	% Very Poorly-Controlled
Gender				
Male	3357	38.2	26.2	35.6
Female	2845	43.6	28.2	28.2
Age				
<45	1026	59.2	22.2	18.6
45–64	3897	38.0	27.8	34.2
≥65	1279	33.9	29.2	36.9
Race/Ethnicity				
White non-Hispanic	4109	44.3	25.0	30.7
Black non-Hispanic	622	31.4	33.6	35.1
Hispanic	938	29.5	33.5	37.0
Asian	286	46.9	25.9	27.3
Other	247	38.5	24.3	37.3
Marital Status				
Never married	961	44.8	27.4	27.9
Married/living with a partner	3978	42.6	26.6	30.8
Widowed, divorced, or separated	1163	32.0	28.1	39.9
Education				
College/post-graduate	3194	52.5	24.1	23.5
Some college	1964	31.7	29.7	38.7
High school or less	970	20.3	31.4	48.3
Smoking Status				
Never smoker	3832	44.0	26.3	29.7
Previous smoker	1791	39.1	26.8	34.1
Current smoker	438	24.2	31.3	44.5

Table 1. Cont.

Characteristics at Wave 4 *	Total *	% Controlled	% Poorly-Controlled	% Very Poorly-Controlled
BMI				
Normal (<25)	1450	54.6	22.7	22.8
Overweight (25–29)	2111	41.8	27.5	30.7
Obese (>30)	2436	31.7	29.2	39.2
Social Integration				
High	5587	42.8	26.9	30.3
Low	411	16.8	28.7	54.5
Depression				
No	4384	50.2	25.9	23.9
Yes	1452	15.8	28.4	55.8
Probable PTSD				
No	4632	50.0	25.9	24.1
Yes	1452	12.4	29.5	58.1
GERS				
No	3450	50.7	25.1	24.2
Yes	2344	27.8	29.0	43.2
Sleep Apnea				
No	4081	49.7	25.6	24.7
Yes	1647	21.9	28.5	49.5
Had at least one regular healthcare provider				
No	415	42.4	28.2	29.4
Yes	5681	40.7	26.9	32.4
Air pollution/irritants as an important trigger				
No	2777	49.2	24.8	26.0
Yes	2926	30.3	29.9	39.8
Dust cloud exposure at 9/11				
No	2587	46.9	25.3	27.8
Yes	3592	36.1	28.5	35.4

* Variable may not add up to total due to missing category. BMI: body mass index; PTSD: post-traumatic stress disorder. GERS: gastroesophageal reflux symptoms.

3.2. Self-Reported Air Pollution/Irritants as Trigger and Asthma Control

Enrollees who reported air pollution/irritants as triggers had elevated odds ratios for poorly-controlled (adjusted odds ratio (AOR): 1.70, 95% CI: 1.45–1.99) and very poorly-controlled asthma (AOR: 2.15, 95% CI: 1.83–2.53), after adjusting for covariates (Table 2).

Table 2. Multivariable odds ratios for association of level of asthma control with air pollution/irritants, controlling for selected sociodemographic factors, WTC dust cloud exposure, physical and mental health co-morbidities among 9/11-exposed individuals with asthma, 2015–2016.

Characteristics at Wave 4 *	Poorly-Controlled	Very Poorly-Controlled
	Adjusted OR (95% CI)	Adjusted OR (95% CI)
Gender		
Female	referent	referent
Male	1.08 (0.91–1.28)	1.52 (1.27–1.82)
Age		
<45	referent	referent
45–64	1.41 (1.13–1.75)	1.53 (1.21–1.94)
≥65	1.78 (1.36–2.33)	2.13 (1.60–2.83)
Education		
College/post-graduate	referent	referent
Some college	1.44 (1.20–1.71)	1.79 (1.50–2.15)
High school or less	1.80 (1.39–2.33)	2.76 (2.14–3.55)

Table 2. *Cont.*

Characteristics at Wave 4 *	Poorly-Controlled	Very Poorly-Controlled
	Adjusted OR (95% CI)	Adjusted OR (95% CI)
Smoking Status		
Never smoker	referent	referent
Former smoker	1.07 (0.90–1.27)	1.19 (1.00–1.42)
Current smoker	2.11 (1.50–2.97)	2.61 (1.86–3.67)
BMI		
Normal (<25)	referent	referent
Overweight (25–29)	1.32 (1.08–1.63)	1.22 (0.98–1.52)
Obese (>30)	1.58 (1.28–1.95)	1.68 (1.35–2.10)
Social Integration		
High	referent	referent
Low	1.60 (1.09–2.37)	1.77 (1.21–2.60)
Depression		
No	referent	referent
Yes	1.46 (1.14–1.87)	2.32 (1.83–2.94)
Probable PTSD		
No	referent	referent
Yes	2.64 (2.04–3.43)	3.39 (2.63–4.37)
GERS		
No	referent	referent
Yes	1.47 (1.24–1.73)	1.72 (1.45–2.03)
Sleep Apnea		
No	referent	referent
Yes	1.38 (1.13–1.68)	1.78 (1.46–2.16)
Dust cloud exposure at 9/11		
No	referent	referent
Yes	1.22 (1.05–1.43)	1.36 (1.16–1.59)
Air pollution/irritants		
No	referent	referent
Yes	1.70 (1.45–1.99)	2.15 (1.83–2.53)

* Non-significant covariates were not reported in the table.

3.3. Asthma Control and HRQoL

All three HRQoL indicators were strongly associated with asthma control level (Table 3). Enrollees with poorly-controlled asthma had higher odds ratios for ≥14 physically or mentally unhealthy days (AOR: 2.12, 95% CI: 1.78–2.52), ≥14 days of activity limitation (AOR: 2.17, 95% CI: 1.70–2.77), and self-rated poor general heath (AOR: 2.66, 95% CI: 2.22–3.18), compared to those with well-controlled asthma. Stronger associations were observed for very poorly-controlled asthma.

3.4. Mental Health, Asthma Control and HRQoL

Consistent with previous WTCHR findings, both depression and PTSD were associated with asthma control level [2]. Enrollees who reported depression or PTSD had higher odds ratios for poorly-controlled (AOR: 1.46, 95% CI: 1.14–1.87; AOR: 2.64, 95% CI: 2.04–3.43) and very poorly-controlled asthma (AOR: 2.32, 95% CI: 1.83–2.94; AOR 3.39, 95% CI: 2.63–4.37), respectively. Moreover, both mental illnesses were associated with ≥14 physically or mentally unhealthy days (AOR: 5.24, 95% CI: 4.22–6.51; AOR 3.08, 95% CI: 2.46–3.86); ≥14 days of activity limitation (AOR: 3.18, 95% CI: 2.58–3.92; AOR: 2.13, 95% CI: 1.72–2.64); and self-rated poor general heath (AOR: 2.65, 95% CI: 2.17–3.24; AOR: 2.04, 95% CI: 1.66–2.51) for depression and PTSD, respectively.

Table 3. Multivariable odds ratios for association of three health-related quality of life indicators with asthma control, controlling for selected sociodemographic factors, WTC dust cloud exposure, physical and mental health co-morbidities among 9/11-exposed individuals with asthma, 2015–2016.

Characteristics at Wave 4 *	≥14 Days of Poor Physical or Mental Health	≥14 Days of Activity Limitation	Fair/Poor General Health
	Adjusted OR (95% CI)	Adjusted OR (95% CI)	Adjusted OR (95% CI)
Sex			
Female	referent	referent	referent
Male	0.81 (0.70–0.95)	1.12 (0.92–1.35)	1.16 (0.99–1.37)
Age			
<45	referent	referent	referent
45–64	1.26 (1.03–1.55)	1.35 (1.03–1.77)	1.58 (1.28–1.97)
≥65	1.33 (1.03–1.71)	1.92 (1.40–2.63)	1.76 (1.36–2.29)
Race/ethnicity			
White non-Hispanic	referent	referent	referent
Black non-Hispanic	1.05 (0.81–1.35)	1.37 (1.03–1.81)	1.32 (1.03–1.70)
Hispanic	1.13 (0.91–1.40)	1.05 (0.83–1.33)	1.40 (1.13–1.73)
Asian	1.10 (0.77–1.59)	0.76 (0.46–1.25)	2.46 (1.72–3.52)
Other	1.11 (0.76–1.63)	1.32 (0.87–2.01)	1.48 (1.01–2.17)
Marital Status			
Never married	referent	referent	referent
Married/living with a partner	0.87 (0.71–1.07)	0.71 (0.55–0.90)	0.78 (0.64–0.97)
Widowed, divorced, or separated	1.11 (0.87–1.43)	0.93 (0.71–1.23)	0.91 (0.71–1.17)
Highest Education Attainment			
College/post-graduate	referent	referent	referent
Some college	1.29 (1.09–1.51)	1.47 (1.22–1.78)	1.40 (1.19–1.65)
High school or less	1.47 (1.18–1.84)	1.94 (1.53–2.46)	1.90 (1.53–2.37)
BMI			
Normal (<25)	referent	referent	referent
Overweight (25–29)	1.09 (0.90–1.32)	0.98 (0.77–1.25)	1.29 (1.05–1.58)
Obese (>30)	1.17 (0.96–1.42)	1.11 (0.87–1.41)	1.50 (1.22–1.83)
Social Integration			
High	referent	referent	referent
Low	1.80 (1.25–2.59)	1.51 (1.12–2.04)	1.95 (1.40–2.70)
Depression			
No	referent	referent	referent
Yes	5.24 (4.22–6.51)	3.18 (2.58–3.92)	2.65 (2.17–3.24)
Probable PTSD			
No	referent	referent	referent
Yes	3.08 (2.46–3.86)	2.13 (1.72–2.64)	2.04 (1.66–2.51)
GERS			
No	referent	referent	referent
Yes	1.46 (1.25–1.70)	1.57 (1.32–1.87)	1.72 (1.48–2.00)
Sleep Apnea			
No	referent	referent	referent
Yes	1.55 (1.30–1.85)	1.52 (1.25–1.83)	1.81 (1.53–2.14)
Asthma Control			
Controlled	referent	referent	referent
Poorly-controlled	2.12 (1.78–2.52)	2.17 (1.70–2.77)	2.66 (2.22–3.18)
Very poorly-controlled	3.60 (3.02–4.30)	4.37 (3.48–5.50)	4.92 (4.11–5.89)

* Non-significant covariates were not reported in the table.

4. Discussion

4.1. Main Findings

More than half of WTC Health Registry enrollees who have asthma had poorly- or very poorly-controlled symptoms. Consistent with other studies in various populations [7,8], our study found that air pollution/irritants were the most prevalent asthma trigger, and poor asthma control worsened the HRQoL of asthmatic patients. Additionally, our study found that those who identified air pollution/irritants as their asthma trigger were more likely to have poorly- or very poorly-controlled asthma than those who did not report air pollution/irritants as their trigger. Our findings underscore the importance of reduction in indoor and outdoor air pollution exposure, in combination with optimal asthma control, to improve HRQoL among those who were exposed to 9/11 disaster.

4.2. Air Pollution/Irritants and Asthma Control

Consistent with existing knowledge, our study supports the premise that air pollution/irritants are significantly associated with poorer asthma control [5,7,9]. This relationship persists independent of other possible and known risk factors, including 9/11 dust cloud exposure. Higher pollutant levels such as increased daily NO_2 and O_3 have been associated with increased asthma-related emergency department visits after the WTC attacks [9]. Air pollutants may not only increase the frequency and intensity of symptoms but may also promote airway sensitization to airborne allergens in predisposed persons [6]. WTC-dust exposed asthmatic patients may be likely to have poorer asthma control when exposed to certain environmental triggers that recall the WTC attack, such as air pollution/irritants.

Measures reducing indoor and outdoor air pollution/irritants exposure, such as high-efficiency particulate air filtration system, can improve indoor air quality by reducing levels of $PM_{2.5}$ and particle count [26,27]. In addition, educating enrollees about trigger identification and avoidance may prevent exacerbations and help to improve overall asthma management [13,28–30]. Other sociodemographic factors, including older age, lower education level, and higher BMI also contributed to poorer asthma control, consistent with existing literature [2,10,30–32]. This highlights the possible prevention of asthma exacerbation through lifestyle modification focusing on maintaining normal BMI among asthmatic persons.

4.3. Asthma Control and HRQoL

Our findings are also congruent with the existing literature that poorer asthma control is associated with worse HRQoL [10,14,33]. This association continued to be significant after adjusting for known covariates, suggesting that perceived well-being is a complex interplay between the pathophysiological manifestations of asthma, socio-demographic factors, and physical and mental health comorbidities. A previous study also suggested that increased severity of asthma was linked to lower HRQoL among the poorly controlled [33]. In addition, people with poorly controlled asthma and poor HRQoL are more likely to have an asthma attack or been admitted to hospital more than once in the previous 12 month [14]. Since the frequency of asthma attack and asthma-related hospitalization are long-term outcome indicators for asthma [34,35], future studies looking at these outcomes may be helpful to understand how different level of asthma control affects the overall disease outcome.

4.4. Mental Health, Air Pollution/Irritants, and Asthma Control

Our study also supported previous findings that mental health is an important factor for asthma severity, exacerbation and HRQoL [7,15,30,36]. A previous study showed that the effect of air pollution/irritants on asthma control was heightened among WTC workers with panic disorder and PTSD [8]. The air pollution trigger was also found to be associated with anxiety in another study [36], suggesting those with comorbid anxiety might be more susceptible to exacerbation when exposed to air pollution/irritants. Moreover, anxiety and depression were reported to be associated with lower HRQoL among asthmatic patients [15,30,32,36]. Mental illness constitutes a substantial component of asthma disease manifestation. It is necessary to include mental health management in any control measures targeted to improve disease outcome and HRQoL among asthmatic patients.

4.5. Strength and Limitations

The data in this study were self-reported, and we did not have quantitative assessment of asthma control, which requires clinical measurement of pulmonary function such as peak expiratory flow (PEF) and forced expiratory volume (FEV). However, such data may not be essential to our analysis since spirometric lung function may be largely unrelated to perceived asthma triggers [36], though it might support the reliability of our asthma control outcome. A strength of this study was that it included a large sample size and data were available on a wide range of comorbid health conditions. There is a high level of agreement on risk factors of asthma control with previous studies of WTC-exposed populations [2,8], supporting the reliability of our findings.

The asthma triggers information in this study was also self-reported. Given the subjectivity of trigger perception and one's physiological response to it, the validity of self-reported air pollution/irritants was in question. There are publicly available data on air quality from the air monitoring stations, such as the air quality index from the Environment Protection Agency, which provides information on level of specific pollutants such as O_3, sulfur dioxide or NO_2 by geographic area. Future studies integrating such local monitoring environmental data [37,38] with patients' geospatial information such as residential address, may be helpful to validate the accuracy of self-reported air pollution/irritants as trigger.

Given the complexity of treatment regimens and our lack of clinical information on enrollees, we did not account for medication use and treatment adherence, which are both known to play an important role in asthma severity and control [39]. Since self-rated severity of disease has been associated with HRQoL or asthma-related quality of life [10,13,30,33,35,36], future studies that consolidate medication and treatment adherence information to assess asthma severity maybe useful to better understand their role in the relationship of asthma triggers, severity and control, as well as between asthma triggers and HRQoL.

5. Conclusions

Asthma control is closely associated with the perception of asthma trigger exposure, especially to air pollution. Awareness of appropriate preventive measures against air pollution/irritants exposure, and ensuring compliance with these measures may improve asthma control. Asthma control is also closely associated with HRQoL. Optimal asthma control, in combination with treatment for mental health conditions and lifestyle modification advice such as maintaining healthy weight by encouraging diet modification and physical activity, may subsequently lead to improved HRQoL for asthmatic persons exposed to the WTC disaster.

Author Contributions: All authors made substantial contributions to the conception or design of the work; and interpretation of data for the work. J.Y. conducted data analysis and drafted the manuscript with input from S.M.F., J.L., S.O., and J.E.C. All authors edited and finalized the manuscript.

Funding: This research was funded by Cooperative Agreement Numbers 2U50/OH009739 and 5U50/OH009739 from the National Institute for Occupational Safety and Health (NIOSH) of the Centers for Disease Control and Prevention (CDC); U50/ATU272750 from the Agency for Toxic Substances and Disease Registry (ATSDR), CDC, which included support from the National Center for Environmental Health, CDC; and by the New York City Department of Health and Mental Hygiene (NYC DOHMH). Its contents are solely the responsibility of the authors and do not necessarily represent the official views of NIOSH, CDC or the Department of Health and Human Services.

Acknowledgments: We gratefully acknowledge the participation of all Registry enrollees. We thank Charon Gwynn, James Hadler, Mark Farfel, Robert Brackbill, Sean Locke, and Sandhya George for their helpful comments and thorough review of the manuscript.

Conflicts of Interest: The authors declare no conflict of interest.

References

1. Nurmagambetov, T.; Kuwahara, R.; Garbe, P. The Economic Burden of Asthma in the United States, 2008–2013. *Ann. Am. Thorac. Soc.* **2018**, *15*, 348–356. [CrossRef]
2. Jordan, H.T.; Stellman, S.D.; Reibman, J.; Farfel, M.R.; Brackbill, R.M.; Friedman, S.M.; Li, J.; Cone, J.E. Factors associated with poor control of 9/11-related asthma 10–11 years after the 2001 World Trade Center terrorist attacks. *J. Asthma* **2015**, *52*, 630–637. [CrossRef] [PubMed]
3. Price, D.; Dale, P.; Elder, E.; Chapman, K.R. Types, frequency and impact of asthma triggers on patients' lives: A quantitative study in five European countries. *J. Asthma* **2014**, *51*, 127–135. [CrossRef]
4. Ritz, T.; Steptoe, A.; Bobb, C.; Harris, A.H.; Edwards, M. The asthma trigger inventory: Validation of a questionnaire for perceived triggers of asthma. *Psychosom. Med.* **2006**, *68*, 956–965. [CrossRef] [PubMed]
5. Vernon, M.K.; Wiklund, I.; Bell, J.A.; Dale, P.; Chapman, K.R. What do we know about asthma triggers? A review of the literature. *J. Asthma* **2012**, *49*, 991–998. [CrossRef]
6. Amato, M.D.; Cecchi, L.; Annesi-Maesano, I.; d'Amato, G. News on Climate Change, Air Pollution, and Allergic Triggers of Asthma. *J. Investig. Allergol. Clin. Immunol.* **2018**, *28*, 91–97. [CrossRef]
7. Goksel, O.; Celik, G.E.; Erkekol, F.O.; Gullu, E.; Mungan, D.; Misirligil, Z. Triggers in adult asthma: Are patients aware of triggers and doing right? *Allergol. Immunopathol. (Madr.)* **2009**, *37*, 122–128. [CrossRef]
8. Morales-Raveendran, E.; Goodman, E.; West, E.; Cone, J.E.; Katz, C.; Weiss, J.; Feldman, J.M.; Harrison, D.; Markowitz, S.; Federman, A.; et al. Associations between asthma trigger reports, mental health conditions, and asthma morbidity among world trade center rescue and recovery workers. *J. Asthma* **2018**, 1–8. [CrossRef]
9. Sharma, K.I.; Abraham, R.; Mowrey, W.; Toh, J.; Rosenstreich, D.; Jariwala, S. The association between pollutant levels and asthma-related emergency department visits in the Bronx after the World Trade Center attacks. *J. Asthma* **2018**, 1–7. [CrossRef]
10. Gonzalez-Barcala, F.J.; de la Fuente-Cid, R.; Tafalla, M.; Nuevo, J.; Caamano-Isorna, F. Factors associated with health-related quality of life in adults with asthma. A cross-sectional study. *Multidiscip. Respir. Med.* **2012**, *7*, 32. [CrossRef]
11. Chen, H.; Gould, M.K.; Blanc, P.D.; Miller, D.P.; Kamath, T.V.; Lee, J.H.; Sullivan, S.D.; TENOR Study Group. Asthma control, severity, and quality of life: Quantifying the effect of uncontrolled disease. *J. Allergy Clin. Immunol.* **2007**, *120*, 396–402. [CrossRef]
12. Archea, C.; Yen, I.H.; Chen, H.; Eisner, M.D.; Katz, P.P.; Masharani, U.; Yelin, E.H.; Earnest, G.; Blanc, P.D. Negative life events and quality of life in adults with asthma. *Thorax* **2007**, *62*, 139–146. [CrossRef]
13. Luskin, A.T.; Chipps, B.E.; Rasouliyan, L.; Miller, D.P.; Haselkorn, T.; Dorenbaum, A. Impact of asthma exacerbations and asthma triggers on asthma-related quality of life in patients with severe or difficult-to-treat asthma. *J. Allergy Clin. Immunol. Pract.* **2014**, *2*, 544–552. [CrossRef]
14. Upton, J.; Lewis, C.; Humphreys, E.; Price, D.; Walker, S. Asthma-specific health-related quality of life of people in Great Britain: A national survey. *J. Asthma* **2016**, *53*, 975–982. [CrossRef]
15. Geraldo Jose Cunha, A.; Zbonik Mendes, A.; Dias Wanderley de Carvalho, F.; Aparecida Ribeiro de Paula, M.; Goncalves Brasil, T. The impact of asthma on quality of life and anxiety: A pilot study. *J. Asthma* **2018**, 1–6. [CrossRef]
16. Brackbill, R.M.; Hadler, J.L.; DiGrande, L.; Ekenga, C.C.; Farfel, M.R.; Friedman, S.; Perlman, S.E.; Stellman, S.D.; Walker, D.J.; Wu, D.; et al. Asthma and posttraumatic stress symptoms 5 to 6 years following exposure to the World Trade Center terrorist attack. *JAMA* **2009**, *302*, 502–516. [CrossRef]
17. Farfel, M.; DiGrande, L.; Brackbill, R.; Prann, A.; Cone, J.; Friedman, S.; Walker, D.J.; Pezeshki, G.; Thomas, P.; Galea, S.; et al. An overview of 9/11 experiences and respiratory and mental health conditions among World Trade Center Health Registry enrollees. *J. Urban Health Bull. N. Y. Acad. Med.* **2008**, *85*, 880–909. [CrossRef]
18. National Asthma Education and Prevention Program. Expert Panel Report 3: Guidelines for the Diagnosis and Management of Asthma. National Heart, Lung, and Blood Institute. Available online: https://www.ncbi.nlm.nih.gov/books/NBK7232/ (accessed on 28 May 2019).

19. Moriarty, D.G.; Zack, M.M.; Kobau, R. The Centers for Disease Control and Prevention's Healthy Days Measures-population tracking of perceived physical and mental health over time. *Health Qual. Life Outcomes* **2003**, *1*, 37. [CrossRef]

20. Center for Disease Control and Prevention, National Center for Chronic Disease Prevention and Health Promotion. Division of Population Health Health-Related Quality of Life (HRQOL). Available online: https://www.cdc.gov/hrqol/syntax.htm (accessed on 3 May 2019).

21. Blanchard, E.B.; Jones-Alexander, J.; Buckley, T.C.; Forneris, C.A. Psychometric properties of the PTSD Checklist (PCL). *Behav. Res. Ther.* **1996**, *34*, 669–673. [CrossRef]

22. Ventureyra, V.A.; Yao, S.N.; Cottraux, J.; Note, I.; De Mey-Guillard, C. The validation of the Posttraumatic Stress Disorder Checklist Scale in posttraumatic stress disorder and nonclinical subjects. *Psychother. Psychosom.* **2002**, *71*, 47–53. [CrossRef]

23. Kroenke, K.; Strine, T.W.; Spitzer, R.L.; Williams, J.B.; Berry, J.T.; Mokdad, A.H. The PHQ-8 as a measure of current depression in the general population. *J. Affect. Disord.* **2009**, *114*, 163–173. [CrossRef]

24. Spitzer, R.L.; Kroenke, K.; Williams, J.B.; Lowe, B. A brief measure for assessing generalized anxiety disorder: The GAD-7. *Arch. Intern. Med.* **2006**, *166*, 1092–1097. [CrossRef]

25. Cohen, S.; Underwood, L.G.; Gottlieb, B.H. *Social Support Measurement and Intervention: A Guide for Health and Social Scientists*; Oxford University Press: Oxford, UK, 2000.

26. Huang, G.; Zhou, W.; Qian, Y.; Fisher, B. Breathing the same air? Socioeconomic disparities in PM$_{2.5}$ exposure and the potential benefits from air filtration. *Sci. Total Environ.* **2019**, *657*, 619–626. [CrossRef]

27. Leas, B.F.; D'Anci, K.E.; Apter, A.J.; Bryant-Stephens, T.; Lynch, M.P.; Kaczmarek, J.L.; Umscheid, C.A. Effectiveness of indoor allergen reduction in asthma management: A systematic review. *J. Allergy Clin. Immunol.* **2018**, *141*, 1854–1869. [CrossRef]

28. Bobb, C.; Ritz, T.; Rowlands, G.; Griffiths, C. Effects of allergen and trigger factor avoidance advice in primary care on asthma control: A randomized-controlled trial. *Clin. Exp. Allergy* **2010**, *40*, 143–152. [CrossRef]

29. Rojano, B.; West, E.; Goodman, E.; Weiss, J.J.; de la Hoz, R.E.; Crane, M.; Crowley, L.; Harrison, D.; Markowitz, S.; Wisnivesky, J.P. Self-management behaviors in World Trade Center rescue and recovery workers with asthma. *J. Asthma* **2018**, 1–11. [CrossRef]

30. Sundh, J.; Wireklint, P.; Hasselgren, M.; Montgomery, S.; Stallberg, B.; Lisspers, K.; Janson, C. Health-related quality of life in asthma patients—A comparison of two cohorts from 2005 and 2015. *Respir. Med.* **2017**, *132*, 154–160. [CrossRef]

31. Tarraf, H.; Al-Jahdali, H.; Al Qaseer, A.H.; Gjurovic, A.; Haouichat, H.; Khassawneh, B.; Mahboub, B.; Naghshin, R.; Montestruc, F.; Behbehani, N. Asthma control in adults in the Middle East and North Africa: Results from the ESMAA study. *Respir. Med.* **2018**, *138*, 64–73. [CrossRef]

32. Pate, C.A.; Zahran, H.S.; Bailey, C.M. Impaired health-related quality of life and related risk factors among US adults with asthma. *J. Asthma* **2018**, 1–9. [CrossRef]

33. Correia de Sousa, J.; Pina, A.; Cruz, A.M.; Quelhas, A.; Almada-Lobo, F.; Cabrita, J.; Oliveira, P.; Yaphe, J. Asthma control, quality of life, and the role of patient enablement: A cross-sectional observational study. *Prim. Care Respir. J.* **2013**, *22*, 181–187. [CrossRef]

34. Calciano, L.; Corsico, A.G.; Pirina, P.; Trucco, G.; Jarvis, D.; Janson, C.; Accordini, S. Assessment of asthma severity in adults with ever asthma: A continuous score. *PLoS ONE* **2017**, *12*, e0177538. [CrossRef] [PubMed]

35. Siroux, V.; Boudier, A.; Anto, J.M.; Cazzoletti, L.; Accordini, S.; Alonso, J.; Cerveri, I.; Corsico, A.; Gulsvik, A.; Jarvis, D.; et al. Quality-of-life and asthma-severity in general population asthmatics: Results of the ECRHS II study. *Allergy* **2008**, *63*, 547–554. [CrossRef] [PubMed]

36. Ritz, T.; Wittchen, H.U.; Klotsche, J.; Muhlig, S.; Riedel, O.; sap-NEEDs Study Group. Asthma Trigger Reports Are Associated with Low Quality of Life, Exacerbations, and Emergency Treatments. *Ann. Am. Thorac. Soc.* **2016**, *13*, 204–211.

37. Jayawardene, W.P.; Youssefagha, A.H.; Lohrmann, D.K.; El Afandi, G.S. Prediction of asthma exacerbations among children through integrating air pollution, upper atmosphere, and school health surveillances. *Allergy Asthma Proc.* **2013**, *34*, e1–e8. [CrossRef] [PubMed]

38. Nishimura, K.K.; Galanter, J.M.; Roth, L.A.; Oh, S.S.; Thakur, N.; Nguyen, E.A.; Thyne, S.; Farber, H.J.; Serebrisky, D.; Kumar, R.; et al. Early-life air pollution and asthma risk in minority children. The GALA II and SAGE II studies. *Am. J. Respir. Crit. Care Med.* **2013**, *188*, 309–318. [CrossRef] [PubMed]
39. Gemicioglu, B.; Bayram, H.; Cimrin, A.; Abadoglu, O.; Cilli, A.; Uzaslan, E.; Gunen, H.; Akyildiz, L.; Suerdem, M.; Ozlu, T.; et al. Asthma control and adherence in newly diagnosed young and elderly adult patients with asthma in Turkey. *J. Asthma* **2018**, 1–9. [CrossRef] [PubMed]

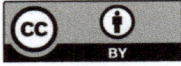

MDPI

St. Alban-Anlage 66

4052 Basel

Switzerland

Tel. +41 61 683 77 34

Fax +41 61 302 89 18

www.mdpi.com

International Journal of Environmental Research and Public Health Editorial Office

E-mail: ijerph@mdpi.com

www.mdpi.com/journal/ijerph

www.ingramcontent.com/pod-product-compliance
Lightning Source LLC
Chambersburg PA
CBHW051718210326
41597CB00032B/5524